ADVANCED IMMUNOLOGY

ADVANCED IMMUNOLOGY

DAVID MALE MA, PhD
Lecturer in Neuroimmunology
Department of Neuropathology
Institute of Psychiatry
London, UK

BRIAN CHAMPION BSc, PhD
Senior Biologist
Department of Immunobiology
Glaxo Group Research Limited
Greenford, Middlesex, UK

ANNE COOKE BSc, PhD
Wellcome Trust Senior Lecturer
Department of Immunology
The Middlesex Hospital Medical School
London, UK

J.B. Lippincott Company   Philadelphia

Gower Medical Publishing London · New York

Distributed in USA and Canada by:
J. B. Lippincott Company
East Washington Square
Philadelphia, PA 19105
USA

**Distributed in UK and Continental
Europe by:**
Harper & Row Ltd
Middlesex House
34-42 Cleveland Street
London W1P 5FB, UK

**Distributed in Australia and
New Zealand by:**
Harper & Row (Australasia) Pty Ltd
PO Box 226
Artarmon, NSW 2064
Australia

**Distributed in Southeast Asia, Hong Kong,
India and Pakistan by:**
Harper & Row Publishers (Asia) Pte Ltd
37 Jalan Pemimpin 02-01
Singapore 2057

Distributed in Japan by:
Igaku Shoin Ltd
Tokyo International
PO Box 5063
Tokyo
Japan

**Distributed in Philippines/Guam,
Middle East, Latin America and Africa by:**
Harper & Row International
10 East 53rd Street
New York, NY 10022
USA

Project Editor: Helen Hadjidimitriadou
Design and Illustration: Celia Welcomme
Linework: Marion Tasker

Origination in Italy by Trilogy
Typesetting by Informat and Ampersand Typesetting Ltd, UK
Typeface: Optima and Univers
Produced by Mandarin Offset. Reprinted in Hong Kong in 1989.

ISBN: 0-397-44641-1 (Lippincott/Gower)

Library of Congress Catalog Card Number: 65-40058
Library cataloging in Publication Data available.

British Library Cataloguing in Publication Data:
Male, David K.
    Advanced Immunology.
    1 Immunology
    1. Title II Cooke, Anne
    574.2'9

Preface

This book is designed for people who already have a knowledge of basic immunology, and who want to understand the process involved in immune reactions in greater depth. We have concentrated on the central areas of immunology, namely, immune recognition, cooperation between immunologically active cells and the development of immune reactions. Particular emphasis has been placed on those subjects which are less well covered in introductory textbooks, and on recent studies concerning the molecular basis of immune recognition and cellular interactions. In order to keep the text to a manageable length, we have not reiterated basic data which may be found elsewhere, on the assumption that readers will be familiar with them.

The book is divided into four main sections, preceded by an introductory chapter; this constitutes a concise summary of basic immunology, necessary for the understanding of subsequent chapters, but some readers may prefer to omit it.

The first section is concerned with the molecules involved in immune recognition and the functional cell surface molecules of lymphocytes. The second section deals with how lymphocytes recognize natural, synthetic and microbial antigens on antigen-presenting cells and target cells. This is followed by a group of chapters detailing the processes of cellular activation, cooperation between immunocompetent cells, and regulation of immune responses. The final section considers how lymphocytes and antigen-presenting cells traffic through tissues in health, during the development of immune responses and in inflammatory reactions.

To explain various points, we have selected particular experiments from research papers, and we would like to acknowledge the work of the many immunologists and molecular biologists whose work we have presented in our accompanying figures. These figures are intended to be illustrative, and many equally good studies have not been mentioned. We have included those details of the experimental design which are necessary in order to follow the points, but have usually omitted basic methodology. Readers who wish to examine the precise techniques used in the experiments are referred to the lists of additional reading at the end of each chapter, where they may find the original sources of each study together with a number of useful reviews.

It is inevitable, in the writing of any textbook relating to areas of research which are fast-developing, that certain sections will become slightly dated even during the months of writing and producing such a text. In immunology today this is particularly true especially in research relating to the definition of surface antigens and lymphokines.

David Male
Brian Champion
Anne Cooke

Nomenclature

During the preparation of this book there has been a change in the nomenclature of lymphocyte surface molecules which are now referred to as CD antigens. The system simplifies the naming by giving the same CD designation to equivalent molecules in different species, and replaces the previous 'T' series. Designations are as follows:

CD1: T6 Thymocyte differentiation marker
CD2: T11 Sheep erythrocyte receptor of T cells
CD3: T3 Molecular complex associated with the T cell antigen receptor
CD4: T4 (L3T4 in mouse). Marker of T helper subpopulation
CD5: T1 T cell marker
CD6: Fcμ receptor of T cells
CD7: T cell marker
CD8: T8 (Ly2,3 in mouse). Marker of T cytotoxic/ suppressor subpopulation
CD25: TAC Activated T cell IL-2 receptor

In this book, the larger fragment of complement C2 is referred to as C2b, in common with the large fragments of other complement components. Although this usage is not uncommon, it has not been approved by the WHO complement nomenclature committee which designates this fragment as C2a.

Contents

INTRODUCTION

1 The Basis of Immunity

The immune system has evolved to protect us from the numerous potential pathogens which are present in the environment. The basis of immunity is the immune system's ability to recognize foreign molecules (antigens) and react to them, while at the same time tolerating molecules of the body's own tissues. This chapter provides a concise summary of the structure and function of the immune system. While much of the information is presented in the form of statements, the various aspects will be expanded upon and discussed in subsequent chapters.

Broadly speaking, an individual's reaction to a pathogen consists of a non-adaptive or innate response, and an adaptive immune response. The innate response is not improved by repeated encounters with any particular pathogen. By contrast, the adaptive response has two important characteristics, namely specificity and memory. The adaptive immune system can specifically recognize a pathogen when it first encounters it, and if reinfection with that particular pathogen occurs it will mount an enhanced response. Immune recognition and the immune reactions that ensue are central to the subject of immunology and the defence against microorganisms. Where the system breaks down, the same system and types of immune reaction can lead to immunopathological damage.

CELLS OF THE IMMUNE SYSTEM

Adaptive immunity is effected primarily by leucocytes; that is, lymphocytes and phagocytes which are derived from bone marrow stem cells (Fig.1.1; see overpage). These cells recirculate through the body via the blood, tissues and lymphoid system. The leucocytes can also interact with and recruit other types of cell to sites of immune reactions. Phagocytes are primarily responsible for taking up particles, including pathogens, and breaking them down in their phagolysosomes. Lymphocytes are responsible for recognizing and differentiating the various antigens which the immune system encounters. Although phagocytes are sometimes viewed as the mediators of innate immunity and lymphocytes of adaptive immunity, both of these cell types cooperate and interact with each other in the development of an immune response. For example, many phagocytes can process antigens in such a way that they can be recognized by lymphocytes. This is termed 'antigen presentation'. Molecules secreted by lymphocytes, including lymphokines and antibody, enhance the ability of phagocytic cells to take up antigenic material and eliminate it.

Lymphocytes
Lymphocytes constitute 20% of blood leucocytes and most are capable of recognizing antigens. Lymphocytes are of two main types, namely B cells which develop in the bone marrow or fetal liver and may differentiate into antibody-producing plasma cells, and T cells which differentiate in the thymus and serve a number of functions. These include helping B cells to make antibody, killing virally infected cells, regulating the level of the immune response, and stimulating the microbicidal and cytotoxic activity of other immune effector cells, including macrophages. Communication between the cells is effected either by direct cell/cell contact, or by soluble factors.

Each lymphocyte carries a surface receptor which is capable of recognizing a particular antigen. Although each lymphocyte carries only one type of receptor and therefore can only recognize one type of antigen, different lymphocytes have different receptors, so that the lymphocyte population as a whole can recognize a wide range of antigens. The antigen receptors are generated during lymphocyte development by the process of somatic mutation and recombination acting on a relatively small number of initial germline genes (see Chapters 2 and 3). The antigen receptors used by B and T cells are different. The B cell antigen receptor is a form of membrane-bound antibody (surface immunoglobulin - sIg), this being a cell surface form of the antibody which it will ultimately secrete. The T cell antigen receptor is generated from a different set of genes which appear to encode the cell surface receptor only. Indeed, T and B cells recognize antigen in different forms: B cells can recognize an unmodified antigen molecule, either free in solution or on the surface of other cells, whereas T cells only recognize antigen when it is presented to them in association with molecules encoded by the major histocompatibility complex (MHC). The function of presenting antigen to lymphocytes in a form which they can recognize is performed by a miscellaneous group of cells, collectively called antigen-presenting cells (APC).

The basis of the adaptive immune response is that of clonal recognition and response. As stated above, each lymphocyte recognizes only one antigenic structure. When antigen enters the immune system, it binds only to those lymphocytes which have a receptor capable of recognizing it. Only those cells which have been stimulated by antigen respond; the response is usually manifested by the proliferation and further differentiation of responding cells. This may be accompanied by the release of mediators, such as lymphokines, monokines, interleukins and antibodies.

When the immune system first encounters an antigen, there will be relatively few lymphocytes available with a complementary antigen receptor which can make an immune response, but during the initial (primary) response to that antigen the responding population will expand and develop. If the antigen is encountered again, there will be a larger population of cells available to react to it, and these cells will already have undergone several steps of their differentiation pathway. This clonal expansion and differentiation underlies the observation that the secondary

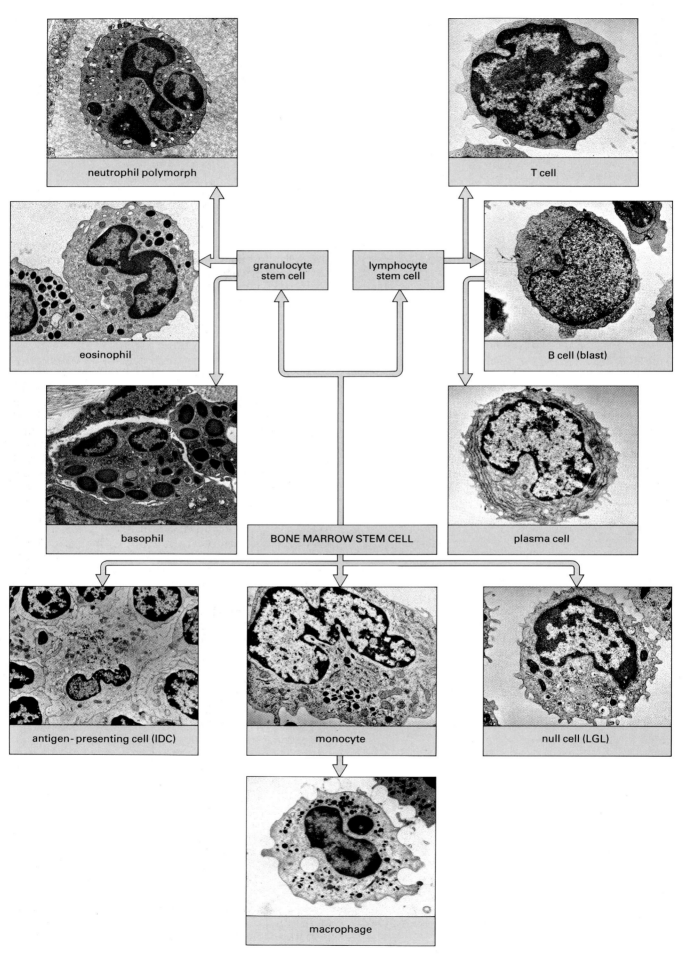

neutrophil polymorph

T cell

granulocyte stem cell

lymphocyte stem cell

eosinophil

B cell (blast)

basophil

BONE MARROW STEM CELL

plasma cell

antigen- presenting cell (IDC)

monocyte

null cell (LGL)

macrophage

immune response is faster to develop, and usually more effective, than the primary response.

Lymphocytes stimulated by antigen (primed) may either differentiate fully into immune effector cells, or they may form the expanded pool of cells (memory cells) which can respond to a secondary challenge with the same antigen.

B Cells

B cells are responsible for the antibody formation. They recognize antigen by their endogenously synthesized cell surface immunoglobulin, which is the characteristic marker of B cells. Other molecules present on the B cells are MHC class II molecules, complement receptors (CR1 and CR2), and other molecules, such as the Lyb series of antigens in mice, whose functions are only partly known. Some B cells occasionally carry markers more usually associated with T cells, such as Ly1 (mouse) or T1 (human). B cells must also carry receptors for the various molecules which are used in signalling, including receptors for the Fc region of antibody, for fragments of complement C3, and for B cell growth and differentiation factors. The latter have not yet been fully characterized.

To produce an antibody response, most B cells require both the presence of antigen and help from antigen-specific T cells. Such antigens which cannot induce B cells to produce antibody without T cell help are called T dependent (T_{dep}) antigens. A number of antigens can, however, stimulate B cells directly, without T cell help. These are known as T independent (T_{ind}) antigens. The majority of protein antigens are T dependent, while many of the T independent antigens are large polymeric molecules with multiple identical antigenic determinants, including carbohydrate and other non-protein antigens. Other T_{ind} antigens include molecules with the ability to activate B cells independently of their antigen specificity (polyclonal B cell activator). The antibody response to T dependent antigens generally matures in a secondary immune response, so that it consists of a greater proportion of IgG and has a higher average affinity for antigen than in the primary response. The response to T independent antigens does not usually mature in this way and remains predominantly IgM. There is some evidence in mice that different subsets of B cells occur which are responsible for the recognition of T_{dep} and T_{ind} antigens, and these may be differentiated by the Lyb5 surface marker.

Activated B cells proliferate, mature under the influence of T cells, and ultimately differentiate into plasma cells. Plasma cells have a greatly expanded cytoplasm, extensive endoplasmic reticulum, and a protein synthesis system which is almost entirely devoted to the production of secreted antibody.

T Cells

T cells are lymphocytes which develop and differentiate in the thymus before seeding the secondary, peripheral lymphoid tissues. T cells recognize antigen and MHC molecules via a receptor molecule distinct from, but related to, immunoglobulin. This receptor is associated with a glycoprotein, T3, which is present on all mature human T cells, and an equivalent molecule has recently been identified in association with the mouse T cell receptor. In man the markers T1 and T11 are also present on all T cells, while in mice the molecule Thy1 is the characteristic T cell marker. Activated T cells also carry MHC class II molecules (except mouse T cells) and express receptors for the lymphokine interleukin 2 (IL-2). This allows them to respond to signals from other T cells. MHC class II and IL-2 receptors are absent from the surface of resting T cells. Other markers differentiate T cell subsets.

There are three main types of T cell, which can be distinguished according to function and surface proteins. These are the helper (T_H), suppressor (T_S) and cytotoxic (T_C) T cells. Additionally, T cells are often defined according to particular functions. For example, the T cells responsible for reactions of delayed hypersensitivity (T_D) consist mainly of helper T cells.

T_H cells are stimulated by a combination of an antigen and an MHC class II molecule on the surface of an antigen-presenting cell. They cooperate with B cells in the production of an antibody response to T_{dep} antigens, are involved in the maturation of T_C cells, and also interact with macrophages and other cells by secreting lymphokines. T_H cells are characterized by the surface marker T4 in humans or its equivalent (L3T4) in the mouse. In mice the T_H population also carries the marker Ly1. The T4 molecule appears to be involved in the recognition of MHC class II molecules.

The cell surface markers of cytotoxic and suppressor T cells are similar in that there has been no surface molecule detected so far which reliably differentiates them. Despite this, the two populations are thought to be distinct because of functional differences. T_C and T_S cells in man express the molecule T8 which is involved in the recognition of class I MHC molecules. Mouse T_C and T_S cells express the Ly2/3 alloantigens, which appear to be functionally similar to T8.

Fig. 1.1 Morphology and lineage of leucocytes and antigen-presenting cells. The electron micrographs indicate the morphology of the cells involved in the immune response and the way in which they are derived from the bone marrow stem cell. T and B cells are both derived from lymphocytic stem cells following differentiation in the primary lymphoid organs. They both have large nuclei and a thin rim of cytoplasm containing relatively few mitochondria and polysomes. After activation, lymphocytes appear as blast cells (in this instance a B cell blast is shown), where the cytoplasm is expanded and contains more endoplasmic reticulum and Golgi apparatus. B cells may ultimately develop into plasma cells which are entirely devoted to antibody synthesis. Null cells have many of the attributes of lymphocytes, but appear to arise by a separate differentiation pathway. Mature null cells appear as large granular lymphocytes (LGL). The blood monocyte typically has a horseshoe-shaped nucleus and a variety of enzyme-containing granules. After emigration from the blood stream, they mature into macrophages with increased metabolic and phagocytic capacities. Other antigen-presenting cells (APC) are also thought to be derived from bone marrow stem cells. These are exemplified here by the interdigitating cell (IDC) seen in the T cell area of a lymph node. It is in close contact with a number of the surrounding lymphocytes. The neutrophil is a short-lived phagocyte with a polymorphic nucleus and numerous cytoplasmic granules containing proteolytic enzymes. The granules of the eosinophil contain a central crystalloid core, while the large electron-dense granules of the basophil contain a variety of inflammatory mediators. The eosinophil and neutrophil are actively phagocytic, whereas the basophil is not; indeed the basophil may be more closely related to the tissue mast cell, with which it shares functional similarities.

T_S

Ly2 and Ly3 are markers almost invariably expressed together and linked so closely that a crossover between the loci has not yet been observed.

Different subsets of mouse T cells also express the Qa markers, which are structurally similar to MHC class I molecules. Their function is uncertain, although it has been suggested that they are developmental differentiation proteins. T cells also carry a variety of 'internal' markers which may be used to identify them, for example, the characteristic dotted distribution of the enzyme α-naphthyl acid esterase (ANAE). More recently it has been suggested that expression of the polypeptide chains of the T cell antigen receptor differs between the various T cell subpopulations, although this still requires some further clarification.

Null Cells

Some lymphocytes seem to express neither T nor B cells surface markers, while others have an ambivalent mixture of lymphocyte and macrophage surface proteins, such as the T3 surface protein of T cells and the macrophage marker identified by antibody OKM1. These cells are referred to as nonT/nonB, null or third population cells. This population appears to be a distinct lineage, where the cells carry T cell markers at an early stage of differentiation and acquire the macrophage markers later. When mature, these cells assume the appearance of large granular lymphocytes. Most of them have receptors for the Fc portion of IgG, and this population is particularly effective at killer (K) or natural killer (NK) cell activity. K cells are leucocytes which can recognize target cells coated with specific antibody: they bind via their Fc receptors and subsequently kill the target cells. NK cells recognize determinants on some tumours and virally infected cells and can also kill them, although antibody is not required for recognition in this case. Although K and NK cell activities are functionally distinct, both functions may be performed by the same cell.

Phagocytes

Phagocytic cells include the neutrophil polymorph, blood monocyte and the various cells of the reticuloendothelial system distributed throughout the body. Among the latter are the tissue macrophages, Kupffer cells of the liver, microglial cells of the brain and mesangial phagocytes of the kidney. Phagocytes recognize material to be taken up via their cell surface receptors. These include receptors for activated complement components (C3b, C3bi and C3d) and for the Fc portion of IgG, which become attached to antigenic particles. By facilitating recognition and uptake of phagocytosable material, IgG and complement act as opsonins.

Polymorphs are short-lived cells, constituting about 70% of blood leucocytes which are produced in large numbers by the bone marrow. They spend about 36 hours in the circulation before migrating into the tissues, where they phagocytose material and die. By contrast, the blood monocyte is a long-lived cell which develops into the tissue macrophage. Macrophages are more metabolically active than monocytes. They also are more strongly phagocytic due to the increased density of their surface receptors, and they have a larger battery of lysosomal enzymes. They are capable of presenting antigen to lymphocytes in a form which they can recognize, recirculating through the lymphatic system (recirculating macrophages), and thus carrying antigen from the periphery to the regional lymph nodes where they can stimulate appropriate immune responses. The most important surface receptors and markers of lymphocytes and macrophages are summarized in Figure 1.2.

Cell	Receptors		Other markers
B cell	sIg - antigen receptor		DR-MHC class II
	CR1, CR2, IL-2*, Fc†		
T cell	Ti/T3 -antigen receptor IL-2* (TAC)		T11, T10, DR*
TH	"		T1, **T4**
Tc/Ts	"		**T8**
Null	Fc, IL-2, CR3		OKM1, **HNK1** T8†, T10†, T11†
Macrophage	Fc, CR1, CR3		**OKM1**, DR

Fig. 1.2 Receptors and surface markers of human lymphocytes and phagocytes. This table shows the more important cell surface markers and receptors of the cells indicated. The marker which is most frequently used to identify the particular cell type is indicated in bold type. The receptors CR1 - CR3 are for activation products of complement C3. * = Activated cells; † = Some cells only.

Antigen-Presenting Cells

Cells which can present antigen to lymphocytes in an immunogenic form are collectively termed antigen-presenting cells (APC). This group includes several cell types derived from bone marrow stem cells, such as the Langerhans cell of the skin which recirculates to lymph nodes where it becomes the dendritic cell seen in T cell areas of the node. Also within the lymph node are the follicular dendritic cells and marginal zone macrophages, as well as the recirculating macrophages mentioned above. In special circumstances, many other cell types can be induced to act as antigen-presenting cells, including endothelial, endocrine and epithelial cells. The function of antigen presentation depends both on the way in which the cells process the antigen and on their cell surface molecules. For example, Langerhans cells present antigen on their surface in association with class II MHC molecules. This is recognized by TH cells. Follicular dendritic cells, on the other hand, take up immune complexes via their C3b receptors and these complexes are particularly effective at stimulating B cells. It has recently become apparent that B cells themselves can present their specific antigen to TH cells. In this case, the surface immunoglobulin molecules may serve to concentrate antigen which is subsequently processed before associating with class II MHC molecules. These cellular interactions which depend on recognition of MHC and/or antigen are termed cognate interactions, to distinguish them from those interactions which do not require specific immune recognition (for example, most lymphokine effects). The major groups of APCs are listed in Figure 1.3. The ways in which different antigens are presented to different types of lymphocytes largely determine the type of immune response which the antigen will evoke.

CELL		Area of secondary lymphoid tissue	Recirculation	Fc/C3 receptor	MHC class II	Present to
Marginal zone macrophages		Lymph node: marginal zone sinus. Spleen: marginal zone	–	+	–	B cell (T_{ind} response)
Follicular dendritic cells		Follicles and B cell area	–	+	–	B cells
Langerhans cell becomes interdigitating dendritic cell		Skin → Lymph node: paracortex	+	±	+	T cells
Macrophages		Lymph node: medulla	+	+	+	T cells and B cells
Interdigitating cells		Thymus	–	–	+	Thymocytes

Fig. 1.3 Antigen-presenting cells. This table indicates the location of antigen-presenting cells within the secondary lymphoid tissues. Some of the cells recirculate, including the Langerhans cell which appears as the dendritic cell of lymph nodes. Fc and C3 receptors permit the cell to take up antigen in the form of immune complexes, while the presence of MHC class II molecules on the cell surface permit it to present antigen to T_H cells.

THE LYMPHOID SYSTEM

Leucocytes and the majority of auxiliary cells are derived from bone marrow stem cells. The B cells mature in the bone marrow and T cells mature in the thymus, hence these are called primary lymphoid organs. The lymphocytes recirculate via the tissues and secondary lymphoid organs back into the circulation. Secondary lymphoid organs include the spleen, the accumulations of lymphoid tissue associated with mucosal surfaces, as well as the lymph nodes which punctuate the network of lymphatic vessels. Within each of these organs there is an orderly arrangement of lymphocytes in particular areas depending on their type and function (Fig. 1.4). For example, T cells predominate in the paracortex of the lymph node, while B cells are more abundant in the germinal centres of the cortex. The spatial organization of the lymphocytes is mirrored by that of the antigen-presenting cells. There is a similar functional/structural relationship in the spleen, where lymphocytes are present as focal aggregations around the arterioles. These collections of cells constitute the periarteriolar lymphatic sheaths (PALS) or white pulp (Fig. 1.4).

Lymphocytes migrate from the blood into the tissues across a specialized region of endothelium, the high endothelial venule (HEV). The endothelial cells of these venules are columnar and lymphocytes pass into the tissue by moving between these cells. High endothelial venule regions also occur in lymph nodes and other secondary lymphoid tissues, so that lymphocytes may reach a lymph node in two ways: either via the afferent lymphatics from the tissues, or by direct immigration from the blood.

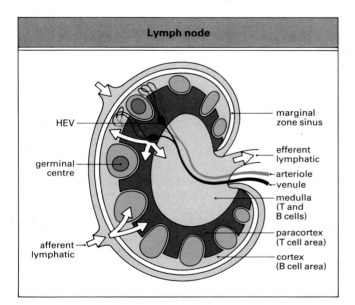

Lymph node

HEV
marginal zone sinus
efferent lymphatic
germinal centre
arteriole
venule
medulla (T and B cells)
paracortex (T cell area)
afferent lymphatic
cortex (B cell area)

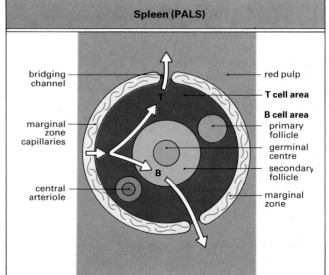

Spleen (PALS)

bridging channel
red pulp
T cell area
B cell area
marginal zone capillaries
primary follicle
germinal centre
secondary follicle
central arteriole
marginal zone

Fig. 1.4 Secondary lymphoid tissues. Lymph nodes and the spleen are part of the secondary lymphoid tissue. Each is divided into functional areas depending on the type of lymphocytes which occur there. The traffic of cells through the organs is also indicated.
Lymph Node. Lymphocytes and recirculating antigen-presenting cells may enter lymph nodes via the afferent lymphatics, and lymphocytes can also arrive by traversing the high endothelial venules (HEV). B cells tend to localize in the cortex and T cells in the paracortex. All cells

leave the lymph node via the efferent lymphatic.
Spleen. Most of the lymphoid tissue in the spleen is arranged around arterioles forming periarteriolar lymphatic sheaths (PALS). This is the white pulp of the spleen. Lymphocytes enter the white pulp from the network of capillaries in the marginal zone. T cells traverse the PALS and re-enter the circulation by passing across bridging channels in the marginal zone before entering the red pulp. B cells may divert to the B cell areas and are particularly abundant in germinal centres.

Chains of lymph nodes lie along the draining lymphatic vessels, but they are particularly concentrated in the neck, axilla, groin, the mesentery and on either side of the spine. The majority of the lymphatic vessels from the trunk and lower limbs ultimately drain into the right thoracic duct, which returns the lymph to the circulation. This circulation of lymphoid cells is referred to as lymphocyte traffic. The arrangement of the lymphatic system ensures that antigen is directed to the regional lymph nodes. When antigen first arrives at the lymph nodes of an immune individual, there is an immediate shut-down of the traffic through the node. Immune reactions within the node are accompanied by expansion of particular regions of the node. For example, antigens which stimulate a strong T cell response induce paracortical proliferation.

In short, one of the functions of the lymphatic system is to bring antigen into contact with lymphocytes which are capable of recognizing it. For this reason, the recirculation of antigen-presenting cells mentioned above is also most important in ensuring that antigen encounters lymphocytes and does so in a suitable form.

THE DEVELOPMENT OF T CELLS AND B CELLS

Lymphoid stem cells start to colonize the thymus in waves late in fetal life. These pre-T cells lack the majority of surface markers associated with T cells which develop during the thymic differentiation. They do, however, possess some of their characteristic enzymes, including terminal deoxyribonucleotidyl transferase (Tdt) and acid phosphatase. The majority of thymocytes lie within the cortex, where there is considerable cell proliferation. More mature cells are present in the relatively sparsely populated medulla. This sparsity might be related to the considerable cell death which is known to occur within the thymus. The T3 and T11 molecules, which are related to antigen-specific and antigen-non-specific T cell activation respectively, both appear on cortical thymocytes along with the T6 differentiation marker. T4 and T8, which are the characteristic markers of the helper and suppressor/cytotoxic populations respectively, appear simultaneously on cortical thymocytes, but one or the other marker is lost from either cell type before it leaves the thymus as a mature, functionally committed cell. Other receptors subsequently appear on mature T cells in the periphery. These include the Fc receptors for immunoglobulin (IgM and IgG) and for IL-2 (TAC in humans). Activated T cells may also express class II MHC molecules. Therefore, the process of thymic differentiation involves:
A. The acquisition of T cells' antigen-specific receptors.
B. Considerable cell death, which is thought to be associated with the loss of self-reactive clones or clones lacking functional receptors.
C. Differentiation into the various T cell subpopulations. Even after T cells have departed for the periphery, they may still be influenced by factors released from the thymus (thymic hormones; see Chapter 4).

In birds, B cells develop in a special organ called the bursa of Fabricius, for which there is no mammalian equivalent. In mammals, it is thought that B cells complete their differentiation steps in the bone marrow. B cells initially acquire surface immunoglobulin of the IgM class, which acts as their antigen receptor. During subsequent development, B cells may change the class of their surface immunoglobulin, but their antigen specificity does not alter. Surface Ig is present on all B cells, but is not expressed when they terminally differentiate into plasma cells. Mature B cells lose their internal Tdt which is present in lymphocytic stem cells, but they may develop receptors for Fc of IgG and for C3, as well as expressing MHC class II molecules. Antigen-activated B cells develop receptors for lymphokines, including B cell growth and differentiation factors and IL-2, which allow them to respond to signals from T cells; some of these receptors are not yet fully characterized.

IMMUNE RECOGNITION MOLECULES

Antibody

Antibody or immunoglobulin (Ig) is the immune recognition molecule generated by B cells. Antibodies are of two basic forms: membrane and secreted Ig. Membrane Ig acts as the B cell antigen receptor and is an integral membrane protein. Each B cell can also produce a secreted Ig with identical antigen specificity to that of its receptor.

There is enormous heterogeneity in the population of antibody molecules, although each one is constructed from a basic unit consisting of two identical heavy polypeptide chains and two identical light chains. These are crosslinked and stabilized by interchain disulphide bonds and by secondary interactions. Both heavy and light chains are folded into globular domains - regions of folded polypeptide and with a particular globular tertiary structure. Each domain consists of about 110 amino acids and contains several loops of anti-parallel β-pleated sheets stabilized by intrachain disulphide bonds. The domain structure which is seen in antibody polypeptides appears to be representative of a basic building block for many of the molecules involved in immune recognition, including the T cell receptor and MHC-encoded class I and II molecules. This is illustrated in Figure 1.5.

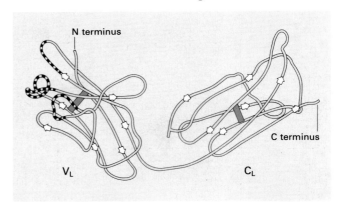

Fig. 1.5 The domain structure of an immunoglobulin light chain. Light chains are composed of two domains, one constant and one variable, but the overall structures are essentially similar, since they contain three or four sections of anti-parallel β-pleated sheet which is stabilized by secondary bonds and an intrachain disulphide bond between cysteine residues. The hypervariable loops which form part of the antigen-combining site are exposed at the extreme (left) end of the variable domain. Analogous domain structures occur in many of the other molecules involved in immune recognition (by inference from their related amino acid sequences).

Fig. 1.6 Antibody structure. All antibodies are assembled from units consisting of two identical heavy and two identical light chains crosslinked by disulphide bonds (red). The arrangement of bonds seen in human IgG1 is illustrated here. The chains are divided into globular regions, termed domains, which are stabilized by β-pleated sheet and intra-chain disulphide bonds. Antigenic determinants (epitopes) bind to the combining site (paratope) generated by the N-terminal domains of light and heavy chains. These domains are extremely variable between different antibodies (V domains) and contain the antibody-idiotypic determinants. The constant (C) domains are encoded by the heavy and light chain isotypes. The molecule can be fragmented into Fab and Fc by digestion with papain. It is found that a number of cells in the body have receptors for the Fc region, and thus antibody can act as a flexible adapter between antigen and those cells. The hinge region of the molecule confers segmental flexibility on the molecule, thus permitting the Fab arms to bind to separate antigenic determinants.

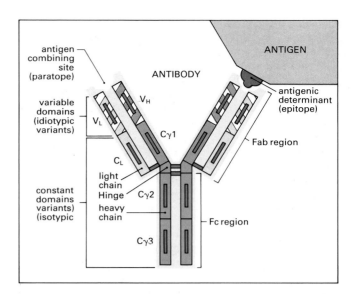

The N-terminal domains of one heavy and one light chain form an antigen-binding site, and these domains are highly variable between different antibodies (V domains). The remaining domains are less variable (Constant - C domains), and some of these C domains are involved in interactions between antibody and receptors (Fc receptors) on the body's cells. Thus, antibody can act as a bifunctional adapter which can crosslink antigen and cells.

The structure of an antibody molecule is illustrated in Figure 1.6.

Antibodies are divided into the different classes and subclasses according to the type of heavy chain they contain. In man there are nine different types of heavy chain (subclasses), each encoded by a separate gene in the heavy chain gene stack. These are IgM, IgG1, IgG2, IgG3, IgG4, IgA1, IgA2, IgD and IgE, which are grouped into the

	Properties					Functional interactions in humans								Human subclasses		Mouse subclasses	
	Subunits	H chain domains	Size	Serum half life (human) days	Complement fixation	Platelet binding	Mast cell and basophil sensitization	Transplacental transfer	Transepithelial transfer	Opsonization for macrophages; neutrophils; eosinophils	Sensitization for K cells	Binding to lymphocytes	Subclasses	Serum concentration mg/ml	Subclasses	Serum concentration mg/ml
IgM	5	5	19s	5.1	++	−	−	−	(+)	−	−	T†	μ	1.5	μ	0.6-1.0•
IgG	1	4	7s	23*	+*	+	−_	+*	(+)	+*	+*	T†B	γ₁	9	γ₁	4.6-6.5
													γ₂	3	γ₂ₐ	1.0-4.2
													γ₃	1	γ₂ᵦ	1.2-2.0
													γ₄	0.5	γ₃	0.1-0.2
IgA	1,2 or more	4	7s or 11s	5.8	−	−	−	−	++	−	−	T†B†	α₁	3	α	0.26-0.4
													α₂	0.5		
IgD	1	4	7s	2.8	−	−	−	−	−	−	−	−	δ	0.03	δ	−‡
IgE	1	5	8s	2.3	−	−	++	−	−	−	−	T†B†	ε	0.05x10⁻³	ε	0.1x10⁻³

•The range of mouse subclasses varies greatly between strains and at different ages
* Some subclasses only
† Some subsets of cells only
‡Serum levels of mouse IgD are very low or undetectable

Fig. 1.7 Characteristics and functions of antibody classes. Antibodies of different classes are formed from one or more basic subunits of two light and two heavy chains. The heavy chain determines the antibody class, and the number of domains in the heavy chain may be four or five depending on the class, one of which is variable and the others constant. Antibody effector functions relate largely to the cells and effector systems with which the Fc regions interact. (* = Only some of the subclasses are effective in this function. + = Only some subpopulations of the cells named have receptors for this antibody class). Complement, platelets, mast cells and basophils mediate inflammatory responses. Macrophages and neutrophils phagocytose and destroy antigenic particles opsonized by antibody. Eosinophils and K cells engage target cells via antibody bound to their Fc receptors, while the receptors for antibody on T and B cells are thought to be involved in immune regulation.

five different classes according to similarities in their overall structure. Since there is a copy of each subclass in a haploid genome, the heavy chain subclasses are isotypes. There are two different classes of light chain, namely kappa (κ) and lambda (λ). The functions of the various classes are reflected in their cellular binding activities and in their ability to activate effector systems, such as complement (Fig. 1.7; see previous page).

Many of the effector functions of antibody are mediated via their binding to Fc receptors on cells. Different classes of antibodies bind to different types of Fc receptor and mediate different immunological functions. Receptors for IgG are found on phagocytic cells where they facilitate uptake of antigenic particles coated with the antibody. Receptors for polymeric IgA are present on the serous side of a number of epithelial cells, where they are involved in the transfer of IgA across the cells to the mucosal surface and thence into secretions. IgE receptors are present on mast cells and these permit the cell to become sensitized with antigen-specific IgE. When antigen binds to the IgE the cells are triggered to release a number of inflammatory mediators, and this is one means by which the immune system can trigger inflammatory reactions. Fc receptors also occur on killer cells permitting them to recognize potential target cells, and another group of Fc receptors occurs on T and B cells. The latter are also class-specific and involved in the control of immune responses. From this it may be seen that different antibody classes subserve different functions, and the type of immune response which occurs to an antigen will be affected by the antibody classes directed towards it (see Fig. 1.7).

The immunoglobulin chains are encoded by genes at three separate loci on different chromosomes. One locus encodes the heavy chain isotypes and there are separate loci for the κ and λ light chains, although a B cell only ever transcribes from one of these light chain loci. The genes encoding immunoglobulin V domains are generated during B cell ontogeny by a process of somatic recombination, involving the joining of separate gene segments, which is described in Chapter 2. This process yields an enormous diversity of different heavy and light chain V regions, so that the immune system's B cell population can generate a very large number of different immunoglobulin antigen receptors to specifically recognize different antigens.

It must be emphasized, however, that any one B cell only ever uses one heavy chain and one light chain recombined variable domain, so that it only has one specificity of antigen receptor. It follows from this that only one allele of the heavy chain and one allele of the light chain are expressed by a particular cell: an example of allelic exclusion. Different B cells will, therefore, use one or other of the maternal or paternal alleles but, taken as a whole, the expression of immunoglobulin chain alleles within an individual is codominant.

Individual B cells can switch the type of heavy chain which they express, while still retaining antibody of the same antigen specificity. This is possible because the genes encoding the C domains (determining antibody class) and the genes encoding the V domains (determining antibody specificity) are separated in the genome by introns and are only spliced together when the mRNA is processed. The B cell controls which class will be expressed by altering the C region genes used to make the primary RNA transcript. This in turn can be adjusted either during transcription or at the level of the DNA itself. The process of class switching is

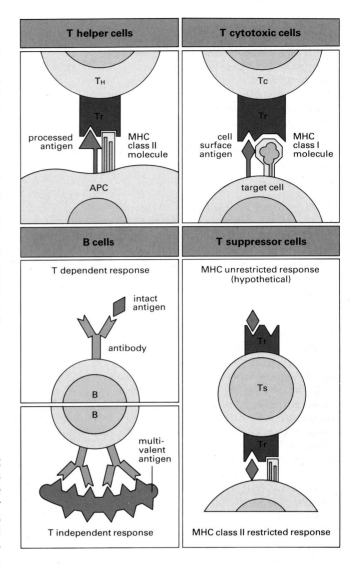

Fig. 1.8 Immune recognition. Immune recognition is dependent on three separate types of molecules. T helper cells (TH) recognize antigen on the surface of APCs when it is presented in association with MHC class II molecules. Cytotoxic T cells (Tc) use a similar type of antigen receptor; however, they usually recognize antigen only when it is presented in association with MHC class I molecules, such as would be present on a virally infected target cell. B cells recognize antigen via their cell surface immunoglobulin which can bind to unmodified antigen. A number of multivalent antigens can stimulate B cells directly without the requirement for T cell help, but help is necessary to produce a response to the majority of protein antigens. In some cases, suppressor T cells (Ts) appear to recognize antigen and MHC molecules, but this is not always the case. Whether or not they use the same type of antigen receptor as other T cells is still not clear.

an important event in B cell development and maturation, and is reflected in the switch from IgM synthesis in the primary immune response to the synthesis of other classes in the secondary response.

The enormous heterogeneity in the population of antibody molecules in an individual may be divided into two types:
1. Idiotypic variability is related to the different V domains,

each one generated by a separate recombinational event. Each antibody molecule has a set of antigenic determinants associated with its V domains. These are termed idiotopes, and the set of idiotopes constitutes the idiotype of an antibody.

2. Isotypic variability is due to the different sets of germline genes which encode the different C regions and produce the different antibody classes and subclasses.

There is also intraspecies variation in the different antibody isotypes, and this is referred to as allotypic variation (cf. blood groups and other allotypically variant sets of molecules).

T Cell Antigen Receptor

Like B cells, T cells also recognize antigen using a receptor which is generated by a process of recombination from a set of germline genes, to produce a wide diversity of receptors capable of binding different antigens. The molecular structure and development of the T cell antigen receptor is discussed fully in Chapter 3. Unlike B cells, T cells do not recognize antigen alone: they recognize antigen in association with molecules encoded by the major histocompatibility complex (MHC). The majority of T helper cells recognize antigen in association with class II MHC molecules, such as would occur at the surface of antigen-presenting cells. Indeed, antigen-presenting cells bearing class II molecules are particularly effective at stimulating T_H cells. The majority of cytotoxic cells recognize a combination of antigen and MHC class I molecule, as occurs on the surface of virally infected cells. In fact, the prime physiological function of Tc cells may be to eliminate virally infected cells.

Some T suppressor cells also are antigen-specific. In some experimental protocols they appear to recognize antigen in association with MHC molecules, although in other experiments they are able to recognize antigen alone. The recognition of antigen by T and B cells is summarized in Figure 1.8.

The way in which T_H and Tc cells recognize antigen/MHC is genetically restricted. That is, T cells which develop in an animal with a particular MHC haplotype and are primed to respond to antigen in that individual, are subsequently only normally capable of recognizing antigen in association with MHC molecules of that haplotype. In other words, there is a restriction on the type of MHC molecules a T cell will react to. The principle of genetic restriction can be used to examine the immune response. For example, if it is necessary for the MHC class II molecules of an antigen-presenting cell and a responding T cell to be of the same haplotype, this implies that the class II molecules are involved in the interaction between the APC and the T cell.

Some T cells can also recognize allogeneic MHC molecules. The T cells recognize the allogeneic molecules as an equivalent signal to antigen plus self MHC, and this underlies the (non-physiological) reactions which occur to foreign tissue grafts that express allogeneic MHC molecules.

The Major Histocompatibility Complex (MHC)

Although the MHC was first identified through its role in graft rejection, this is not its physiological role. As indicated above, the true function of the MHC lies in the process of antigen recognition by T cells.

Three types of molecule are associated with the MHC: class I, class II, and some complement components (class III). Class I molecules, present on the surface of all nucleated cells, are involved in the recognition of target cells by cytotoxic T cells. Target cells in this context may be virally infected tissue cells, or graft cells expressing non-self MHC antigen. Class I molecules consist of an MHC-encoded glycoprotein chain which is associated with β_2-microglobulin. The MHC-encoded chains are highly polymorphic, while β_2-microglobulin is not. There are several loci within the MHC which encode class I molecules, and outside the MHC there are other loci which encode molecules with very similar structures (for example, the Qa locus in the mouse).

The function of class II molecules is to present antigen to T helper cells. MHC class II molecules are present on a limited variety of APCs. Each class II molecule consists of two MHC-encoded polypeptides, both of which are polymorphic. The number of gene loci within the MHC which encode class II molecules varies greatly between

Molecule		Peptides	Approximate molecular weight	Number of domains	Chromosome	
					man	mouse
sIg B cell receptor		heavy chain (9 isotypes)	50-75 kD	4 or 5 tm	14	12
		κ or λ	25 kD	2	2	6
			25 kD	2	22	16
Ti T cell receptor		α	43 kD	2 tm	14	14
		β	40 kD	2 tm	7	6
MHC class I		α	45 kD	3 tm	6	17
		β₂ microglobulin	12.5 kD	1	15	2
MHC class II		α	32 kD	2 tm	6	17
		β	28 kD	2 tm	6	17

Fig. 1.9 Molecules involved in immune recognition. This table lists the characteristics of the B and T cell antigen receptors and the MHC molecules. The characteristics given are those of human molecules, but they are similar in all species. The peptides appear to have arisen from a common ancestral gene, and there is structural homology between the domains of all these molecules. The T cell receptor and MHC molecules consist of one of each of the peptides described, while the surface Ig of B cells consists of the four chain structure shown in Fig.1.6. tm indicates that the peptide traverses the plasma membrane, and thus has a transmembrane and intracytoplasmic segments as well as the extracellular domains.

species. For example, the mouse has two such loci, but in humans there are many more. The structure of class I and II MHC molecules and their gene organization is discussed further in Chapter 5.

A number of the complement system components, including C2, C4 and factor B, are encoded within the MHC, both in man and mouse. These are referred to as class III MHC molecules. Although the complement system is involved in several immune reactions, the function of the complement components is quite dissimilar to that of the class I and II molecules, and it may be wholly coincidental that they are genetically linked to each other in the MHC. Evidently, strong evolutionary pressure has maintained a genetic linkage between class I and class II molecules in species as diverse as man and mouse. Therefore, any genes such as those encoding class III molecules which lie between class I and II loci would be passed on in the linkage group.

The nature and specificity of the processes involved in immune recognition are further detailed in Chapters 6-8. The molecules involved in immune recognition are summarized in Figure 1.9 (see previous page).

CELLULAR IMMUNE RESPONSE INTERACTIONS

The immune response results from the interactions of the various cell types described above. The main steps of this process are:

A. The uptake, processing and presentation of antigen to T and B cells, which is effected both by recirculating APCs and those resident in secondary lymphoid organs.

B. The interactions which occur between T helper cells and the various effector cells, including macrophages, B cells and cytotoxic T cells. These interactions may be effected by direct cellular interaction, or may be mediated by soluble factors - lymphokines and monokines.

C. The level and type of the response is then regulated by T suppressor cells as well as by APCs, TH cells and antibody. Finally, the immune system interacts with other cells, such as granulocytes, mast cells, fibroblasts and endothelial cells and with the serum enzyme systems to produce inflammatory reactions aimed at eliminating the source of the antigen and, if this is due to a pathogen, minimizing the damage that it causes. These interactions are introduced below and discussed fully in later chapters.

Cell Cooperation in the Immune Response

Since B cells and T cells recognize antigen in different ways using different types of receptor, it is not surprising that they recognize different parts of the same antigen. In experimental systems, these parts are differentiated as hapten and carrier determinants. B cells recognize antigenic determinants (epitopes) present on the intact antigen, but T cells usually recognize processed antigen which may be a small denatured fragment of the original antigen, presented in association with MHC molecules. The way in which the antigen is presented to a T cell depends on the MHC molecules of the APC. An individual's MHC haplotype plays a major part in determining the level and specificity of the immune response. Different haplotypes present antigen in different forms, and since the MHC haplotypes vary between individuals, the antigen/MHC complex presented to the T cells and the ensuing response also vary.

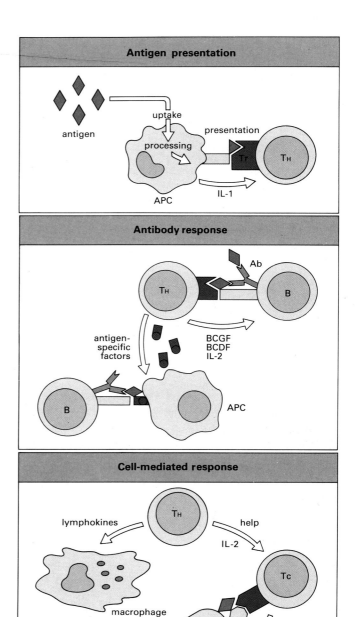

Fig. 1.10. Cellular cooperation.
Antigen presentation. Antigen taken up by antigen-presenting cells (APCs) is processed and presented to TH cells. The APC also stimulates the T cells by releasing monokine interleukin-1 (IL-1) which, among other things, induces IL-2 receptors on the T cell.
Antibody response. TH cells help B cells to make antibody either by direct interactions with the B cells across an antigen bridge, or by releasing factors which may act by first binding to APCs. The interaction between the T helper cells and B cells is also effected by the lymphokines IL-2, B cell growth factor (BCGF) and differentiation factor (BCDF).
The cell-mediated immune response involves cooperation between TH cells and the effector cells - macrophages and cytotoxic T cells. This is again mediated by a variety of lymphokines. Cytotoxic T cells and macrophages can both damage target cells and tissues: macrophages by the release of enzymes and other inflammatory mediators, and Tc cells by direct antigen-specific cytotoxicity.

Some individuals have a characteristically high level of response to particular antigens, while others have a low response. Hence these are called high and low responders. High responders to some antigens may be low responders to others, and vice versa. Although the overall level of immune response is determined by a large number of genes (immune response genes), the MHC class II molecules are particularly important in this respect. Indeed, the MHC class II gene locus was initially identified as a region containing immune response (Ir) genes. MHC class II genes are not only involved in the interactions between APCs and T helper cells, but also in the cooperation between T cells and B cells in the production of an antibody response to T_{dep} antigens. There is evidence that T cell help may be transmitted either in direct cell/cell contact, or by lymphokines, of which there is a considerable number.

Lymphokines and Monokines

Activated T cells and macrophages release a number of molecules which act as signals for other cells, and these are essential for the development of the immune response. Factors released by lymphocytes are termed lymphokines and those from monocytes and macrophages are monokines. This group of chemical messengers includes the interleukins and some of the interferons. Macrophages release interleukin 1 (IL-1) which acts on T cells to produce, among other effects, the release of IL-2 and expression of IL-2 receptors. IL-2 acts on T cells to cause the proliferation of cells which have previously been activated by an antigen/MHC signal. T cells also release lymphokines which act on B cells, the so-called B cell stimulating factors (BSFs). Since T cells can cooperate with B cells in an antigen-specific fashion, there is some debate as to whether T cells release antigen-specific factors (see Chapters 10 and 11). Alternatively, T cells may cooperate directly with B cells, with the carrier-specific T cell being linked to the hapten-specific B cell by antigen acting as a bridge. The antigen may bridge the T cell and B cell receptors, but it is more probably associated with class II molecules on the B cell surface. The cooperative interactions which occur within the immune system are summarized in Figure 1.10.

In vivo the role and specificity of the lymphokines is even more difficult to investigate, since many lymphokines only act as short range signalling molecules within the confines of particular areas of lymphoid organs. Microenvironmental effects may, thus, limit the extent of lymphokine effects. Several lymphokines are involved in the activation of the microbicidal powers of macrophages. There are a large number of different lymphokines and it is likely that the mixture of lymphokines released by, for example, T cells depends not only on the type of cell, but also on its stage of development and its point in the cell cycle. Since the expression of receptors on responding cells also fluctuates, this leads to precise and subtle regulation of immune reactions.

REGULATION OF IMMUNE RESPONSES

Immune responses are controlled by the interactions described above and by the action of T suppressor cells. Because antigen is the initial signal for all immune reactions, the elimination of antigen such as occurs following the resolution of an infection limits further stimulation of the immune system. Thus, the action of the system as a whole can be seen as being directed towards the elimination of antigen, producing a feedback inhibition of further activation of the antigen-specific cells. Within this system there are a number of smaller scale regulatory interactions. For example, the production of antibody feeds back on antigen-specific B cells (probably via their Fc receptors) to limit their further proliferation. As indicated above, T cells are crucial in regulating the level of the response. In addition to the T helper cells which are specific for antigen, there is a second group of T helper cells active in some responses. These are idiotype-specific T cells which are responsible for selectively expanding the populations of B cells carrying particular idiotypes. In effect, T cell help can act at two levels. Initially, antigen-specific T cells expand the population of antigen-specific B cells, and this may be followed by selective expansion of particular subpopulations of the B cells (for example, those expressing a particular idiotype), as will be described in Chapter 13.

Antibody responses and many cell-mediated reactions are also modulated by T suppressor cells which, like T helper cells, may be antigen-specific, idiotype-specific or non-specific, termed Ts1, Ts2 and Ts3 respectively. The activation signal for Ts1 cells is, naturally enough, antigen itself, but the generation of the idiotype-specific Ts2 population depends on the idiotype expressed on B or T cells. Suppressor cells can act on both the generation of the immune response and on the effector cells (as explained in Chapters 10 and 12).

IMMUNE EFFECTOR MECHANISMS

The first step in many immune reactions is the recognition of antigens which are carried on the surface of invading organisms, but this is only preliminary to the reactions which follow, aimed at eliminating the source of the antigen. To achieve this, the immune system recruits a number of other effector systems in the body's defence and the end result is inflammation. Of prime importance in this respect is the complement system, consisting of about twenty normal serum proteins. The functions of this system include the attraction of cells to the site of inflammation (chemotaxis), increasing the local blood supply and increasing vascular permeability, so that there is an increased flow of serum proteins across the vascular endothelium and into the tissues. Inflammation can also be triggered by the activation of mast cells sensitized with antigen-specific IgE, causing the release of the mast cell granule contents and inducing the synthesis of a group of inflammatory mediators derived from arachidonic acid, the leukotrienes, thromboxanes and prostaglandins (Fig. 1.11; see overpage).

Inflammatory reactions may be acute with a preponderance of neutrophils, or, if the antigenic stimulus is persistent, a chronic reaction may develop. Sites of chronic inflammation usually contain considerably more lymphocytes and macrophages. In either case, the development of the lesion is dependent on the interplay between the immune system and the other inflammatory effector systems, which is signalled by the various soluble factors, including antibody, lymphokines and activated serum enzyme system peptides, as will be expanded upon in Chapter 15.

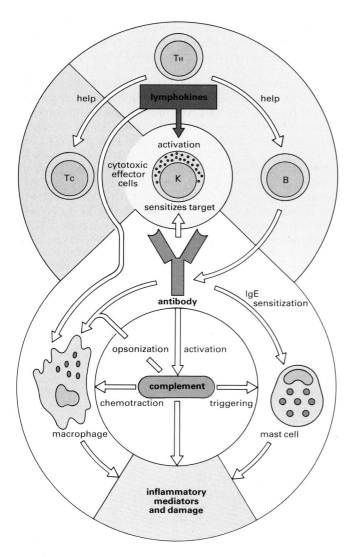

Fig. 1.11 Immune effector mechanisms. The immune system can activate a variety of inflammatory effector systems. The cells with antigen specificity interact with other cells by the release of antibody and lymphokines. Antibody sensitizes target cells for K cell-mediated cytotoxicity, and can also act as an opsonin for macrophages and other phagocytes with Fc receptors (e.g. neutrophils). Antibody in association with antigen can activate the classical complement pathway. This in turn releases a number of chemotactic peptides and can lead to the deposition of complement on the surface of the activating material: complement also acts as an opsonin. IgE antibody sensitizes mast cells, which release a wide variety of inflammatory mediators when triggered by antigen. Lymphokines and some of the complement peptides also serve to activate cells at sites of inflammation.

MODES OF IMMUNE RESPONSE

The type of reaction produced by the immune system in response to an antigen usually determines the way in which it will subsequently react to the same antigen. Generally speaking, the system tolerates all the potential antigens on the body's own tissues, while reacting against external antigens. The type of response produced to the external antigens depends to a great extent on the way in which the antigen is processed and presented to the different lymphocyte populations and this, in turn, depends on the nature of the antigen and its route of entry into the body. So, any single antigen might stimulate an antibody response if injected parenterally, but induces T cell-mediated sensitization if applied to the skin. Similarly, an antigen which induces no response when soluble may be immunogenic when aggregated. However, once an antigen has elicited one type of response, subsequent antigenic challenge will usually produce the same type of response, due to the selective expansion of particular subpopulations of lymphocytes. Similarly, if an antigen has once induced immunological tolerance, particularly in the neonatal period, the condition of tolerance often persists on subsequent exposure to the antigen.

The secondary response to most antigens is usually greater than the primary response and usually shows maturation. This is seen in the class switching from IgM to IgG and other isotypes which occurs in the antibody response and is often accompanied by an increase in the affinity of the antibodies. This indicates that the enhanced secondary response is not merely due to its being generated by an expanded responding B cell population, but that the response is produced by cells which have undergone additional differentiation steps. Similar considerations apply to the secondary responses of T cells.

TOLERANCE

Tolerance is the specific lack of an immune reaction to a particular antigen, which may be induced naturally or by particular injection schedules. Tolerance may occur as an active process due to ongoing suppression of potentially reactive cells, or may be due to the functional deletion of those cells. The two conditions may be distinguished since active suppression by T suppressor cells can be transferred to a non-tolerant individual, whereas tolerance due to clonal deletion cannot.

The most marked example of tolerance is that of tolerance to self tissues. During their development, lymphocytes pass through a stage at which they are highly susceptible to the induction of tolerance, with a relatively low dose of antigen. It is much more difficult to render mature cells tolerant, and virtually impossible to tolerize cells which have already been primed with antigen. Since the whole immune system is immature in the earliest stages of neonatal life, a newborn animal is particularly susceptible to the induction of tolerance. The functional deletion of self-reactive clones at this early stage of life is thought to be one way of developing self-tolerance. Self-reactive cells are not usually destroyed as they can be found in the circulation of an adult animal, and self-tolerance can be broken by experimental manoeuvres. Strictly speaking, it is only really necessary that T cells are self-tolerant, since most B cells require both antigen and T cell help as their activation signal. There are extra checks on self-reactivity which are mediated by T suppressor cells, thus, self-tolerance may also be established by deletion or active suppression; these concepts will be discussed in more detail in Chapter 12. Breakdown of self-tolerance occurs surprisingly frequently. However, it is only in a limited number of cases that the autoimmune reactions become chronic, and in those instances autoimmune disease may ensue.

SUMMARY

The adaptive immune system is responsible for recognition and reaction to antigens, and forms the main line of defence against invading pathogens. Lymphocytes are responsible for the function of recognition, while phagocytes and other effector systems may be recruited subsequently. The type of immune reaction which is generated depends not only on the antigen, but on how it enters the body and on the way in which it is presented to the lymphocytes by the various antigen-presenting cells. Recognition of antigens is dependent on three groups of molecules, the antigen receptors of T cells and B cells (sIg) and on the class I and class II molecules encoded by the major histocompatibility complex (MHC). These three gene loci generate molecules with an enormous amount of polymorphism, capable of recognizing whatever antigens may arise.

The cooperation between the various cells involved in the immune response may take place either by direct cellular interaction, or by soluble mediators. Interactions can be either antigen-specific or non-specific, but the structural organization of the lymphoid system means that even antigen-non-specific signals will have limited and localized effects.

Although problems may occur when the immune system reacts against its own tissues or where inappropriate hypersensitivity reactions occur, these should always be viewed in relation to the observation that a functional immune system is vital in host defence.

FURTHER READING

Golub E.S. (1981) *The Cellular Basis of the Immune Response.* Sinauer Associates, Massachusetts.

Lachmann P.J. & Peters D.K. (1981) *Clinical Aspects of Immunology.* 4th edn. Blackwell Scientific Publications, Oxford.

McConnell I., Munro A. & Waldmann H. (1981) *The Immune System: a Course on the Molecular and Cellular Basis of Immunity,* 2nd edn. Blackwell Scientific Publicatons, Oxford.

Nisonoff A. (1982) *Introduction to Molecular Immunology.* Sinauer Associates, Massachusetts.

Roitt I.M. (1984) *Essential Immunology,* 5th edn. Blackwell Scientific Publications, Oxford.

Roitt I.M., Brostoff J. & Male D.K. (1985) *Immunology.* Gower Medical Publishing Ltd, London.

Stites D.P., Stobo J.D., Fudenberg H.H. & Wells J.V. (1984) *Basic and Clinical Immunology,* 5th edn. Lange Medical Publications, Los Altos, California.

Taussig M.J. (1984) *Processes in Pathology and Microbiology.* Blackwell Scientific Publications, Oxford.

MOLECULES OF THE IMMUNE SYSTEM

2 Antibody

The three sets of molecules involved in immune recognition are a) the antibodies, b) the T cell receptor and c) the MHC-encoded cell surface molecules. Of these, antibodies were the first to be identified as factors present in the gamma globulin fraction of serum, which were capable of neutralizing a number of infectious organisms. Since antibodies, unlike the other receptor molecules, can be produced in both membrane and secreted forms, they can be prepared in relatively large quantities and this has led to the elucidation of their structure by biochemical and crystallographic means. Consequently, antibodies are the best characterized of the receptor molecules, and much of what is known of the structure of the T cell receptor and MHC molecules is derived by comparison and inference from the known antibody structures.

Antibodies are produced by B cells in two distinct forms: as cell surface antigen receptors of other B cells or, if the B cell is stimulated to differentiate into an antibody-secreting cell, as soluble antibody in the extracellular fluids. The quintessential role of antibodies is as bifunctional molecules, which bind antigen via their antigen-combining sites and then crosslink the antigen to cells of the immune system. The protein structure of antibodies reflects this function since they have highly variable (V) domains, which can interact with the vast diversity of antigens, and relatively constant portions formed by constant (C) domains which interact with cells and effector systems of the body. Again, the dual function of antibodies is mirrored in the genetic organisation of antibody genes, where separate exons encode the variable and constant domains which are stitched together by DNA recombinations and RNA splicing.

Antibodies can be divided on the basis of structural differences into classes and subclasses, differing in their Fc regions, so that they can interact with different cells of the immune system and effector systems such as complement. The classes are IgG, IgM, IgA, IgD and IgE, each of which can be produced in a membrane or secreted form, and every one of these classes has been found in different mammalian species studied, although the number of subclasses within each class varies between species. This implies that diversification of subclasses has occurred during the development of mammals, whereas the classes can be traced further back in evolution. For example, IgG is present in birds, and antibodies resembling IgM are present in the most primitive fishes. The diversification of antibody classes and subclasses has occurred concurrently with the development of the advanced immune systems seen in vertebrates. The evolution of different subclasses which can interact with different effector cell types permits the B cell to act as the body's general recognition system, by supplying antigen recognition molecules (antibodies) for the use of other cells.

Surface IgM is the first antibody to appear on the surface of B cells, and secreted IgM is the major component of the primary immune response. The affinity of IgM antibodies is relatively low but this is offset by their multivalency, so that the overall avidity of IgM antibodies is often quite high, especially when binding to antigens which express multiple antigenic determinants (epitopes). This sort of polyvalent antigen includes the polymeric carbohydrates and peptidoglycans present on bacterial cell walls. Many of these antigens induce antibody responses without T cell help (T independent antigens). Generally the affinity of the antibody response to an antigen increases during a response, but this is not true of IgM antibodies, and the affinity of antibodies to T independent antigens also tends to remain stable. The increase in antibody affinity is associated with a switch to IgG production, both at the level of individual B cells and in the overall profile of the antibody response (Fig. 2.1).

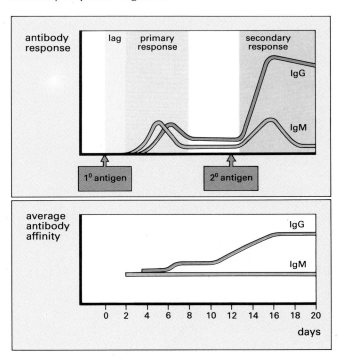

Fig. 2.1 Development of the antibody response. The upper graph shows that, following primary antigenic challenge, there is a lag period before the appearance of specific antibody (typically 2-3 days). IgM appears first in the primary response, followed by IgG. Secondary challenge with T_{dep} antigen produces a much enhanced response with a shorter lag period and a switch to IgG production. The lower graph shows that the affinity of IgM antibodies generally remains little changed by repeated antigenic challenge, whereas the average affinity of IgG antibodies starts to increase (affinity maturation) towards the end of the primary response, and increases further with additional antigenic stimulation. In general, smaller antigen doses produce the most marked affinity maturation, whereas larger doses tend to produce more antibody but of lower affinity.

IgG is the major component of the secondary immune response to T dependent antigens. Most subclasses of IgG can activate complement (IgG1, 2 and 3 in humans), and there are specific receptors to transfer IgG subclasses across the placenta. Fc_γ receptors which mediate opsonic adherence are present on macrophages and neutrophils, and there are also receptors for IgG on B cells and some T cells which are thought to be involved in immuno-regulation. IgG is also the most effective class of antibody for sensitizing targets for antibody-dependent cytotoxicity (ADCC), such as the killing of schistosomules by eosinophils which is effected by linking of the eosinophils to the Fc region of IgG on the target schistosomule. If one considers IgM as the first line of defence to microorganisms, capable of inhibiting pathogens by virtue of its agglutinating ability, then IgG is the second line adapter molecule which permits many other immune effector systems to be brought into play.

IgA is the major immunoglobulin component of secretions, and is transported across epithelia of the gut and salivary glands by a ligand transfer system involving binding to secretory component. It is, therefore, the key adaptive element of the body's exterior defences, where it functions to inhibit pathogen proliferation and prevent reinfection (Fig.2.2).

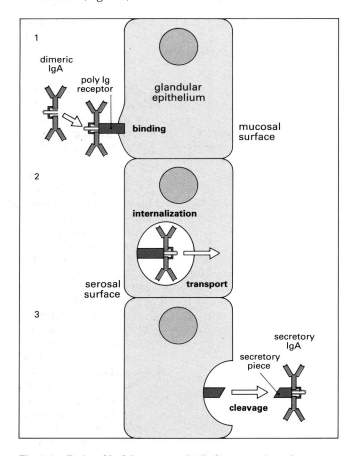

Fig.2.2 Role of IgA in protection of mucosal surfaces.
Dimeric IgA can link to the poly-Ig receptor exposed on the serosal side of glandular epithelia (e.g. the gut). The IgA/receptor complex is internalized and transported to the mucosal surface where it is released by proteolysis. The ligand-binding portion of the receptor remains attached to the IgA dimer by disulphide bonds and constitutes the secretory piece which protects IgA from degradation in the mucosal secretions.

IgE sensitizes mast cells via their Fc receptors, and thus provides a link between the immune system and inflammatory effector systems. It may also be responsible for the sensitization of worms for destruction by eosinophils. The role of IgD is controversial. Some immunologists maintain that it plays an essential role in B cell ontogeny, and in establishing the state of immunity/tolerance to particular antigens. Others consider it an evolutionary relic, which is on its way out. For example, the structure of mouse IgD appears to be degenerate with respect to its structural flexibility, hence in its antigen-binding function.

ANTIBODY GENES AND POLYPEPTIDES

The mRNA for an immunoglobulin chain is formed by linking separate gene segments (exons) encoding the variable and constant domains of each chain. The structure of the immunoglobulin genes is closely related to that of their polypeptide chains: each domain is encoded by a separate exon, and there are additional exons encoding the hinge region and transmembrane portions of the heavy chains (Fig.2.3). The segments of DNA which encode each of the domains are separated from each other by introns. The mRNA encoding each chain is assembled from heteronuclear RNA, by enzymatic splicing to remove the introns and appose the exons coding for the different domains. The gene segment which encodes the V domains lies several kilobases upstream of the C region genes, and a V gene may link to any one of the C genes. Thus, a B cell which initially links its heavy chain V gene to an IgM C gene can subsequently link the same V gene to a different C gene isotype (for example, IgE or IgG1). This process underlies class switching, where a single B cell changes the class of antibody which it produces, while retaining the same antigen specificity (see Chapter 4). Although the B cells of normal individuals carry two genes for each of the Ig gene loci, only one heavy chain allele and one light chain allele are ever expressed by any one cell. This process of allelic exclusion ensures that the individual B cell only produces one specificity of antibody.

Since antibodies were first discovered, there has been fierce debate about how the large range of antigen-binding specificities is produced. This question has recently been resolved. Three theories were proposed to account for the generation of antibody diversity:
1. A very large number of different V domain genes;
2. Somatic mutation of a small number of V genes;
3. Recombination of several small genetic elements at random to form the entire V domain gene.
It is now known that all the theories are correct, as each makes some contribution to variable region diversity.

Although there is only one copy of each of the constant region isotypes on each allele, there are multiple copies of the variable region genes. In addition, the gene segment present in the B cell which encodes the variable domain is assembled during B cell development from two or three separate gene segments by a process of somatic recombination. Heavy chain V region genes are formed by the recombination of a V segment, a D segment and a J segment, while light chain V genes are formed by a V segment and a J segment only. The V segments encode the N-terminal 100 (approximately) amino acids of the V domain. The J segments encode ten (approximately) amino acids lying at the C-terminal end of the V domain and join the V domain to the neighbouring C domain. The D segments present in heavy chains encode a variable number of amino acids (2 +) lying between those encoded by the V segment and those by the J segment. Each set of immunoglobulin genes (λ,κ or heavy chain) has multiple copies of V gene segments, D genes (heavy chains only) and J genes arranged in that order on the chromosome. The actual numbers of V, D, and J genes vary between the different loci and between species. For example, the human heavy chain gene stack is estimated to contain more than 300 separate V gene segments, whereas estimates of the number of mouse V_H genes range from 160 upwards. In mice the κ gene stack contains more than 50 V genes, whereas the region encoding the four λ chain isotypes has only two V genes, each of these being associated with two C and J genes. Ordinarily, though, the numbers of D and J genes are far fewer than the V genes. For example, the genes encoding the mouse heavy chain include 12 D and 4 J genes. A significant proportion of the different V, D and J genes are non-functional pseudogenes. These pseudogenes have structural homologies with their functional counterparts, but they cannot encode polypeptides, either because they lack the necessary recombination sequences on their flanking introns, or because mutation in the DNA has produced frame shifts.

VARIABILITY OF ANTIBODY STRUCTURE

Antibody variability was identified long before its genetic basis was understood, and the terminology which describes variability is, therefore, based on the observed differences of the protein structure of the antibodies, identified by antisera which recognize antigenic determinants on the antibodies. The total heterogeneity of antibodies is derived from three sources:
A. Variability of the different V regions, which is related to their ability to bind different antigens. This is known as *idiotypic variation*.
B. Variability in the constant domains which is determined by the C genes encoding the different classes and subclasses of the heavy chain and the two types of light chain, λ and κ. This is *isotypic variation*: every individual of a species carries the C genes for each one of the isotypic variants.
C. Variations in antibody structure which occur in different individuals of a species, called *allotypic variants*. This means that each variant is present in only a proportion of the members of a species.

Idiotypic Variation (Ids)
Antibody V domains, like any other protein, contain a number of antigenic determinants which can be recognized by specific antisera (anti-Ids). The determinants are idiotopes and the collection of idiotopes expressed by an antibody constitutes that antibody's idiotype (Id). The idiotopes may be formed by either the heavy or the light chain, or may consist of parts of both heavy and light chain. Furthermore, it is possible to distinguish between idiotopes located within the binding site (site-associated Ids) and those outside (site-non-associated Ids). Anti-idiotypic antisera which bind to an idiotype and prevent that idiotype from binding to its antigen do so by preventing the antigen from reaching the combining site, hence they are anti-Id to site-associated idiotopes. This does not mean that the antigen and the anti-Id bind to exactly the same point on the Id, but merely implies that the anti-Id is sufficiently large to prevent the antigen binding to the paratope. Anti-Ids which do not block antigen binding to idiotype are directed to site-non-associated idiotopes. An idiotope which can be detected on two different antibodies is termed a cross-reactive idiotope, and the antibodies which share them are cross-reactive idiotypes (CRI). This is analogous to cross-reactive antigens. CRIs are not usually identical to each other; they merely share some similar idiotopes. One other feature of idiotypic variation is of interest, the observation that particular idiotypes appear to be inherited from one generation to another within a particular strain of inbred animals, that is, they act like isotypes. These are referred to as heritable Ids.

Since there are a large number of genes which may contribute to the formation of the antibody V domains, the nature of idiotypic variation within an individual is very complicated. Considering the V domain as a whole, the framework regions and the first two hypervariable regions are encoded by the V gene segments in the germline, but

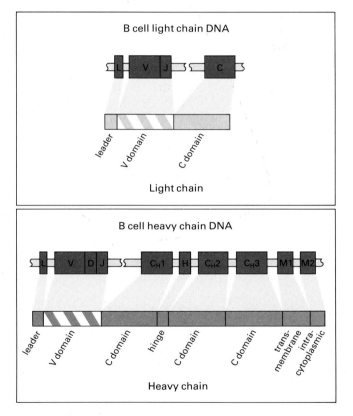

Fig.2.3 The relationship of antibody genes to their polypeptides. In a mature B cell the gene encoding the expressed light chain consists of three exons: an L exon encoding a leader peptide required for translation of the polypeptide across the membrane of the endoplasmic reticulum, an exon formed by the recombination of a V and a J gene, which will encode the variable domain, and a C exon encoding the constant domain. Heavy chains in these cells (here illustrated as membrane IgG1) also have a leader. The variable domain is encoded by an exon formed by the recombination of three separate gene segments, that is a V gene, a D gene and a J gene. There are separate exons for each constant domain, one for the hinge (H), and two for the transmembrane (M1) and intracytoplasmic portions (M2) of the membrane antibody.

the third hypervariable region is formed by the 3' end of the V gene segment, the D gene (heavy chains) and the J gene. Since recombination of the V, D and J genes does not always occur with absolute precision, areas of the third hypervariable region may not be directly encoded by any germline gene at all (Fig. 2.4).

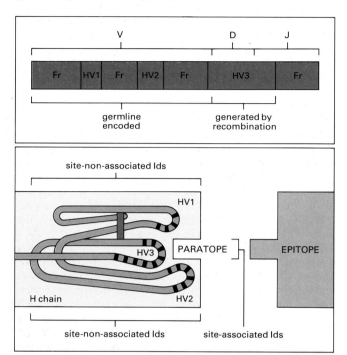

Fig. 2.4 Idiotopes. The upper diagram illustrates the structure of the exon encoding a V$_H$ domain. Two of the hypervariable regions (HV1 and HV2) are directly germline-encoded, while HV3 is produced by recombination of V, D and J genes. Idiotopes are the V region's antigenic determinants, and they may be present in the paratope (site-associated) or outside of it, as illustrated below. Since the residues which form the idiotopes and those which bind the antigen are often different, the determination of whether an idiotope is site-associated depends on the anti-Id preventing the Id binding to antigen. Whether they will interfere in this way is influenced by the affinities and sizes of the anti-Id and antigen. Thus, the discrimination between the two types of idiotope is not absolute. Idiotopes may be encoded by hypervariable or framework regions. The latter are likely to be more common in an individual's total antibody repertoire than those encoded by hypervariable regions.

How, then, does idiotypic variability correspond to the different germline V genes? Before the complexity of the Ig genes was discovered, it was observed that the V regions within an individual fell into a number of structurally similar groups and subgroups, which could be distinguished by their having particular antigenic determinants. This is rather similar to the categorization of antibodies into classes and subclasses according to their C regions. The epitopes which determine the V region groups and subgroups lie within the framework regions of the V domains and are, therefore, site-non-associated idiotopes. It also means that the determinants which identify the different groups and subgroups are encoded by the germline V gene segments. There are approximately ten mouse heavy chain groups and, since there are hundreds

of V$_H$ gene segments, this means that several different V genes encode antibodies of each of the different groups. In other words, there are sets of different V genes which are sufficiently similar to each other to belong to the same serologically identified heavy or light chain group. Sets of structurally related V genes can be identified by Southern blot analysis, since cDNA probes complementary to one member of the group will more readily hybridize to another member of the same group, than to V genes belonging to another group. Using this type of analysis on mouse heavy chain V genes, it was found that the genes belonging to a particular group lie adjacent to each other on the chromosome and are separate from adjoining stacks of V genes belonging to other goups or subgroups. This is illustrated in Figure 2.5.

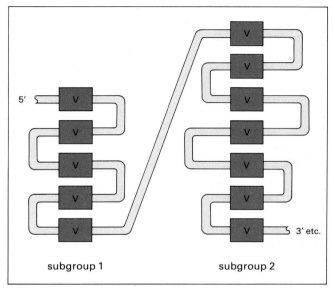

Fig. 2.5 Relation of subgroups to genes. This diagram shows how the V genes which encode Ig polypeptides belonging to different groups and subgroups lie together in the V gene stack. There may be several such stacks in the entire genome, each encoding different groups. The groups and subgroups have similar framework residues. The different V genes in a group have diversified relatively recently and/or a gene correction mechanism maintains V gene homology within each group.

Although members of a group are structurally related, this relationship does not extend as far as their antigen-binding capacities. For example, when four genes of the T15 group were analysed, one (T15 itself) encoded antibody which bound to phosphoryl choline, a second to influenza haemagglutinin, a third to another unidentified antigen, and the fourth was a non-functional pseudogene.

Whereas the first two hypervariable regions of each V domain are germline-encoded, the third is formed by recombination of a V, (D) and J gene at random with the purpose of generating variability to produce many different antigen-combining sites. It might be anticipated that the idiotopes expressed by the third hypervariable region vary at random between different antibodies and among strains, but this is not so, for two reasons. Firstly, elements of the third hypervariable region are germline-encoded (for example, each individual D or J region) and, if a particular idiotope is encoded by one of these elements, then the idiotope will occur on many other antibodies which use the same D or J genes. Secondly, there are some functional constraints on antibody variability. In other words, there frequently are idiotypic similarities between antibodies which bind to the same antigen. If a particular set of amino acids in an antibody's paratope binds efficiently to one particular epitope, then the antigen will selectively stimulate B cells whose immunoglobulin receptors have that particular set of amino acids. If that set of amino acids defines a site-associated idiotope, then antigen will selectively stimulate B cells with that particular idiotype (Fig.2.6).

This reasoning can explain why some idiotypes occur in the immune response of different individuals to the same antigen (recurrent idiotypes). Either different individuals of

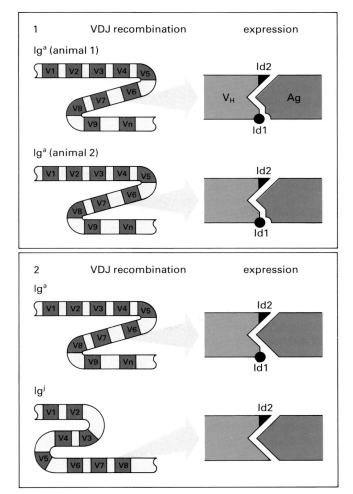

Fig.2.6 Recurrent idiotopes. This diagram illustrates how different antibodies to the same antigen can carry a common cross-reactive idiotope. There are two possible reasons for the recurrence of cross-reactive idiotopes on antibodies to a particular antigen (Ag): 1. Animals of the same Ig haplotype (eg. Ig^a) produce antibodies using the same set of germline V genes. These express the same sets of idiotopes (Id1 and Id2) and act as heritable idiotypes. 2. Animals of different Ig haplotype can also produce antibodies with the same idiotope. They are clearly generated from different sets of V genes in this case, but constraints on the structure of the antibody combining site produces similar idiotopes in the combining site (Id2). The similarities between the two antibodies which create the cross-reactive idiotope may be very limited, sometimes only a few amino acids.

the same strain have the same sets of V, D and J genes and therefore tend to produce antibodies of similar structure or, in different strains where the animals have different sets of V, D and J genes, the antigen itself may selectively stimulate antibodies with similar structures that are complementary to that antigen. The occurrence of heritable idiotypes can be explained in a similar way. If the germline V, D or J genes determine the expression of a particular idiotype, then the idiotype will be transmitted to an individual's offspring and will be expressed by a proportion of the B cells. In this way, the heritable idiotypes are effectively encoded by different V gene isotypes.

Isotypic Variants

The constant region genes are isotypic variants. In the case of light chains, there is one isotypic variant of the kappa chain and several of the lambda chain. For example, there are three functional lambda isotypes in mouse (two major ones) with 70% amino acid homology between their C_1 regions, and there are at least four lambda isotypes in humans. It is thought that each of the different lambda isotypes is encoded by separate genes. The number of heavy chain isotypes varies between species. In man there are nine: μ, δ, γ_1, γ_2, γ_3, γ_4, ϵ, α_1 and α_2, with the μ and α_2 genes lying closest to the V genes. The region also contains three pseudogenes. Mice have eight heavy chain isotypes: μ, δ, γ_3, γ_1, γ_{2b}, γ_{2a}, ϵ and α arranged in that order. Each of these (except δ) is preceded by a sequence important in class switching, and each of the heavy chain isotypes can be produced in membrane or secreted form. The lack of a switching sequence in front of delta precludes B cells from making IgD alone. It is always produced together with at least some IgM. Every one of the C genes has exons encoding the C-terminal transmembrane segments and intracytoplasmic portions of the membrane form of the antibody. Membrane antibody is translated from mRNA which includes these exons, while they are absent in mRNA for secreted antibody. The cell can splice a single heteronuclear RNA, mRNA precursor, in one of two ways, to produce the two types of mRNA, and hence membrane or secreted antibody. The molecular mechanisms which determine this choice are not yet known. This critical stage of differentiation control is likely to keep molecular biologists busy for many years.

The different subclasses of heavy chains appear to have developed in various mammalian species since the divergence of different orders, and so it is unprofitable to compare them in widely divergent species. Nevertheless, in closely allied species they do have similarities. For example, goat and sheep IgG subclasses are very similar both structurally and functionally, and humans seem to share IgG2 and IgG3 with the great apes. In general, however, subclasses given the same designation in different species are not usually functionally related.

The immunoglobulin domains are clearly related to each other and to the MHC-encoded molecules, including β_2-microglobulin as well as the T cell surface marker Thy1 (see Chapter 5). Each of these molecules contains a number of domains with the potential to fold into a structure similar to that of an antibody domain, with regions of β-pleated sheet stabilized by intrachain disulphide bonds in some cases. Generally, the homology between the immunoglobulin C domains of κ, λ and γ is 30-40%, while their homology with α and μ is less. Homologies between the individual domains of the human γ subclasses are greater, up to 80%, and there is some indication that different domains have not diversified at the same rate. With the large numbers of related immunoglobulin domains it is not surprising that some determinants recognized by antibodies to Ig are expressed on different isotypes. This includes determinants recognized by isotype-specific sera, and those recognized by anti-allotypic reagents, indicated below.

Allotypes

The immunoglobulins of individuals of a species express allotypic determinants which are recognized by other individuals lacking the allotype. Human Ig allotypes were originally recognized by rheumatoid sera which contain naturally occurring anti-Ig antibodies, but anti-allotypes raised by deliberate or accidental immunization identify allotypes more accurately as they are usually specific for single allotypes, whereas rheumatoid sera are not. Five sets of allotypic markers are recognized in humans. These are the Gm, Am and Mm systems which are determined by the heavy chain C regions, the Km (=Inv) system determined by the kappa genes, and the Hv system determined by the V_H genes which could be considered a public idiotype marker, that is, a marker present on a large set of different antibodies. Since heavy chains of different classes may combine with kappa chains, the Km allotypes may occur in association with any of an individual's heavy chain allotypes on different antibodies (Fig.2.7).

Allotype system	Location	Comment
Km (= Inv)	κ chains	expressed on IgG1 and IgG3; 3 variants; requires IgG quarternary structure for expression
Hv	heavy chain V domain	one variant
Am	Fc$_\alpha$	two variants of IgA2
Mm	Fc$_\mu$	one variant
Gm	Fc$_\gamma$ and C$_H$1	at least 24 variants 3 associated with IgG1 1 with IgG2, 13 with IgG3 + 7 unassigned

Fig.2.7 Human Ig allotypes. List of five major systems of human Ig allotypes and their gene locations.

The Gm series of heavy chain allotypic determinants are most numerous (at least 24 variants), occurring on IgG constant regions. The majority of the allotypic sites have been localized to the Fc region, but G1m(4) and G1m(17) are determined by the C$_H$1 domain. Since the anti-allotype sera recognize determinants rather than individual isotypes, some of the allotypic markers can occur on different subclasses, while others may only be expressed on one subclass. To indicate this, the nomenclature includes a

figure showing which subclasses each allotype is associated with. For example, G1m(4) and G1m(17) are associated with IgG1, while G3m(5) and G3m(6) occur on IgG3. In some cases, if an individual haplotype carries one Gm allotype it precludes the presence of another (i.e. G3m(5) and G3m(21)), which implies that the allotypes are determined by close or identical amino acid positions. In some cases the presence of the allotype depends on single amino acid changes. For example, G1m(4) has Arg at position 214 of the γ_1 chain, whereas IgG1 antibodies lacking this allotype do not. In other cases the determinant is produced by the three-dimensional structure of the immunoglobulin. For example, the Km light chain determinants are only weakly expressed on free light chains, or on kappa chains associated with γ_2 or γ_4 heavy chains. The majority of allotypes are restricted to a single antibody isotype, but in some cases allotypes can occur on different classes or subclasses also. For example, the allotype of IgG4 nG4m(a) is also present on all IgG1 and IgG3 molecules. Such markers are called isoallotypes.

Although Ig allotypes are of interest to population geneticists, one might wonder whether they have any significance in the operation of the immune system. There have been reports of disease association with particular allotypes (for example, in rheumatoid arthritis), but this may only reflect a tighter linkage to V region idiotypes and the B cell repertoire. The associations are in any case relatively weak when compared with MHC allotype disease association. However, it has been noted that the levels of particular isotypes within an individual are partly dependent on that individual's allotype: individuals who are homozygous for G3m(5) have approximately twice the amount of serum IgG3 than do those who lack the allotype. Heterozygotes have intermediate levels.

Ig allotypes are present in every animal species tested so far. In mice they have been very useful for determining the origin of secreted Ig in experiments where donor cells of one allotype are transferred into a recipient of another allotype. Unfortunately, the nomenclature of the mouse Ig allotypes is extraordinarily confusing. The allotypes of the Ig-1 gene locus encode IgG2a heavy chains, Ig-2 encodes IgA, Ig-3 encodes IgG2b, Ig-4 encodes IgG1, Ig-5 encodes IgD and Ig-6 encodes IgM. There are between two and eight alleles for each of these loci, with greater numbers of recognized allotypic determinants. For example, the eight allotypes of Ig-1 include ten recognized allotypic determinants. Once again, it is doubtful whether this genetic complexity has any more than a marginal effect on the operation of the immune system.

RECOMBINATION OF ANTIBODY GENES

Assembling mRNA for an immunoglobulin polypeptide requires DNA recombination during B cell development and maturation. This occurs in two stages. The first stage involves the recombination of V, D and J segments to form the gene encoding the V_H and V_L domains. This takes place during differentiation of lymphoid stem cells into B cells. The second stage of gene recombination may occur in the C_H genes of differentiated B cells, and is involved in irreversible class switching by the B cell.

Comparison of the immunoglobulin DNA in non-lymphoid cells and in B cells shows that gene rearrangements take place during B cell ontogeny, as evidenced by changes in the restriction enzyme fragments of the Ig genes in mature B cells. The underlying cause of these changes is recombination between the V, D and J gene segments with loss of intervening introns (Fig.2.8). The recombination takes place in a defined sequence, heavy chains first, and then kappa and lambda genes until functional V genes for both heavy and light chains have been generated (see Chapter 4). In heavy chains, DJ recombination precedes VD recombination, and early B cells may transcribe some non-functional D, J, C transcripts. The mechanism which activates the process of recombination of Ig genes only occurs efficiently in B cells, and, appears to be directed by specific recombination sequences flanking the V, D and J exons. These sequences consist of complementary sets of bases which can form loops with the sequences adjoining the next type of gene segment. The particular sequences take the form of a heptamer, then 12 or 23 unpaired bases are followed by a nonamer. These are arranged in such a way that a flanking intron which contains a sequence of 12 unpaired bases will only recombine with an intron containing a sequence with 23 unpaired bases. The converse is also true (Fig.2.9 overpage). The flanking introns ensure that a light chain V segment can only recombine with a J gene, and a heavy chain V segment can only recombine with a D segment. Recombination is thought to occur exclusively on the cis chromosome and requires that the DNA strands are

broken and rejoined to remove the intron. Although the precise mechanism for this is not known, enzymes similar to those involved in DNA repair are implicated. Since the unmatched 12/23 base pairs can be in either orientation on the DNA strands, it is presumably the overall shape of the structure which is important in directing the enzymes to the correct site to effect the recombination. Pseudoalleles of J regions lacking the correct flanking sequences cannot recombine and are not expressed. Since any V_H gene can recombine with any D and any J gene, an enormous diversity of recombined VDJ genes can be formed. A similar argument applies to the light chains.

The recombination mechanism is not perfectly accurate. The exact point of recombination can vary between cells which are using exactly the same combinations of V and J genes. This may produce a limited shift in the RNA reading frame, but provided this is corrected by a compensatory shift in an adjoining recombination, this does not matter. All that it means is that the base sequences at the junction of V and J in these cells will differ slightly, and this in turn often produces polypeptides with different amino acids at the junction. Heavy chain genes also recombine with slight inaccuracies in the VDJ junctions, but in addition extra bases may be inserted into the recombined gene on either side of the D segment. This is seen in heavy chains which contain amino acids in the D, J junction which cannot be explained by any of the possible

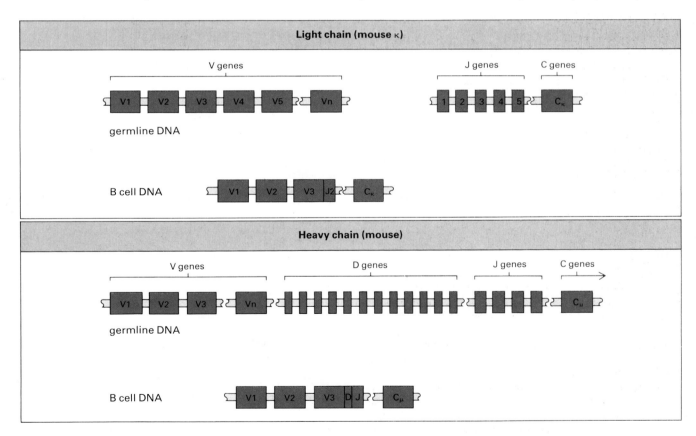

Fig.2.8 Recombination of light and heavy chains. The exon encoding the variable domain of a light chain (mouse kappa) is formed by the recombination of one of many V genes with one of four functional J genes, here illustrated as recombination between V2 and J2. The recombinational event can use any combination of V and J genes, although in mouse the third kappa J gene is a non-functional pseudogene which lacks the necessary flanking introns to

allow it to recombine. The exons encoding the mouse heavy chain are formed by the recombination at random of one of a large number of V genes, with one of twelve D gene segments and one of four J genes, to produce a recombined VDJ gene. The recombined gene segments encoding the variable domains become linked to exons encoding the C domains during mRNA splicing. This recombination takes place early on in B cell development.

D, J combinations in that species. The addition of extra bases in this way means that some of the bases have no origin in the germline. But the addition does not seem to be at random. For example, one group of Ig heavy chains which are present in antibodies to arsonate frequently contain a Ser residue in the VD junction which is encoded by bases inserted during recombination. Surprisingly, only one of the six Ser codons occurs at this point in these antibodies, although several different base insertions would produce the same protein. This implies that there may be constraints on which inaccuracies of recombination are permissible. Certainly, if recombinational inaccuracy produces a frame shift extending over any significant distance, the transcript would encode a non-functional protein, and such proteins are not found *in vivo*. Mutant plasmacytomas with untranslatable mRNA can arise *in vitro*, but this is an experimental contrivance and probably does not relate to physiological B cell development. Nevertheless, the possibilities created by inaccurate recombination are a further source of immunoglobulin V domain diversity.

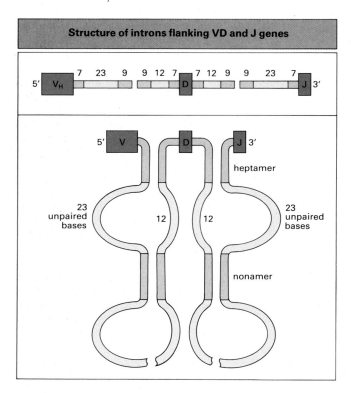

Structure of introns flanking VD and J genes

Fig.2.9 Recombination of heavy chain V, D and J genes. The three exons of heavy chain V genes have a heptamer-23 base pair-nonamer sequence, which corresponds to a sequence on the 5' side of the D genes. Similarly, there are corresponding sequences on the 3' side of D and the 5' side of J. The recombination mechanism is thought to involve looping out of the introns, with hybridization between heptamer and nonamer sequences, leaving unpaired loops of 12 and 23 base pairs which can act as a signal for recombination enzymes. The 12/23 rule states that recombination only occurs when the loops have these numbers of unpaired bases, and by this rule it is impossible for a heavy chain V gene to recombine directly with a J gene, since this would produce two loops of 23 unpaired bases. (Kappa light chain V genes have 12 base pairs on their 3' introns and the J genes have 23 base pairs on their 5', so that V kappa can recombine directly to a J kappa gene.)

SOMATIC MUTATION

At one time immunologists argued whether gene recombination or somatic mutation was the source of antibody diversity. It is now known that both mechanisms operate. Somatic mutation does occur in antibody molecules and it is not confined to the V regions. When a group of different T15.Id⁺ hybridoma antibodies raised to phosphoryl choline were sequenced, it was found that IgM antibodies had sequences directly encoded by the T15 germline DNA, but the IgA or IgG antibodies of the same specificity had sequences containing amino acid changes caused by point mutations in the DNA (see Gearhart, 1982). This implies that a mutational mechanism is activated during class switching which acts on the Ig genes. These mutations are present in both framework and hypervariable regions of the heavy chain V domains. The mutation rate in the Ig genes is very high, so high that the cell could not tolerate it in all its genes. Therefore, the mutational area is of necessity confined to the Ig genes but, interestingly, when the base sequences of the Ig heavy chain genes of mature B cells are examined, the mutations are found distributed throughout both the introns and the exons. In other words, the mutation mechanism which accompanies class switching acts on the general region of the Ig genes, and not at particular places.

This somatic mutation underlies the affinity maturation seen during the maturation of the IgG response to T dependent antigens. The advantages of mutation should be viewed in relation to antigen-driven selection of high affinity B cell clones. In this scheme, the mechanisms of VDJ recombination provide an initial crude antigen-combining site which may be modified and refined by mutation, and mutations which lead to higher affinity antibody on the B cell surface would lead to those B cells with higher affinity antibodies being selectively stimulated by comparison with the original unmutated antibody. Conversely, mutations which lead to lower affinity antibody receptors would bind antigen poorly, and those clones would not be stimulated to divide. It is worth recalling that the first and second hypervariable regions are germline-encoded and so initially they have less potential diversity than the third hypervariable region generated by recombination. Hence the first two hypervariable regions have greater scope for improvement than the third.

Recent data from Berek and colleagues (1985) suggest that the story does not end here. Examination of the amino acid sequences of antioxazolone antibodies which had been generated at different stages of the immune response, revealed that antibodies from the early primary response were effectively encoded by germline genes (when considering one particular idiotypic set). Antibodies from the late primary response used the same sets of heavy and light chain V genes but had, as expected, a number of mutations and increased affinity. However, in the secondary immune response many of the antibodies to oxazolone were generated from completely different sets of V genes, with moderately high affinity. One explanation of this finding is that, in the primary response, the antigen stimulates any major cell population to which it binds, and the affinity of these antibodies increases by mutation. However, in the secondary response, minor B cell populations which can respond to the antigen and have a greater potential for affinity maturation are selectively expanded.

The major population which reacts in the primary reaction has limited scope for improvement. Thus, the way in which an antibody response develops depends not only on the B cell antigen receptors, but also on the proportions of cells carrying the different receptors. As indicated above, antigen receptors are not generated at random, but they are partially constrained by the genes available in the genome.

To summarize this section, binding site diversity may be created by the multiple V, D and J gene and the combinations of these which may occur, along with possible inaccuracies in the recombination process. Somatic mutation can act on initially low affinity antibodies, to increase their binding ability, so that antigen selection preferentially stimulates those B cells. Since the antibody paratope is formed by both heavy and light chains, this is an additional source of diversity. Certain combinations of heavy and light chain may be particularly effective at binding some antigens. For example, $V_\kappa 45.1$ encoded light chain V domains and $V_H 7$ encoded heavy chain V domains frequently occur together in the response to oxazolone. There is evidence, however, that some H and L chain combinations may not be permitted. For example, it is noted that when the H and L chains of different myelomas are dissociated, they preferentially recombine with their homologous partner, indicating a restriction on their binding abilities. The mechanisms mentioned here can comfortably account for the enormous range of antibody paratopes which an individual can generate.

CONSTANT REGION GENES

The heavy chain constant region genes lie 3' to the recombined VDJ gene. Initially, B cells express only surface IgM. The μ gene is the closest C gene to the recombined VDJ, and the earliest functional trancript of the heavy chain genes starts with the leader sequence 5' to the recombined VDJ and extends through the VDJ gene to the C_μ gene, including the long intron between the variable and constant domain genes, which contains an enhancer sequence (see Chapter 4). Each of the constant domains is encoded by a separate exon, and the hinge region and transmembrane segments are also on different exons (Fig.2.11). There are two exons for the transmembrane segments: the first encodes the stretch of hydrophobic amino acids which actually transverse the membrane, and the second encodes the short intracytoplasmic segment. The sequence of the transmembrane section is highly conserved among different antibody classes, which suggests that each of the different antibody isotypes is locked into the membrane in a similar way, to activate the cell by a common pathway. The process of RNA splicing removes the introns between all of these exons during the formation of mRNA, but RNA splicing is also important in:

1. Determining whether mRNA is produced for membrane or secreted Ig;
2. Determining whether a cell will express IgM or IgD;
3. The initial stages of class switching.

The choice between the production of membrane or secreted Ig mRNA is made when the transcript is adenylated. Poly-A is attached to the 3' end of all mammalian RNA molecules which will become mRNA. This process is required for transport of the mRNA from the nucleus to the cytoplasm. The C_μ genes have two polyadenylation sites. One of them lies within the $C_\mu 4$ terminal exon of secreted IgM and the second lies at the 3' end of the second membrane domain. If polyadenylation takes place at the first of these sites, then mRNA for secreted IgM will be produced but, if it occurs at the second site, the RNA is spliced to remove the stop codon at the end of $C_\mu 4$ and the mRNA will include the membrane exons (Fig.2.11 overpage). Although transfection studies have shown that the proximity of the polyadenylation site to the promoter may affect the choice of site, it is uncertain whether this is the physiological mechanism of regulation.

Differential polyadenylation may also determine which Ig class a cell expresses. Long transcripts have been identified from B cell lines which include a recombined VDJ and more than one C gene. In these cases, the mRNA produced from the long transcript again depends on which of the several polyadenylation sites available are selected. For example, the transcript which includes VDJ, C_μ and C_δ is 25kB long and contains five alternative polyadenylation sites. The ways in which B cells vary their Ig RNA splicing are discussed in Chapter 4. The other mechanism by which B cells can switch class involves the second of the DNA recombination processes referred to earlier.

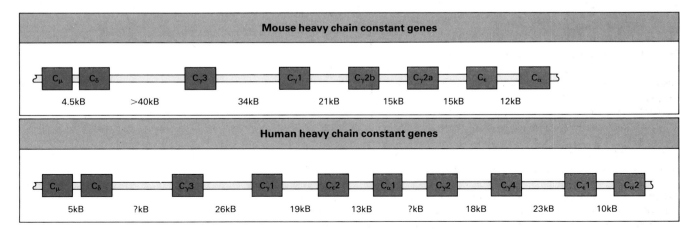

Fig.2.10 C genes. In both mouse and man the C_μ and C_δ genes are proximal to the recombined VDJ gene. These are separated from the other genes by long introns. (Figures indicate the length of introns in kilobases -kB.) In man there is a non-functional pseudogene ($C_{\epsilon 2}$) and the C gene stack seems to have arisen by duplication of a set of four genes. It must be noted that subclasses in man and mouse are not analogous.

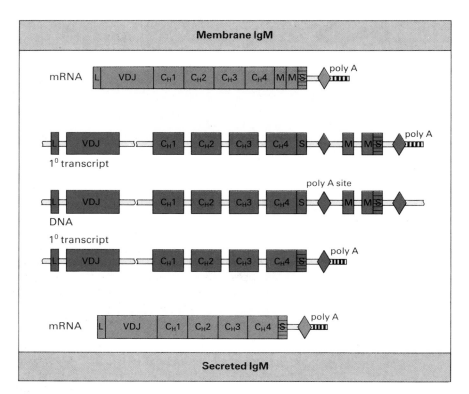

Fig.2.11 Polyadenylation control of gene expression. The DNA for the mouse IgM gene (centre) has two possible translation stop signals (S), one at the end of C_H4 and the other at the end of the second membrane exon (M). It also has two possible polyadenylation sites (here represented by diamond shapes). If the second site is used (upper), a transcript is produced which includes both membrane exons. During splicing, the first membrane exon is spliced to a site within the C_H4 exon to remove the terminal codons of the C_H4 domain containing the stop codon (S). Translation of this mRNA produces membrane IgM. If polyadenylation occurs at the first site following the C_H4 exon there is no further transcription, and splicing produces mRNA for secreted IgM (lower). Translation stops at the terminal codon of the C_H4 domain which has not been removed by splicing in this case.

In many mature B cells which have switched their Ig class expression, there are deletions of C genes between VDJ and the expressed C gene. This only occurs on the chromosome with the functionally rearranged VDJ. Analysis of the base sequences of C genes shows that all of them (in mouse), except delta, have a switching sequence 5' to the first C domain exon. The sequences are of the form $(GAGCT)_nGGGGT$, where the first element is a tandem repeat occurring one to seven times, and the whole sequence is then repeated up to 150 times. This gives a region of DNA 1-10kB long which lies 1-4kB upstream of the exon. The precise mechanism of recombination is uncertain, but it is thought that the similar S sequences cause the genes to be juxtaposed, so that enzymes can break and reconnect the strand to produce the recombination. It is quite possible that in some cases the chromosome carrying the VDJ gene is recombined at this stage to the sister chromatid, such that the final unit contains V genes and recombined VDJ of one parental haplotype and C genes of the other. Recombination of the C genes is effectively an irreversible event, since the intervening sequences are lost from the genome.

PRODUCTION OF ANTIBODY PEPTIDES

The processing of mRNA is thought to be effected by small ribonucleoprotein units. By analogy with other eukaryotic gene systems, the RNA in these units causes the donor and acceptor junctions immediately flanking the exons to be apposed, and then enzymes in the unit cut and rejoin the RNA strands, excising the introns, to leave mRNA. mRNA for immunoglobulin chains leaves the nucleus and becomes attached to ribosomes in the cytoplasm. The process now follows the general course taken by both membrane and secreted proteins, as the H and L chains are translated across the membrane of the endoplasmic

reticulum (ER). Initially, only the leader peptide encoded by the first exon is translated; further translation on that ribosome is blocked, until the translated leader binds to a signal recognition protein.

This protein then docks to a docking protein at a vacant site on the endoplasmic reticulum. The translation block is lifted and the ribosome proceeds to translate the rest of the polypeptide chain across the endoplasmic reticulum. The leader peptide, which is only required to direct the ribosome to the ER, is now enzymatically cleaved from the immunoglobulin chain. Membrane Ig molecules remain locked in the membrane at this stage, while secreted molecules are released into the endoplasmic reticulum. Membrane and secreted antibodies are then directed through different intracellular pathways.

Heavy and light chains are coordinately produced, and surplus chains which do not associate correctly with a partner are degraded within the cell. In developing B cells the production of functional antibody molecules also feeds back to control the process of gene recombination. Antibodies are glycoproteins, and they become glycosylated in the Golgi apparatus. Large carbohydrate units are transferred to acceptor sites on the Ig polypeptide which are subsequently enzymatically remodelled by transglycosylases. All antibody molecules contain some carbohydrate varying between 3-12%. The major carbohydrate units are covalently attached to asparagine (Asn) residues in the Fc region. For example, human IgG1 has units attached to Asn at position 297 in $C_\gamma2$ (Fig. 2.12). Carbohydrate is also attached to the Fab units of some antibodies, and occasionally affects antibody-binding characteristics by limiting the access of the antigen to the antibody paratope. Also, there is often microheterogeneity in carbohydrate units, so that the molecule as a whole is not necessarily totally symmetrical.

The J chain, found in secretory IgA and IgM, is a molecule of 137 amino acids (both in man and mouse) encoded on a different chromosome from the other Ig

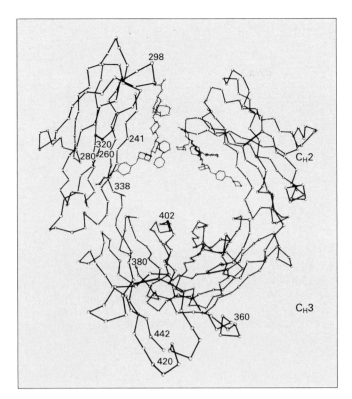

Fig.2.12 Structure of the Fc region. This illustrates the alpha carbon backbone of an IgG Fc region. The C$_H$3 domains are closely paired and linked by non-covalent bonds, but the C$_H$2 domains lie apart and two carbohydrate units (one from each chain) run down the cleft. The C$_H$2 domain contains the C1q binding site and is also mandatory for binding to the majority of Fc receptors. C$_H$3 and C$_H$2 are required together to form the protein-A binding site, and there is evidence that residues in C$_H$3 may also be involved in binding to some Fc receptors. Courtesy of Dr. J. Deisenhofer, adapted from Figure 2 in Biochemistry **20**, page 2365 (1981).

polypeptides. Its primary structure has recently been deduced from a B cell genomic library fragment. The molecule (which has nothing at all to do with J gene segments) is required for the correct polymerization of polymeric Ig (sIgM and polymeric IgA), and is also necessary for the binding of IgA to the secretory component. The J chain forms disulphide bonds with two Ig units, maintaining the correct conformation to facilitate polymerization. Enzymes have been found specifically in IgM-producing cells capable of catalysing the polymerization. Although the incorporation of the J chain is mandatory for the secretion of IgM, it is optional in IgA producers, and IgA producing cells can secrete mixtures of monomeric and polymeric IgA. There is only one J chain per polymer, regardless of the number of immunoglobulin units. In some diseases, like rheumatoid arthritis, monomeric IgM may appear in the serum, but it is not known whether this is due to degradation of the polymer, or to aberrant IgM synthesis. Although X-ray crystallographic data of the J chain structure are not available, the primary structure hints at the possibility of sections of anti-parallel, β-pleated sheet resembling Ig domains. Additionally, a B cell-specific promoter sequence found in the DNA 5' to the heavy and light chains also occurs 5' to the J chain gene. The J chain gene itself consists of a leader exon and three other exons, which is quite dissimilar to the

domain arrangement of Ig genes. There is 77% homology between human and mouse J chains and, interestingly, the C-terminal domains of the IgA and IgM heavy chains in these species also show greater homology than other domains, which indicates constraints on the antibody structure possibly due to the requirement to interact with the J chain. The J chain is synthesized in equal amounts by B cells producing IgM, IgA and IgG. There is considerable degradation of surplus J chains within the cells, but the function of the J chain in cells which do not produce polymeric immunoglobulins is a puzzle.

RELATIONSHIP OF STRUCTURE TO FUNCTION

The modular structure of antibodies reflects their role as bifunctional molecules, with different domains serving different purposes. The V domains generate antigen-combining sites, while the C domains interact with the complement molecules and various Fc receptors.

It is well established that the hypervariable loops of the V domains lie at the paratope. There is a relative lack of secondary bonds within these loops, and the flexibility resulting from this allows some latitude as to the structure of the epitope with which a particular antibody can combine. Although at a superficial level the epitope and the paratope may be said to have complementary shapes, the bond between them is ultimately dependent on the formation of a number of secondary bonds between individual amino acid residues in the paratope and individual residues in the epitope. This can be demonstrated by studying the binding of synthetic antigens to antibodies. By using hexapeptide antigens and substituting single amino acids, it is possible to determine which residues of the epitope are obligate, and which may be substituted by other amino acids without preventing antigen/antibody interaction. In some cases conservative substitution is permissible (i.e. residues with related structures), while non-conservative substitutions are not. This analysis indicates which residues form the bonds and what their nature is. Antibodies may also have particular obligate residues in the combining site. For example, a Ser residue is present in the heavy chain of anti-Ars antibodies mentioned above. This residue is a key feature which forms both parts of the Id, and it is necessary for antigen binding.

Observation of the three-dimensional structure of the paratope shows that, in many cases, the third hypervariable regions formed by VJ and VDJ lie at the centre of the combining site with HV1 and HV2 of heavy and light chains clustered around the periphery. Since HV3 is generated by recombination, and HV1 and HV2 are derived from the germline (initially), HV3 is the region of greatest variability and therefore more likely to generate a suitable set of binding residues for the antigen. Meanwhile, HV1 and HV2 can potentially limit access of antigen to the combining site. Therefore, in this scheme many antigens will bind initially to residues in VJ and VDJ, with the specificity of the interaction modulated by residues in HV1 and HV2. As the immune response develops, mutational mechanisms are activated and residues in HV1 and HV2 are changed, causing refinement of specificity and enhanced affinity. Naturally, many mutations will cause poorer antigen binding, but cells which have generated these mutations are comparatively less able to bind antigen and will not be stimulated into further division.

Functions of Constant Domains

$C_\gamma 1$ domain is closely associated with C_L, and is required for structural integrity of the Fab region and the expression of some of its associated allotypic determinants. The only other function which has been ascribed to this domain is binding of activated C4b and C3b. A labile thioester bond is exposed when C4 and C3 are cleaved, which can covalently attach to molecules in the immediate vicinity of the activation site, but whether complement binding to $C_H 1$ is a specific correlate of $C_H 1$ structure is debatable.

Complement activation via the classical pathway is initiated by binding of C1q to a site in $C_H 2$ of IgG and $C_H 4$ of IgM. Although all the subclasses of human IgG have potential C1q binding sites, the site in IgG4 is inaccessible to C1q because of steric hindrance by the Fab arms. It was once thought that the C1q binding site only became exposed once antigen bound to the antibody's paratope, but this is apparently not so since structural analysis, using nuclear magnetic resonance, of antibodies which have antigen bound to their combining site shows no evidence of allosteric changes extending down to the $C_H 2$ domain. This again emphasizes the structural independence of the different domains. It is now thought that binding of C1q to single antibody molecules is too weak ($1\text{-}5 \times 10^4 M^{-1}$) for there to be any significant level of binding in serum. But when there is a cluster of Fc regions, such as is present on immune complexes, C1q binds with higher avidity, thus activating C1r and C1s (for example, $10^6 M^{-1}$ for dimer complexes and $3 \times 10^9 M^{-1}$ for tetramers). The complement-activating capacity of complexes is therefore critically dependent on their size, larger complexes being much more effective. This scheme does not explain how IgM activates complement, since single molecules of IgM bound to antigen can trigger the entire classical and lytic pathways. In this case, the steric conformation of the whole IgM molecule is thought to be important, in that binding of Fab arms to the antigen (especially in a crab-like configuration) increases accessibility of the complement-activating site for C1q. The hinge region of antibody is critically important in conferring segmental flexibility on the molecule, which permits the two Fab arms to independently bind to epitopes. The hinge region is encoded by exons separate from the exons coding for the domains. Usually there is one hinge exon, but in human IgG3 which has an extended hinge region containing 15 inter-heavy chain S-S bonds, the hinge is encoded by several exons which apear to have arisen by gene duplication.

The carbohydrate which is attached to $C_H 2$ of IgG affects the overall solubility of the molecule and may be involved in the control of its catabolic rate. The glycosylation of antibodies is also necessary for cellular secretion of some of the antibody classes, including human IgE and IgA.

Receptors for Fc recognize sites in $C_\gamma 2$ and $C_\gamma 3$, but it has been quite difficult to pin down the precise residues involved (Fig.2.13). It is generally agreed that different cells express different receptors, with different binding characteristics. In some cases (for example, mouse macrophages), one cell type has several kinds of Fc receptors. Cells carrying receptors for Fc of IgG include neutrophils, macrophages, and cells of the RE system. These have receptors which are involved in phagocytosis of complexes and their degradation. B cells and some T cells also have Fc receptors for IgG, and these may play a role in regulating the immune response. A small population of T cells have receptors for IgM, and it has been proposed that these may be responsible for the augmented response to antigen seen when specific IgM is present. Mast cells and basophils have receptors for IgE, and platelets receptors for IgG. These cell types are involved in the control of inflammation, and their activation by antibody provides a link between the immune system and inflammatory mechanisms (discussed further in Chapter 15). The Fc receptors on K cells (including null cells, some T_γ cells and some monocytes) are required for recognition of target cells

Species/ cell type	Receptor	M^{-1} assoc. constant *	Class/subclass specificity†	Probable function
Human monocyte	IgG	5×10^8	IgG3, IgG1>IgG4>>IgG2	opsonic adherence
Mouse macrophage	IgG FcR1 FcR2 FcR3	2×10^7 5×10^5	IgG2a IgG2b, IgG1, IgG2a IgG3	opsonic adherence
Human polymorph	IgG	10^6	IgG3, IgG1>IgG4>>IgG2	opsonic adherence
Human T cells	IgG	$10^5\text{-}10^7$ ●	IgG1, IgG3>IgG4>IgG2 ● IgG2, IgG3>IgG1>IgG4	immunoregulation
Human platelet	IgG	2×10^7	IgG3, IgG1>IgG2>IgG4	mediates inflammation
Human syncytiotrophoblast	IgG	$1\text{-}4 \times 10^7$	IgG1, IgG3>IgG4>IgG2	transplacental transfer
Human T cells	IgM	2.5×10^9	—	immunoregulation
Human T cells	IgA	?	IgA2 > IgA1	immunoregulation
Human T cells	IgE	$1.2\text{-}13 \times 10^6$	—	immunoregulation
Rat mast cell and basophils	IgE	6×10^9	IgE >>> IgG4	mediates inflammation

* For monomeric antibody, of the class/subclass with highest affinity for that receptor
† Cross-species reactivity occurs, but only homologous binding is described
● In experiments by different groups

Fig.2.13 Fc receptors. This table lists some of the better characterized Fc receptors. Some of these bind to several isotypes but show characteristic patterns of class and subclass specificity. The constant association is a measure of the strength of binding of the receptor for monomeric Ig (of the highest affinity isotype). High affinity receptors, such as the IgE receptor on mast cells, bind monomer strongly, but other Fc receptors, such as the IgG receptor on the human polymorph, bind monomer weakly and only bind to a significant extent when the IgG is complexed. B cells (not listed) appear to share a receptor of the polymorph type, but also have an additional receptor. This is thought to be involved in immunoregulation. The data are based on a consensus of many research papers, and are not definitive (see Burton, 1985, for discussion).

sensitized with antibody. Lastly, but of great importance, are the Fc receptors expressed by the placental syncytiotrophoblasts, which are responsible for transport of IgG across the human placenta. Not all isotypes of IgG bind equally well to each kind of Fc receptor. For example, IgG1 and IgG3 bind most effectively to receptors on macrophages, whereas neutrophils bind all IgG isotypes. In some cases there is evidence of slight reactivity of antibody of one class with receptors for another. There is evidence, for instance, that IgG4 is capable of binding to Fc receptors on mast cells and can trigger them when crosslinked by antigen in an analogous way to IgE. Even if the affinity of the Fc receptors for IgG4 is very low by comparison with IgE, this may still be physiologically significant because of the much greater quantity of IgG4 present compared to IgE. It is evident from the diversity of the immunoglobulin isotypes and the variety of cells carrying Fc receptors, that the antibody genes have evolved in parallel with Fc receptors on different cell types to mediate a wide variety of immunological and inflammatory reactions.

SUMMARY

Antibodies are bifunctional molecules which bind antigen via their V domains and can interact with the body's effector systems via their C domains. The exons for the heavy chain V domains are generated by a process of somatic recombination between V, D and J gene segments, while light chain V domains are formed from V and J segments only. There are large numbers of V genes and several D and J genes, and since these can recombine in many different combinations, this provides the main source of V domain diversity generating a great number of antigen-combining sites. The V exon becomes joined to the C domain exons during the process of mRNA splicing. There are a number of different C genes, each one corresponding to a different immunoglobulin isotype. At different stages of B cell development the V exon can be linked to the C genes for different classes. This process of class switching can be effected either by differential mRNA splicing of the primary RNA transcripts, or by a second series of gene recombinations, affecting the C genes. During class switching, additional refinement of the antigen-combining capacity of the antibody occurs by a process of somatic mutation.

The process of antibody formation and diversification is reflected in the diversity of antibodies found in the serum and on B cells. Each antibody can be produced in a membrane or secreted form. In addition, the variation of antibodies can be analysed serologically under three different headings. Idiotypic diversity refers to the variation expressed in the antibody V domains and depends on the multiple genes and processes of recombination and somatic mutation which generate the V domains. Isotypic diversity depends on the variety of C genes which encode the different classes and subclasses of antibody, present in each individual of a species, while allotypic diversity depends on structural differences between particular isotypes in different individuals.

FURTHER READING

Alt F.W. (1984) *Exclusive immunoglobulin genes.* Nature **316**, 502.

Berek C., Griffiths G.M. & Milstein C. (1985) *Molecular events during maturation of the immune response to oxazolone.* Nature **316**, 412.

Burton D.R. (1985) *Immunoglobulin G: Functional Sites.* Mol. Immunol. **22**, 161.

Cebra J.J, Komisar J.L. & Schweitzer P.A. (1984) *C_H isotype switching during normal B cell development.* Ann. Revs. Immunol. **2**, 493.

Davies D.D. & Metzger H. (1983) *Structural basis of antibody function.* Ann. Revs. Immunol. **1**, 87.

Fudenberg H.H., Pink J.R.L., Wang A.C. & Ferrara G.B. (1984) *The Genetics of Immunoglobulin Molecules,* in Basic Immunogenetics 3rd Edn., Oxford University Press.

Gearhart P.J. (1982) *Generation of immunoglobulin variable gene diversity.* Immunol. Today **3**, 107.

Hahn G.S. (1982) *Antibody structure function and active sites,* in Physiology of Immunoglobulins: Diagnostic and Clinical Aspects. Ritzmann S.E. Alan Liss.

Hay F.C. (1985) *Generation of Antibody Diversity,* in Immunology, Roitt I.M, Brostoff J. & Male D.K., Gower Medical Publishing, London.

Honjo T. (1983) *Immunoglobulin genes.* Ann. Revs. Immunol. **1**, 499.

Koshland M.E. (1985) *The coming of age of the J chain.* Ann. Revs. Immunol. **3**, 425.

Lydyard P.M. & Fanger M.W. (1982) *Characteristics and functions of Fc receptors on human lymphocytes.* Immunology **47**, 1.

Metzger H. (1983) *The receptor on mast cells and related cells with high affinity for IgE.* Contemp. Topics Mol. Immunol. **9**, 115.

Nissonoff A. (1984) *Introduction to molecular immunology.* (Chapters 1-8) Second Edn., Sinauer Associates.

Shimizu A. & Honjo T. (1984) *Immunoglobulin class switching.* Cell **36**, 801.

Tonegawa S. (1983) *Somatic generation of antibody diversity.* Nature **302**, 573.

Wall R. & Kuehl M. (1983) *Biosynthesis and regulation of immunoglobulins.* Ann. Revs. Immunol. **1**, 393.

3 The T Cell Antigen Receptor

The function of antigen recognition is carried out by the T and B lymphocytes. B cells, which may ultimately differentiate into immunoglobulin-producing plasma cells, also use immunoglobulin as their cell surface receptor for antigen. T cells use a different molecule, the T cell antigen receptor, which has been extraordinarily elusive and has only been identified with certainty in the last two or three years. Immunoglobulins recognize and bind to antigenic determinants (epitopes) on free antigens, but most T cells can only recognize antigen when it is associated with MHC molecules. Helper T cells recognize a combination of antigen and MHC class II molecules on the surface of antigen-presenting cells; cytotoxic T cells recognize antigen plus MHC class I molecules on the surface of target cells. Usually, T cells recognize antigen in association with MHC molecules of the animal's own haplotype(s), but allogeneic MHC molecules can also be recognized by T cells, and can induce similar reactions to the antigen/self MHC signal. In man it is found that T_H cells carry the surface molecule T4 (L3T4 is the equivalent molecule in the mouse), which is involved in the recognition of MHC class II molecules, while cytotoxic T cells carry the T8 molecule (Ly2 in the mouse), related to the recognition of class I molecules (Fig.3.1). T cell recognition of antigen is therefore complicated, compared to recognition by B cells. Nevertheless, there are some similarities between B and T cells, since both populations can recognize a wide range of antigens and within each population an individual cell has only one specificity of antigen receptor. Although the T and B cell antigen receptors are distinct proteins encoded by different sets of genes, they appear to have a common evolutionary origin, and still retain some similarities in their gene and protein structures. This chapter describes the characteristics of the T cell antigen receptor, and how receptors of different specificity are generated from an individual's germline genes.

ANTIGEN/MHC RECOGNITION

Since it became known that T cells recognize antigen in association with MHC molecules (Fig.3.2), it has been

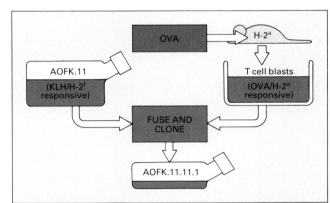

Stimulation of T cells by antigen/MHC	Antigen/MHC			
	OVA/H-2^a	KLH/H-2^a	OVA/H-2^f	KLH/H-2^f
AOFK.11	–	–	–	+
T cell blasts	+	–	–	–
AOFK.11.11.1	+	–	–	+

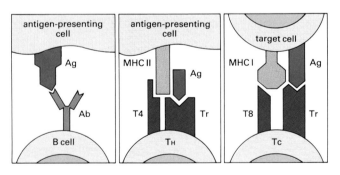

Fig.3.1 Recognition of antigen by T and B cells. B cells recognize antigen through their surface immunoglobulin which acts as an antigen receptor, but T cells recognize a combination of antigen and MHC molecule. T helper cells are stimulated by antigen in association with MHC class II molecules on the surface of antigen-presenting cells, while T cytotoxic cells recognize antigen in association with MHC class I molecules on the surface of target cells. The T cell antigen receptors (Tr) are quite distinct from the antibody receptor of B cells, being encoded by different genes. T cells which recognize class II molecules (in humans) carry the T4 surface protein, and those that recognize class I molecules carry the T8 protein. T4 and T8 appear to be involved in the specific interaction between the T cell and the MHC molecule on the stimulating cell.

Fig.3.2 T cell recognition of an antigen/MHC combination. A clone of T cells was produced (AOFK.11), which responds only to the antigen KLH when presented on antigen-presenting cells of MHC type H-2^f. This line was fused with T cell blasts from an H-2^a mouse immunized with the antigen OVA. A clone was derived from the fusion (AOFK11.11.1), and this was assayed to determine which combinations of antigen and MHC would stimulate it. The clone has a dual specificity: to OVA on H-2^a antigen-presenting cells, like the T cell blasts, and to KLH on H-2^f cells, like AOFK.11. It does not respond to KLH on H-2^a cells or to OVA on H-2^f cells. In effect it recognizes an antigen/ MHC combination, and not antigen and MHC independently. This implies that the T cell antigen receptor recognizes both antigen and MHC. Based on Kappler *et al.*, 1981.

debated whether the antigen receptor itself recognizes both MHC and antigen together, or whether the receptor sees antigen and another molecule sees MHC. These theories are referred to as 'associate recognition' and 'dual recognition' respectively.

Several strands of evidence suggest that the antigen receptor is also the MHC receptor. For example, when hybrid T cells are prepared by fusing together two different T cells each of which is specific for a particular antigen/MHC combination, the hybrid cell reacts to both of the antigen/MHC combinations which stimulate the fusion partners. It does not, however, react to the antigen recognized by one partner in association with the MHC recognized by the other. Experiments on cytotoxic T cells have also concluded that a single receptor is responsible for the specificity of both MHC and antigen recognition. In some experiments, clones of T cells are occasionally found which will recognize one antigen in association with one MHC haplotype, and another antigen in association with another MHC. This is a kind of cross-reactivity between two MHC/Ags as recognized by the T cells, and it further reinforces the view that one receptor recognizes both MHC and Ag.

As stated above, it is known that the T4 and T8 molecules are involved in the recognition of MHC molecules, but T4 and T8 cannot be solely responsible for the function of MHC recognition, for the following reason: each T cell recognizes a particular antigen and a particular MHC haplotype, therefore, to specifically recognize any of the range of different MHC haplotypes the molecule responsible would have to vary for each MHC type, but the T4 and T8 molecules do not vary in this way. Therefore, it is thought that the T4 and T8 molecules must recognize a 'framework' structure on the MHC molecule which is common to many haplotypes. Meanwhile, the antigen/MHC receptor recognizes the allotypic determinants on the MHC molecule (Fig. 3.3). An alternative to the view that the T cell receptor recognizes MHC and antigen is that the

MHC molecule orientates the antigen and that only the antigen is recognized by the T cell. Different MHC haplotypes would associate with and orientate the antigen in different ways, so that the part of an antigen which can be seen by the T cell antigen receptor depends on the MHC haplotype of the stimulating cells. In this way, an MHC molecule determines MHC/antigen specificity without directly interacting with the T cell receptor. These and other theories are discussed fully in Chapter 6.

ISOLATION OF THE T CELL ANTIGEN RECEPTOR

The identification of the T cell antigen receptor followed the development of methods for preparing T cell clones specific for a particular antigen/MHC. Helper T cell clones respond to the correct antigen/MHC stimulus by proliferating and by producing the lymphokine interleukin-2 (IL-2). Cytotoxic T cells may be assayed by their ability to kill target cells of the appropriate allogeneic haplotype, or of their own haplotype if associated with the correct antigen.

Monoclonal antibodies were made to different T cell clones that recognized only the clone to which they were raised, that is, antibodies specific for the idiotype of the particular T cell. The term 'idiotype' is used here in a similar way to the description of a unique set of epitopes on the V domain of an antibody: the idiotype of a T cell (Ti) is the set of epitopes associated with its own individual antigen receptor. The antibodies raised to different T cell idiotypes were found to modulate the response of the T cells to their specific antigen/MHC stimuli. In some cases they would block responses, and in others they would stimulate them. For example, some anti-idiotypes prevent cytotoxic cells from killing their targets, while they can potentiate the ability of these cells to respond to IL-2. The finding that these antibodies specifically affect the response of a particular clone to antigen/MHC, while not affecting others, shows that anti-idiotypes recognize the antigen receptor of that clone.

Using anti-Ti antibodies, the antigen receptor could then be isolated and identified. The cell surface molecules of the T cell clone were radioactively labelled and the membrane fraction prepared from the cells. The antigen receptor was then separated from other molecules by immunoprecipitating it with the anti-Ti antibodies. The labelled peptides in the precipitate could then be subjected to biochemical analysis. Examination of the peptides in precipitates from different mouse T cell clones using SDS polyacrylamide gel electrophoresis, showed that the receptor consisted of a glycoprotein of 80-90 kD which could be dissociated under reducing conditions into two peptides of 43 and 40 kD. This shows that the entire molecule consists of a pair of disulphide-linked peptides of similar size. These peptides are referred to as the α and β chains of the receptor. Although each anti-Ti antibody only recognizes its own clones, the receptors isolated from different clones are all similar. The α and β chains are structurally quite distinct. The α chain has an isoelectric point of 5.0 - 5.5, whereas that of the β chain is 6.5 - 7.0 depending on the clone from which the receptor was isolated.

T cell receptors isolated from human clones also possess a molecule of molecular weight 90 kD consisting of disulphide-linked α and β chains, but the human α and β

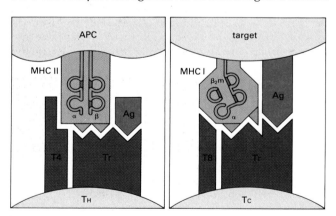

Fig.3.3 Recognition of MHC polymorphic determinants. Since the T cell receptor recognizes a specific combination of antigen and MHC molecule, it is proposed that the receptor binds to allogeneically variable sites on the MHC molecule (pink), which occur in the N-terminal domains of the α and β chains of the class II molecule (left) and on the α_1 and α_2 domains of the MHC-encoded α chain of the class I molecule (β_2 microglobulin is encoded outside the MHC). Meanwhile, the molecules T4 and T8, which are involved in the MHC class restriction of the T cells, interact with 'framework' regions on the MHC molecules. Based on data from Meuer et al., 1984.

chains are slightly larger and more readily separated in SDS gel electrophoresis, as they differ more in molecular weight than do mouse α and β chains.

In humans, a third molecule is associated with the antigen receptor. This is the cell surface molecule T3, recognized by the monoclonal antibody OKT3 (Fig. 3.4).

	Ti	T3	T4	T8
CT4ᵢᵢ	29,000	30,000	118,000	–
CT8ᵢᵢᵢ	42,000	48,000	–	175,000
Peripheral T cells	not tested	25,000	30,000	60,000

Fig.3.5 Occurrence of T cell surface proteins. The number of antigen/MHC receptors (Ti) and cell surface molecules T3, T4 and T8 per T cell in various T cell populations were evaluated by immunofluorescence using a fluorescence-activated cell sorter. The cell line CT4ᵢᵢ carries the antigen T4 but not T8; conversely, CT8ᵢᵢᵢ carries T8 but not T4. In each case, the number of cell surface T3 molecules is very similar to the number of antigen receptors (Ti) detected by anti-idiotypic antibodies, suggesting that T3 and Ti are coordinately expressed by these cells. There are considerably more of the T4 and T8 molecules on these cells, indicating that they are independent of the T3/Ti complex. Although anti-idiotypic antibodies were not available to test the incidence of Ti on peripheral cells (NT), it appears that the activated cell lines express more of the other surface molecules than are present on normal T cells. Data from Meuer et al., 1984.

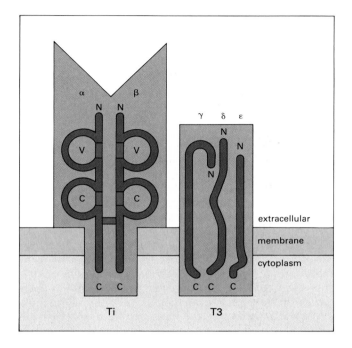

Fig.3.4 Peptide structure of the human T cell receptor. The T cell receptor is a complex of the Ti molecule which binds antigen/MHC and the T3 molecular complex. Ti consists of a disulphide-linked heterodimer formed of α and β chains. Each of these chains consists of variable (V) and constant (C) domains stabilized by intrachain disulphide bonds (red), a short 'hinge-like' segment, and transmembrane and intracytoplasmic portions. The Ti portion of the molecule is polymorphic and carries the T cell idiotype. The T3 complex consists of three non-covalently associated peptides, each of which probably traverses the cell membrane. They are monomorphic and appear to transduce the activation signal from Ti to the cell itself. The monoclonal antibody OKT3 recognizes primarily the δ chain.

Recent data show that there is an equivalent molecule associated with the mouse α and β chains. OKT3 recognizes T3 molecules on the surface of all T cells, unlike specific anti-Ti antibodies. T3 appears on T cells in the thymus at the time they develop immunocompetence, and OKT3 antibody is able to inhibit antigen recognition by T cell clones. For these reasons, it was thought that T3 might form part of the T cell receptor, a constant part present on all cells. It has since been found that the number of T3 molecules present on the surface of T cell clones is always similar to the number of Ti-bearing molecules detected by specific fluoresceinated anti-Ti and anti-T3 antibodies, as occurs with other molecules which are expressed coordinately (Fig. 3.5). Furthermore, removal of T3 molecules from the cell surface results in concomitant removal of molecules reacting with anti-Ti.

Immunoprecipitation of human T cell surface molecules with anti-T3 results in the isolation of a monomorphic peptide of molecular weight 20 kD. If, however, this is performed under gentle conditions, it is found that five separate peptide chains are recovered. Two of these correspond to the α and β chains identified by anti-Ti antibodies, and the other γ, δ and ε chains are associated non-covalently with the α/β heterodimer. The model of this five peptide Ti/T3 complex is presented in Figure 3.4; the characteristics are shown in Figure 3.6.

One puzzling finding is that, whereas immuno-precipitation with anti-T3 results in coprecipitation of Ti, it has been much more difficult to perform the experiment the other way around. Recently, however, precipitations with anti-T cell idiotype have succeeded in isolating other peptides of the Ti/T3 complex. Interestingly, the isolated

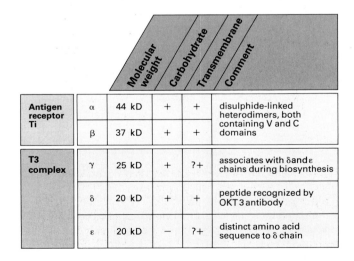

		Molecular weight	Carbohydrate	Transmembrane	Comment
Antigen receptor Ti	α	44 kD	+	+	disulphide-linked heterodimers, both containing V and C domains
	β	37 kD	+	+	
T3 complex	γ	25 kD	+	?+	associates with δ and ε chains during biosynthesis
	δ	20 kD	+	+	peptide recognized by OKT3 antibody
	ε	20 kD	–	?+	distinct amino acid sequence to δ chain

Fig.3.6 Peptides forming the T cell receptor. Under appropriate conditions, five separate peptides are present in isolates of the human T cell receptor. The disulphide-linked α and β heterodimer is associated with the γ, δ and ε peptides of the monomorphic T3 molecule.

complex from the mouse includes a number of peptides which are not seen in humans. The evidence suggests that the association of Ti and T3 is rather loose and may vary in different conditions. It is not known whether this observation is important. Possibly the T3 molecule dissociates from the T cell idiotype once the antigen receptor has become crosslinked by anti-T cell idiotype. If this is so, then T cell activation might be regulated at this level. However, the result could also be due to peculiar conditions related to the antibodies used to isolate the receptor peptides and the location of their epitopes with respect to each other.

The Ti Molecule
The α and β chains form the part of the receptor complex responsible for antigen/MHC recognition. The α chain is unusual in that its N terminus is blocked, probably by a cyclized glutamine residue (mouse). Peptide mapping of the two chains from different clones of the same strain has indicated that there are some peptides common to all clones, while other peptides vary between different clones. This supports the view that both α and β chains of the receptor, like immunoglobulin chains, consist of variable (V) and constant (C) portions. Interestingly, it seems to be much more difficult to raise antibodies to the constant region of the T cell receptor than to the constant region of immunoglobulins, hence the use of anti-T cell idiotype antibodies in most of the immunoprecipitation experiments described above. It is possible to produce xenogeneic antibodies which recognize all the different T cell receptors of mouse clones, but as mouse/anti-mouse T cell receptor C region antibodies have not been found, it must be assumed either that there is little allotypic variation in the T cell receptor, or that it is a very weak immunogen in mice.

With the recent rapid advances in molecular biology, it has become as simple to derive amino acid sequences of proteins from the mRNA as to isolate and sequence the protein. Consequently, our knowledge of the primary structure of the α and β chains of the T cell receptor is largely derived from gene sequences, and identity is confirmed by their correspondence to the smaller number of

sequences (as well as partial sequences) obtained by conventional protein analysis. The α and β chains both have homologies in their amino acid sequences to each other and to immunoglobulins, which implies that each chain consists of an N-terminal variable domain, a constant domain, a short segment containing the interchain disulphide bond, followed by a segment of hydrophobic residues which traverse the membrane, and an intracytoplasmic segment (see Figs. 3.4 and 3.7). This structure has been inferred by analogy with immunoglobulin heavy and light chains, since there is insufficient material available to make a crystallographic analysis of the tertiary structure. In particular, the conserved cysteine residues which form the intradomain disulphide bonds in immunoglobulin chains are also present in the domains of the α and β chains, enclosing peptide loops of about 65 amino acid residues.

Analysis of the variable domains of the β chains, using a method which predicts the tertiary structure of a protein based on its primary structure (developed by Chou and Fathman), indicates which areas will form a β-pleated sheet. The predicted areas of the β chain correspond well with the equivalent areas of immunoglobulin domains which are known to form a β sheet. Thus, it seems that despite the numerous amino acid differences between the T cell receptor and immunoglobulin domains (50-85%), the overall domain structure is probably similar for both classes of antigen receptor.

The transmembrane segments of both α and β chains contain a conserved stretch of hydrophobic amino acid residues ending with a lysine residue. It is unusual to find such a charged residue in a transmembrane segment, however, this lysine could form ionic bonds with other peptides of the Ti/T3 complex. Both α and β chains contain carbohydrate which accounts for the difference between the observed molecular weights and those predicted from amino acid composition alone. There are four potential N-glycosylation sites on the mouse α chain and four or five on the β chain, although they are probably not all glycosylated as some lie in unsuitable areas of the molecule, such as the transmembrane segment. The α and β chains in both human and mouse appear to be assembled

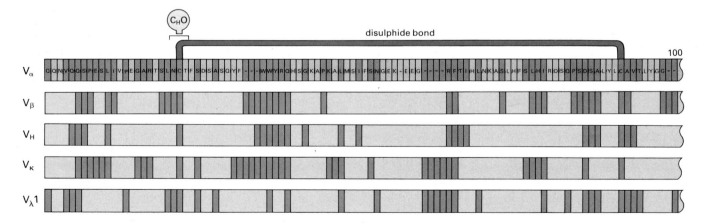

Fig.3.7 Amino acid homologies in peptides of Ti and IgG. The amino acid sequences of the mouse V_α and V_β peptides of the T cell receptor are compared with those of immunoglobulin heavy (V_H) and light chains (V_κ, V_λ) for the first hundred amino acids of the variable domains. Areas with the most homology between the peptides are indicated in red. Note that the cysteine residues which form the

intradomain disulphide bond are highly conserved in all peptides. The position of an N-glycosylation site on the V_α chain is also indicated. While the homology between these peptides is much less than between immunoglobulin chains, it is sufficient to indicate that both the T cell receptor and the immunoglobulins have a common evolutionary origin. Data from Chien *et al.*, 1984.

from V, D and J segments (see below). Mention should also be made of another gene which is present in T cells in rearranged form, which has not been previously referred to. Analysis of T cell clones shows that there are genes for another T cell receptor-like chain called the gamma (γ) chain. This is similar to the α and β chains but quite distinct from the γ chain of T3. Genes for this peptide are found in both man and mouse, and it occurs in a rearranged form in cytotoxic T cell clones of mouse and all T cell subpopulations of human. This indicates that the peptide is important in T cell function. However, it is expressed in much smaller amounts than either the α or β chains, and appears early on in T cell development. Its restriction to cytotoxic T cell clones of mice is very intriguing. This has led to speculation that it is required for the early thymic development of cytotoxic T cells, or that it is involved in associate recognition of class I MHC molecules; in fact, there is no certainty that this chain links to either the α or β chain, or even that it forms a T cell antigen receptor molecule. This peptide, therefore, remains a challenging enigma, as it is almost certainly an important component of some T cell function.

The T3 molecule

Immunoprecipitation experiments have established that the idiotype-bearing part of the antigen receptor is associated non-covalently with the T3 molecule. The OKT3 antibody recognizes a glycosylated peptide of molecular weight 20 kD. This peptide is monomorphic in that peptide maps and isoelectric points from different clones are identical. The δ chain is associated with two other peptides: the γ chain which is glycosylated, and the ε chain which is not. Unlike the other peptides, the ε chain is readily labelled with hydrophobic reagents, which suggests that the chain itself contains hydrophobic sequences possibly associated with a transmembrane segment. These three peptides appear to be synthesized together, and they only become associated with the α and β chains of the antigen receptor on the cell surface; they are closely, but non-covalently, linked. The amino acid sequence of the δ chain has been derived from a gene clone and a partial sequence of the peptide. All three peptides have distinct primary structures, and the δ chain has a transmembrane section which contains an aspartic acid residue. It has been suggested that this residue could interact with the lysine in the transmembrane portion of the α and β chains. Enzymatic degradation of the γ and ε chains suggests that they also have transmembrane segments.

As mentioned above, treatment of T cells with anti-T3 antibody can trigger proliferation. This reaction is dependent on Ca^{++}, and some immunologists believe that the T3 complex may act as an ion channel to effect the passage of Ca^{++} across the membrane. In this case, the hydrophobic chain would be a candidate for the channel itself. The δ chain undergoes proteolytic degradation at its C terminus, although it is uncertain whether the processing is part of the physiological organization of the T3 complex or is related to cellular activation.

It is notable that the DNA for the human T3 δ chain hybridizes to an mRNA expressed in mouse T cells, suggesting that a mouse T3-like molecule is present even though raising antibodies to it has been very difficult. The δ chain is unrelated to any known peptide sequence, and there is only one copy in the genome. Like the α and β chains of T cell idiotype, the gene for δ is expressed only in T cells.

GENES OF THE α, β AND γ CHAINS

The genes for the T cell receptor were originally isolated from T cell lines by identifying genes which were expressed in T but not in B cells, and had become rearranged from the germline configuration (Fig.3.8).

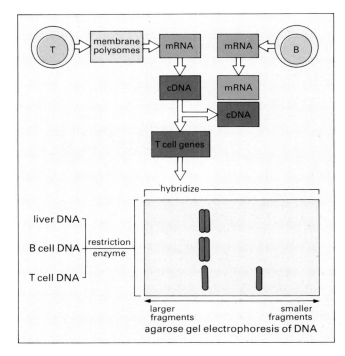

Fig.3.8 Identification of T receptor genes. Membrane polysomes were isolated from a T cell line, under the assumption that the T cell receptor mRNA would be translated across the endoplasmic reticulum; mRNA from these polysomes was used to make cDNA. The cDNA was hybridized to mRNA from B cells, thus removing the cDNA of genes encoding proteins which are also produced by B cells, leaving T cell-specific genes. The final step was to look for genes which became rearranged in T cells. To do this, DNA was prepared from liver cells and B and T cells. This was digested with a restriction enzyme which breaks the DNA at specific points (dependent on the nucleotide sequence). The various fragments of DNA were separated on an agarose gel, and the fragments carrying particular genes were identified by hybridizing to radiolabelled T cell cDNA. Some T cell cDNA gave hybridization patterns (red), although the overall appearance has been idealized and simplified. The T cell-specific genes are present on fragments of a particular size in both liver and B cell DNA, but in T cells the gene is present on two different DNA fragments. One corresponds to the band seen in liver and B cells, but there is also a smaller DNA fragment bearing the gene, showing that the latter has been rearranged in T cells. Since one band corresponds to that seen in liver (germline), this shows that only one copy of the gene has become rearranged in the T cell. Some T cells have rearranged both maternal and paternal genes, and so lack the germline band. The rearranged T cell genes were sequenced, and their amino acid sequence was derived. Some of the genes were then found to encode the α and β chains of the receptor whose amino acid sequence had been identified by conventional protein chemistry. See, for example, Hedrick *et al.*, 1984.

The genes for the mouse β chain which is encoded on chromosome 6 were isolated first. The gene organization bears a remarkable resemblance to that of the Ig heavy chain genes, in that each mRNA is the product of a recombined VDJ gene and a constant region gene (Fig.3.9). There is a similar tandem pair of β chain constant region genes in the human genome. The genomic arrangement of the α, β and γ chains of mouse is illustrated in Figure 3.10. Although the β chains were discovered first, our knowledge of both α and γ chains has increased greatly within the last year; consequently the following discussion compares the recent data with the fully established information on the β chains.

V Genes

The V_T region genes which have been sequenced so far show much greater sequence variability than immunoglobulin V domains. The amino acid sequence homology for different V_β region clones varies between 18-50%. The V genes of an immunoglobulin subfamily have about 75% sequence homology and there are, for example, 4-50 genes in each family. By contrast, the eleven known mouse V_β genes represent eight subfamilies: six with only one member, one with two members and one with three members. It has also been possible to estimate the total number of V genes by looking for the frequency of known V region sequences in thymocytes, which have been

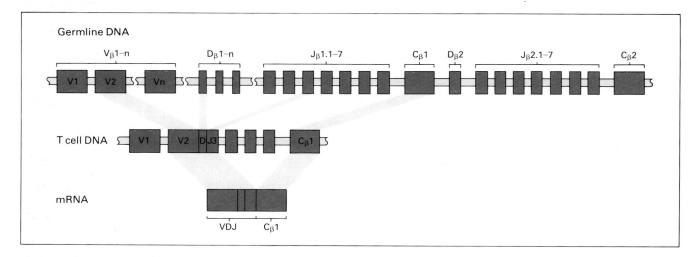

Fig.3.9 Recombination of mouse β chain genes. The mouse β chain gene is assembled from variable (V), diversity (D) and joining (J) chain segments which recombine during T cell development to form a gene segment encoding the variable region of the β chain. This recombined VDJ segment is transcribed along with the adjoining constant (C) region gene and the intervening introns. The gene segments for the variable and constant regions of the receptor are eventually spliced together to produce messenger RNA for the β chain. In the germline gene series, indicated at the top on the diagram, there is a set of variable gene segments and two sets each of D and J genes accompanying their own constant region gene. The diagram shows recombination of $V_\beta 2$ with the first D and third J segment of the $C_\beta 1$ gene. This is only one of the many possible combinations which can occur. It should be noted that the seventh J segment of $C_\beta 1$ lacks the necessary 5' recombining sequences, so that it is not expressed (pseudogene). It is presumed that all the other D and J segments are potentially functional, although not all have been detected in receptor peptides. The data have been compiled by Robertson, 1984.

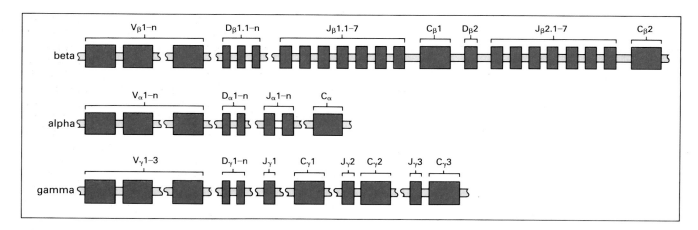

Fig.3.10 Genes which rearrange in mouse T cells. Three genes rearrange in mouse T cells: these are the α and β chains of the T cell receptor, and the γ chain whose function is unknown. All three appear to have V, D and J gene segments, although D segments have not all been fully characterized. The β chain has two tandem constant region pseudoalleles, while there are three separate γ chain constant region genes. Each of these tandem genes is accompanied by its own set of J genes, with which it can recombine. There is only one α chain constant domain, but the α gene has a very large number of J gene segments. Data compiled by Winoto et al., 1985.

recombined to a DJ segment. Several V sequences occur at a frequency of about 10%, again suggesting that there are perhaps only eleven V genes. However, some known V region sequences have not been found in a recombined form, after looking through a large number of thymocyte gene sequences. This implies that some V genes recombine much less frequently than others, and therefore there

is still the possibility that there are two types of V genes: a small number which are expressed relatively frequently, and another set which could be much larger, but where each member only recombines rarely to form a functional gene. In another study, analysis of the V_β gene sequences in 22 thymocyte clones showed that 11 were repeats of others. Statistical analysis of the data places an upper limit of 21 V_β genes. This is a rather modest number by comparison with, for example, the immunoglobulin heavy chain genes.

There is also significant variability at the level of the V_β gene segments in humans. Here it has been shown that a V_β gene probe from a human T cell line hybridizes with at least six different genomic DNA restriction fragments from that line, and to nine fragments from another line. This technique only indicates the minimum possible number of V genes.

The location of the variability within the V gene segments has been estimated by making Kabat and Wu plots of the relatively few V sequences available (Fig.3.11). As indicated above, there is much greater variability than for immunoglobulin sequences. The V_T sequences have variability distributed throughout their entire length, but the regions corresponding to the hypervariable segments of immunoglobulins are particularly variable, and these presumably also form the antigen/MHC binding sites of the T cell receptor. This is based on the reasonable assumption that the T cell receptor V domain folds in a similar way to the immunoglobulin V domain. It has been suggested that there are additional hypervariable regions in the V_T sequences, but this is probably an artefactual appearance created because the overall homology between different V_T sequences is low, and the number of sequences available for comparison is small. Since the T cell receptor appears to recognize both antigen and MHC, it was originally suggested that the additional variable segments are involved in the interaction with the MHC molecules, but this now seems unlikely. The rapid divergence and more extensive sequence variability of the V_T genes may relate to the fact that the T cell receptor recognizes Ag plus MHC, so that the variation in the T cell receptor is linked to the divergence of the MHC allotypes.

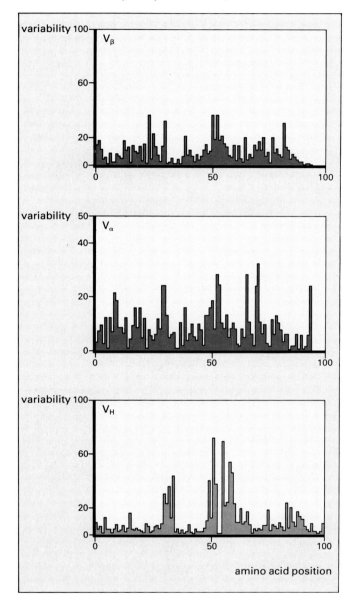

Fig.3.11 Variability of mouse β gene V domains. Using the derived amino acid sequences of mouse β and α chains it is possible to determine which amino acids show greatest variability between the different peptides. Variability is plotted according to the method of Kabat and Wu. It is found that the T cell receptor's β (top) and α (centre) chains have much greater variability than immunoglobulins. The regions which correspond to the hypervariable regions seen in immunoglobulins are discernible by comparison with a similar plot of immunoglobulin heavy chain V regions (bottom). The additional variability seen in the T cell receptor relates in part to their overall high level of variability and the limited number of genes present. It does not necessarily suggest that other regions of the T cell receptor have hypervariable regions related to their function. Based on data of Barth *et al.* (1985) and Arden *et al.* (1985).

D and J Genes

There are two sets of diversity (D), joining (J), and constant (C) genes on each allele of the mouse β chain gene, which is reminiscent of the two tandem sets of genes for the mouse λ chain. The D_β region genes lie about 650 base pairs upstream of the J_β cluster and recombine with V and J segments during T cell development. The recombination with the J gene appears to precede recombination with a V gene, since a large proportion of thymocytes are found which have recombined a DJ segment but lack VDJ recombination. RNA transcripts are made from the recombined DJ segments directed by a promoter immediately upstream from the D genes. Although the DJC transcript cannot produce a functional receptor peptide, the product may have some function within the cell, since the promoter site has been conserved during evolutionary development. Similar incomplete transcripts of Ig_H genes are seen in immature B cells. The DJ recombination point may vary between different cells, even using the same combination of D and J, thus producing additional combining site diversity. Additional nucleotides may also be inserted into the junction during recombination, producing a peptide in which one or more amino acids are

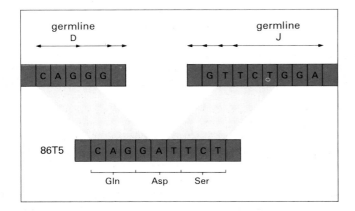

86T5 · C · A · G · G · A · T · T · C · T

Gln   Asp   Ser

Fig.3.12 Diversity created during recombination. This diagram illustrates the recombinational event between the D_β segment and the J_β segment which has occurred in T cell receptor clone 86T5, derived from the germline sequences indicated above. The GAT codon which encodes aspartate is derived from one nucleotide 3' to the D gene, one nucleotide 5' to the J gene, and from an additional nucleotide (A) inserted during the recombinational event. The same D and J segments may, thus, generate different amino acid sequences following recombination. Based on data from Kavaler *et al.*, 1984.

the necessary 5' recombination sequence. The sequence homology and spacing of the J genes in each set is similar in such a way that the two sets of J and C genes have probably arisen by gene duplication of the entire stretch of chromosome. There is considerable variation in the spacing between the heptamer of the flanking sequences and the expected start of the J region. This means that the J segments vary in length and may encode 16-18 amino acids.

The organization of the J regions of the mouse and human α chains is most unusual. In the mouse, the region containing J gene segments extends over more than 40 kilobases upstream of the single C_α gene. This region contains at least 18 J genes and pseudogenes. Similarly in humans, the region is very extended (more than 20 J genes) and research workers are still walking up the chromosome, hoping to come across the D_α gene segments which are supposed to exist.

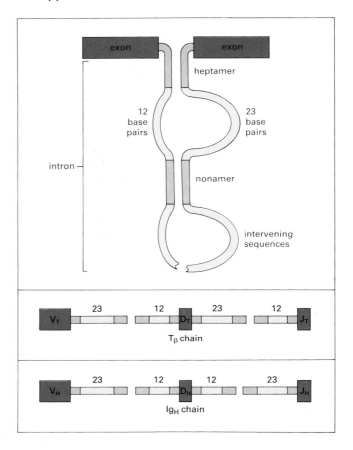

not directly encoded by the germline gene (Fig.3.12). In fact, this diversification mechanism appears to be particularly active in the T cell receptor genes, since VD recombinations occur with equal probability in all reading frames, whereas the immunoglobulin VD recombinations more frequently occur in the orthodox reading frame. Naturally, the orthodox reading frame must be restored by the DJ recombination to leave the J and C genes in the proper frame for translation.

Again, by contrast with immunoglobulins, the contribution of somatic hypermutation (which is an essential element of immunoglobulin affinity maturation) is apparently very limited. The hypermutation mechanism is for B cells only.

The sequences flanking the V, D and J segments have the recombination signal sequences of heptamer-12 or 23 base pairs-nonamer, which are also seen in the flanking sequences of immunoglobulin V, D and J genes (Fig.3.13). Following the proposal of Early and colleagues, it appears that a gene segment, which is flanked by heptamer-12 base pairs-nonamer, may only recombine with a segment flanked by heptamer-23 base pairs-nonamer. This is called the 12/23 rule.

Examination of the D_T region genes shows that each D segment is flanked on one side with a recombination signal including 12 base pairs, and on the other by a sequence with 23 base pairs. This means that it is theoretically possible for a V_T segment to recombine with a J_T segment omitting the D_T. This situation contrasts with that seen in immunoglobulins, where the D segments are flanked on both sides by sequences which include 12 base pairs. At least one example of a recombined T cell β chain VJ gene lacking a D segment has been found. The gene arrangement also theoretically permits the recombination of two or more D segments in a single β chain.

Each DJ recombination occurs within one set of tandem genes. There are seven J_β genes within each set of the tandem genes, but the seventh is not functional as it lacks

Fig.3.13 Recombination of V, D and J gene segments. V, D and J gene segments are flanked by specific sequences which permit them to recombine with each other. The flanking sequences consist of a heptamer, 12 or 23 base pairs and a nonamer which can base pair to the flanking sequence of another gene, as indicated. It is thought that the combination of 12 unpaired bases on one flanking sequence and 23 on the other is important in providing the recombinational signal. The V, D and J sequences of the T cell β chain have the flanking sequences shown below, which theoretically permit VJ as well as VDJ recombination according to the 12/23 base pair rule. The arrangement is interestingly different from that of the immunoglobulin heavy chains, shown at the bottom, which precludes a VJ recombination omitting a D segment. Based on data from Kavaler *et al.*, 1984.

C Genes

The two mouse C region β chain genes are comprised of four exons C_T1-C_T4. The first exon encodes the C region domain, while the remaining exons encode a short 'hinge-like' region, a transmembrane segment and an intracytoplasmic portion (Fig. 3.14).

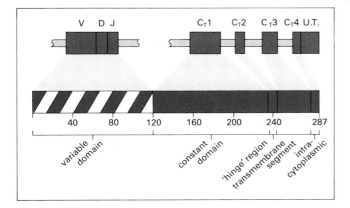

Fig. 3.14 Arrangement of mouse β chain exons. The arrangement of the exons of the $β_1$ C region gene is indicated in relation to the peptide structure of the mouse β chain. This consists of four exons (C_T1-C_T4) which encode the C domain, the hinge region, a transmembrane segment and an intra-cytoplasmic portion respectively. The C_T gene also contains a stretch of untranslated nucleotides (U.T.) before the poly-adenylation signal. The amino acids which correspond to the region boundaries are indicated. The recombined VDJ region is transcribed together with the C region exons to form RNA which is eventually spliced together to form mRNA. The gene arrangement of the other β constant gene is similar. Data from Gascoigne et al., 1984.

Thus, the gene organization is very similar to that of immunoglobulin heavy chains. The two β constant genes have a high degree of amino acid homology, with only four differences in the entire sequence. There is also considerable homology between the human and mouse genes indicating strong evolutionary pressure to conserve the structure. The C_T2 exon encodes the hinge-like region which contains the interchain disulphide bonds and links the α and β chains. The mouse β chain 'hinge' exon has some similarity to the hinge of IgG1 but, unlike that of IgG1, it is too short to confer much segmental flexibility on the molecule.

Interestingly, human peripheral T cells predominately express $C_β2$, while the level of expression of the two $C_β$ chains is identical in thymocytes. By contrast, in mouse (BALB/c) thymocytes the expression of $C_β1$ is 30-fold higher than that of $C_β2$. Nevertheless, the $C_β2$ gene is found to be expressed more frequently in functional T cell lines and hybrids. It had been suggested that one of the $C_β$ isotypes might be expressed in helper cells and the other in cytotoxic cells, but this is not so: either isotype has been found expressed in both cell types. Possibly, then, the change in preponderance of particular $C_β$ isotypes is a maturational change, or there is selective death of cells carrying one isotype in the thymus.

The general structure of the $C_α$ gene appears to be similar to that of the β chains with which it shares 12-60% homology. It also has four exons. Like the β genes, α genes are only found rearranged in T cells.

Both human and mouse $C_α$ gene probes hybridize to one genomic fragment only, indicating that there is only one $C_α$ gene in the genome. The mRNAs for the α and β chains are expressed at similar levels in mature lymphocytes, as is found for the mRNAs of other proteins encoded by separate genes which are coordinately expressed. However, the level of expression of the α chain is much lower in thymocytes suggesting that the β chain may be transcribed earlier in T cell development.

When the α and β chains were first isolated, based on their rearrangement and expression in T cells, other genes which also fulfilled these criteria were found. Although these genes were initially confused with the genes encoding the α chain, it is now known that the peptides encoded by the other genes lack N-glycosylation sites - α chain peptides contain three N-linked carbohydrate moieties. Furthermore, these genes are only expressed in a proportion of T cells. This peptide is now termed the T cell γ chain or T cell rearranging γ chain ($TRC_γ$) in humans, to distinguish it from the γ chain of T3. There are three $V_γ$ and three $C_γ$ genes in the mouse, located in tandem on chromosome 13. These genes are on chromosome 7 in humans and consist of two tandemly arranged $C_γ$ genes about 16 kilobases apart. In humans, the genes are rearranged in helper as well as cytotoxic T cells, whereas only mouse cytotoxic T cells have rearranged γ chains. Another difference between mouse γ chains and human $TRC_γ$ is that the human genes show a greater diversity of rearrangement patterns, indicating that there are more $V_γ$ genes in humans. At present the function of these genes is unknown. The fact that they are rearranged in T cells but not in other cells, and that they have some homology with α and β genes of the T cell receptor, indicates a function which could be related to antigen- or MHC-specific immune interactions.

NATURE OF THE ACTIVATION SIGNAL

While the function of the α and β chains of the receptor is clearly to act as the antigen/MHC receptor, the role of the T3 complex is less well understood, although it is certainly involved in T cell activation. This molecule differs in man and mouse, with the mouse molecule being structurally more complicated. Mouse T3-equivalent contains three monomeric glycoproteins (21-28 kD) and a new family of homodimers and heterodimers associated with the T cell receptor complex. A peptide of molecular weight 28 kD is the murine equivalent to the human T3 δ chain. The smallest peptide (21 kD) becomes phosphorylated following T cell stimulation with Con A, again suggesting a role in cell activation. Using human cells, anti-T3 antibodies can, under appropriate conditions, produce T cell proliferation and IL-2 secretion. In this case the anti-T3 acts as a polyclonal T cell activator, but in most cases an additional factor is required along with the anti-T3 to produce activation, such as the presence of plastic adherent cells (primarily macrophages), IL-2 or the ester phorbol myristate acetate. This implies that the signal transduced by the Ti/T3 complex is only a part of the total activation signal. Normally, the T cell requires additional signals from antigen-presenting cells to initiate cell division. By using a T3-negative mutant of the human cell line 'Jurkat', it has been shown that T3 is necessary for cellular activation, and that the T cell mitogen PHA may act on T cells via the

	Ca^{++}	EGTA
Ag/MHC	34,356	4895
Anti-T3-seph	25,200	347
Anti-Ti-seph	23,098	1091
Anti-Ti'-seph	735	623
IL-2	52,538	44,629

Fig.3.15 Role of calcium in T cell activation. A T cell line (AC3) was stimulated either in the presence of calcium ion (Ca^{++}) or without calcium in the presence of the chelating agent EGTA (0.75mM). The results are expressed in terms of ^{3}H-thymidine incorporation. Provided that calcium is present, the cells are activated by the appropriate Ag/MHC combination or by anti-T3 or anti-Ti coupled to sepharose particles (seph). Antibody to an irrelevant T cell idiotype (anti-Ti') does not stimulate the cells. The cells are also capable of responding to IL-2, whether calcium is present or not. This implies that Ca^{++} is essential for the signal transduced by the Ti/T3 complex, but not for the signal produced by IL-2. Data from Weiss *et al.*, 1984.

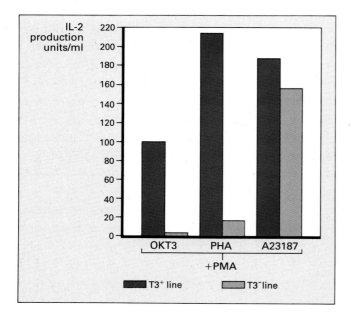

Fig.3.16 T3 transduces the first T cell activation signal. A mutant variant of the T cell line Jurkat was isolated which lacked T3. This T3$^-$ variant and the normal T3$^+$ line were stimulated with anti-T3 (OKT3), the mitogen phytohaemagglutinin (PHA) and the calcium ionophore A23187 in the presence of phorbol myristate acetate (PMA) which provides a second signal to the cell. Stimulation was assessed by IL-2 production. The T3$^-$ variant is unable to respond to OKT3 and only weakly to mitogen, but it can respond if a Ca^{++} influx is generated by A23187. Neither OKT3 nor PMA alone stimulated the normal T3$^+$ cells, and PHA alone produced a very weak activation, similar to that seen on the T3$^-$ cells. The data indicate that the T3 is responsible for the first activation signal of a Ca^{++} influx, and that this signal can also be produced by PHA, possibly by its action on the carbohydrate portion of the T3 glycoprotein. Data from Weiss *et al.*, 1984.

Ti/T3 complex (Fig.3.15). (PHA can crosslink cell surface molecules carrying appropriate carbohydrate side chains).

The signal passed by T3 depends on Ca^{++} flux across the membrane. This can be demonstrated by chelating extracellular Ca^{++}, in which case cellular activation by the use of anti-T3 is blocked. (An alternative activation sequence of human T cells, which is antigen-non-specific and is transduced via the T11 molecule, is also Ca^{++} dependent). The importance of Ca^{++} is confirmed by the observation that intracellular Ca^{++} concentrations rise immediately after activation by anti-T3, and that the calcium ionophore A23187 can substitute for anti-T3 in inducing cell activation (Fig.3.16).

Anti-T3 antibodies can also induce T cells to express IL-2 receptors, and since IL-2 can act as the second signal to induce proliferation, one could envisage a physiological system where antigen/MHC stimulation transduced via Ti/T3 induces IL-2 receptors allowing a T cell to become responsive to the proliferation signal.

One aspect of the signalling is more difficult to explain, that is, the observation that anti-T3 antibodies inhibit the action of cytotoxic T cells even after these cells have engaged their targets. This may be due to the antibodies interfering with the interaction between Ti and T3 and so with the activation of the cytotoxic cell to deliver a lethal hit. In this respect it is interesting that when liposomes containing membrane proteins of cytotoxic cells were fused to non-cytotoxic cells, these became capable of killing target cells. Thus, the cytotoxic function of T cells depends primarily on their membrane proteins which must include Ti and T3. Clearly, the manner in which Ti and T3 are associated under normal conditions and after antigen binding will be most important in determining how the activation signal works for helper and cytotoxic T cells.

SUMMARY

The T cell antigen receptor recognizes both antigen and MHC molecules. The receptor itself is a complex of an antigen/MHC binding portion which carries the T cell idiotype (Ti) and the T3 molecular complex which transduces the initial activation signal to the T cell. The Ti portion consists of a disulphide-linked heterodimer with an α and a β chain. Both of these chains traverse the membrane and each has an N-terminal variable domain and a constant domain adjoining the cell membrane. The variable domains are formed by the recombination of three genes (V, D and J). The genome contains several copies of each of these genes, all varying slightly, and since different V genes can recombine with different D and J genes, a very large number of different chains may be generated during T cell ontogeny. Additional variability in the α and β chains is provided by slight variations at the recombination sites.

The T3 complex consists of three peptides which are closely, but non-covalently, associated with each other and with Ti. During cellular activation via the Ti/T3 complex there is an influx of Ca^{++} which makes the cell responsive to a second signal triggering proliferation and lymphokine secretion.

FURTHER READING

Acuto O., Hussey R., Fitzgerald K., Protentis J., Mewer S., Schlossman S. & Reinherz E. (1983) *The human T cell receptor: Appearance in ontogeny and biochemical relation of α and β subunits on IL-2 dependent clones and T cell tumours*. Cell **34**, 727.

Arden B., Klotz J.L., Siu G. & Hood L. (1985) *Diversity and structure of the genes of the α family of mouse T-cell antigen receptor*. Nature **316**, 783.

Barth R.K., Kim B.S., Lou N.C., Hunmkapiller T., Sobieck N., Winote A., Gershenfeld H., Okada C., Hausburg D., Weissman I.L. & Hood L. (1985) *The murine T-cell receptor uses a limited repertoire of expressed V$_β$ gene segments*. Nature **316**, 517.

Borst J., Alexander S., Elder J. & Terhost C. (1983) *The T3 complex on human T-lympocytes involves 4 structurally distinct glycoproteins*. J. Biol. Chem. **258**, 5135.

Borst J., Coligan J., Oettgen H., Pelsane S., Malin R. & Terhost C. (1984) *The δ and ε chains of the human T3/T cell receptor complex are distinct polypeptides*. Nature **312**, 455.

Chien Y., Becker D., Lindsten T., Okamura M., Cohen D. & Davies M. (1984) *A third type of murine T-cell receptor gene*. Nature **312**, 31.

Chien Y., Gascoigne N., Kavaler J., Lee N. & Davis M. (1984) *Somatic recombination in a T-cell receptor gene*. Nature **309**, 322.

Elsen P., Shepley B., Borst J., Coligan J., Markham A., Orkin S. & Terhost C. (1984) *Isolation of cDNA clones encoding the 20K T3 glycoprotein of the human T cell receptor complex*. Nature **312**, 413.

Gascoigne R.J., Chien Y., Becker D.M., Kavaler J. & Davis M.M. (1984) *Genomic organization and sequence of T cell receptor β-chain constant and joining region genes*. Nature **310**, 387.

Hannum C., Kappler J., Trowbridge, Marrack P. & Freed J. (1984) *Immunoglobulin-like nature of the α chain of a human T-cell antigen/MHC receptor*. Nature **312**, 65.

Hayday A.C., Diamond D.J., Tanigawa G., Heilig J.S., Folson V., Saito H. & Tonegawa S. (1985) *Unusual organisation and diversity of T cell receptor α chain*. Nature **316**, 828.

Hedrick S.M., Cohen D., Nielsen E. & Davis M. (1984) *Isolation of cDNA clones encoding T cell specific membrane-associated proteins*. Nature **308**, 149.

Heileg J., Glimcher L., Kranz D., Clayton L., Kranz D., Clayton L., Greenstein J., Saito H., Maxam A., Birchoff S., Eisen H. & Tonegawa S. (1985) *Expression of the T-cell specific α gene is unnecessary in T cells recognising class 2 MHC determinants*. Nature **317**, 68.

Hood L., Kronenberg M. & Hunkapiller T. (1985) *T cell antigen receptors and the immunoglobulin supergene family*. Cell **40**, 225.

Kappler J.W., Skidmore B., White J. & Marrack P. (1981) *Antigen inducible, H-2 restricted, interleukin-2 producing T cell hybridomas*. J. Exp. Med. **153**, 1198.

Kavaler J., Davis M. & Chien Y. (1984) *Localization of a T cell receptor diversity-region element*. Nature **310**, 421.

Le Franc M.-P. & Rabbitts T.H. (1985) *Two tandemly organised human genes encoding the T cell receptor and constant-region sequences show multiple rearrangement in different T cells*. Nature **316**, 464.

McIntyre B. & Allison J. (1983) *The mouse T cell receptor: Structural heterogeneity of normal T cells defined by xenoanti-serum*. Cell **34**, 739.

Meuer S., Acuto O., Hercent T., Schlossmann S. & Reinherz E. (1984) *The human T cell receptor*. Ann. Rev. Immunol. **2**, 23.

Meuer S., Cooper D., Hodgdon J., Hussey R., Fitzgerald K., Schlossman S. & Reinherz E. (1983) *Identification of the receptor for antigen and histocompatibility complex on human inducer T lymphocytes*. Science **222**, 1239.

Oettgen H.C., Kappler J., Tax W. & Terhost C. (1984) *Characterization of the two heavy chains of the T3 complex on the surface of human T lymphocytes*. J. Biol. Chem. **259**, 12039.

Oettgen H.C., Pettey C.L., Malay L. & Terhorst C. (1986) *A T3-like protein complex associated with the antigen receptor on murine T cells*. Nature **320**, 272.

Patten P., Yokota T., Rothbard J., Chien Y., Arai K. & Davis M. (1984) *Structure, expression and divergence of T cell receptor β-chain variable regions*. Nature **312**, 40.

Reinherz E., Meuer S., Fitzgerald K., Hussey R., Hodgdon J., Acuto O. & Schlossman S. (1983) *Comparison of T3-associated 49- and 43- kilodalton cell surface molecules on individual human T cell clones: Evidence for peptide variability in T-cell receptor structures*. Proc. Natl. Acad. Sci. (USA) **80**, 4104.

Robertson M. (1984) *Receptor gene rearrangement and ontogeny of T lymphocytes*. Nature **311**, 305.

Saito H., Kranz D., Takagaki Y., Hayday A., Eisen H. & Tonegawa S. (1984) *Complete primary structure of a heterodimeric T cell receptor deduced from cDNA sequences*. Nature **309**, 757.

Saito H., Kranz D., Takagaki Y., Hayday A., Eisen H. & Tonegawa S. (1984) *A third rearranged and expressed gene in a clone of cytotoxic T lymphocytes*. Nature **312**, 36.

Sims J.E., Tunnacliffe A., Smith W.J. & Ralstads T.H. (1984) *Complexity of human T-cell antigen receptor β-chain constant and variable region genes*. Nature **312**, 541.

Siom G., Yagüe J., Nelson J., Marrack P., Palmer E., Augustin A., Kappler J (1984) *Primary structure of human T cell receptor α-chain*. Nature **312**, 771.

Siu G., Kronenberg M., Strauss E., Haars R., Mak T. & Hood L. (1984) *The structure, rearrangements and expression of D gene segments of the murine T cell antigen receptor*. Nature **311**, 344.

Weiss A., Imboden J., Shoback D. & Stolso J. (1984) *Role of T3 surface molecules in human T cell activation: T3 dependent activation results in an increase in cytoplasmic free calcium*. Proc. Natl. Acad. Sci. (USA) **81**, 4169.

Weiss M., Daley J., Hodgdon J. & Reinherz E. (1984) *Calcium dependency of antigen-specific (T3-Ti) and alternative (T11) pathways of human cell activation*. Proc. Natl. Acad. Sci. (USA) **81**, 6836.

Winoto A., Mjolsness S. & Hood L. (1985) *Genomic organisation of the genes encoding the mouse T-cell receptor α chain*. Nature **316**, 832.

Yanagi Y., Chan A., Chin B., Minden M. & Mak T. (1985) *Analysis of cDNA clones specific for human T cells and the α and β chain of the T cell receptor heterodimer from a human T-cell line*. Proc. Natl. Acad. Sci. (USA) **82**, 3430.

Yanagi Y., Yoshikai Y., Legett K., Clark S., Aleksander I. & Mak T. (1984) *A human T cell-specific cDNA clone encodes a protein having extensive homology to immunoglobulin chains*. Nature **308**, 145.

Yoshikai Y., Anatamou D., Clark S., Yanagi Y., Slangster R., Van den Elsen P., Terhost C. & Mak T. (1984) *Sequence and expression of transcripts of the human T-cell receptor β-chain genes*. Nature **312**, 521.

Yoshikai Y., Clark S.P., Taylor S., Sohn Y., Wilson B.I., Minden M.D. & Mak T. (1985) *Organisation and sequences of the variable, joining and constant regions of the human T cell receptor α chain*. Nature **316**, 837.

4 The Development of Lymphocytes

The key function of lymphocytes is the recognition of antigen or, in the case of T cells, antigen/MHC. Lymphocytes generate their antigen receptors at an early stage of their development. Rearrangement of the genes for the T cell receptor occurs in the thymic cortex, and the gene products are expressed before the cells reach the medulla. Surface immunoglobulin, the B cell antigen receptor, is seen on B cells present in the haemopoietic tissue of the fetus. The process of VDJ recombination often produces aberrant rearrangements, and the observed high frequency of these non-functional rearrangements indicates that many lymphocytes cannot complete this stage of their development. Once the cells have produced their antigen receptor and completed the first stages of development in the primary lymphoid tissues, they become responsive to antigen and seed the secondary lymphoid tissues. The developmental stages which follow depend on the range surface receptors expressed by the cells, and on the signals they receive. The surface receptors in turn depend on the subpopulation into which the cell has differentiated (for example, T helper, T suppressor) and its state of development. Seen as a whole, the development of lymphocytes includes two main waves of proliferation. The first occurs as the precursor cells develop in the primary lymphoid tissues and the second as the cells proliferate in response to antigen. The nature of the initial differentiation and the signals for antigen-induced proliferation are outlined below.

THE DEVELOPMENT OF B CELLS

B cells develop initially in the fetal liver, but in adult life they are produced in the bone marrow. Broadly speaking, their development occurs in three phases of which the first is commitment to the B cell lineage. This is accompanied by rearrangement of heavy and light chain genes in a determined sequence and the expression of mIgM, the initial antigen receptor. At this stage the cells may differentiate into one of the B cell subsets (see below). In the second phase, the cells populate the secondary lymphoid tissues and some may switch to produce Ig of different classes. Finally, the cells can be triggered by antigen and become responsive to differentiation and proliferation signals from T cells and antigen-presenting cells.

It has been shown that B cells expressing different immunoglobulin isotypes arise from common precursors. Treatment of neonatal animals with anti-μ antiserum causes deletion of mIgM-bearing B cells and leads to the subsequent absence of cells producing IgG and IgA, whereas treatment with anti-γ does not affect the generation of B cells expressing IgM. This shows that IgM-bearing cells develop into B cells expressing other classes.

Nevertheless, there is evidence for the existence of different subclasses of B cells. In mice there are at least two functionally distinct populations of B cells, one which can respond to all T independent antigens, and the other to only some of them. The subset which can respond to all T_{ind} antigens is distinguished in mice by the differentiation antigens Lyb3, Lyb5 and Lyb7, as well as by expression of the M-locus antigen. Much of what is known about the different subsets has been derived from studies in the CBA/N mouse which lacks this subset of B cells. This strain has an X-linked defect which prevents expression of the Lyb5$^+$ B cells. However, the locus on the X chromosome does not itself encode the markers mentioned above, but appears to control the differentiation of this subset. The two subsets can be distinguished by their ability to respond to T independent antigens, based on the observation that the CBA/N strain which lacks the Lyb5$^+$ subset fails to respond to a number of T_{ind} antigens which are referred to as T_{ind} type 2 antigens. T_{ind} antigens are typically high molecular weight molecules, frequently with repeating epitopes, and some have the inherent ability to induce polyclonal B cell activation (Fig.4.1).

T_{ind} antigens	Class	Polymer	B cell mitogenesis
Polymerized flagellin	2	+	−
Pneumonococcal polysaccharide SIII	2	+	+
Dextran	2	+	−
Dextran SO₄	1/2	+	+ +
Ficoll	2	+	−
Levan	2	+	−
Polyvinyl pyrrolidone (PVP)	2	+	+
LPS	1	−	+ + + +
PPD	1	−	+ + +
Poly I: Poly C	2	+	+ +
Nocardia extract	1	−	+ +
Brucella abortus	1	−	+

Fig. 4.1 T independent antigens. The T independent antigens listed here may be classified into type 1 which can stimulate both Lyb5$^+$ and Lyb5$^-$ B cells, and type 2 which can only stimulate Lyb5$^+$ cells. Dextran sulphate holds an equivocal position. Many of these antigens are large polymers, and many have the ability to induce polyclonal B cell activation. While most of the polyclonal B cell activators are type 1, this is not universally true.

Generally speaking, the type 2 T_{ind} antigens do not have mitogenic activity, but there are several important exceptions to this rule. For example, LPS, PPD and *Brucella abortus* are type 1 antigens with polyclonal B cell stimulatory properties, but poly I.C., which is similarly mitogenic, fails to induce an antibody response in CBA/N mice, hence it is a type 2 antigen. The Lyb5$^+$ subset also responds to stimulation with anti-Ig.

The Lyb3, Lyb5$^+$ set can be observed by immunofluorescence with specific antisera and constitutes 40-50% of splenic B cells in the adult mouse. This set of cells appears late in development, being absent at the time of birth and rising to normal levels over two months. Additionally, it is characterized by relatively low levels of IgM and high levels of IgD and Ia, thereby appearing as a more mature B cell. Based on observations in the nude mouse it is thought that both Lyb5$^+$ and Lyb5$^-$ cells arise from a common Lyb5$^-$ precursor, but the development of Lyb5$^+$ cells requires T cells, whereas that of the Lyb5$^-$ population does not (Fig. 4.2).

Characteristic		Lyb5$^-$ B cells	Lyb5$^+$ B cells
Present in CBA/N		+	−
Antigen reactivity	T_{dep}	+	+
	T_{ind} type 1	+	+
	T_{ind} type 2	−	+
Development		early	late
Response to TRF		−	+
Associated surface Ig		high IgM, low IgD	low IgM, high IgD
Tolerizability		high	low
Associated surface receptors		?	Lyb3, Lyb7, Mls complement receptors

Fig. 4.2 B cell subsets. This table summarizes the main characteristics of the Lyb5$^+$ and Lyb5$^-$ subsets of mouse B cells. The Lyb5$^+$ population is formed relatively later in development and is less easily tolerized. The surface receptors with which it is associated are characteristic of more mature B cells. Despite these differences, it is not possible to determine with certainty whether these constitute two distinct lineages, or whether they are subsequent stages on a differentiation pathway. They are, however, functionally distinct.

The ability to respond to T dependent antigens is not limited to one of the B cell subsets, and both sets respond equally well to type 1 T_{ind} antigens. It is noted, however, that the quality of the response to T_{dep} antigens in the CBA/N strain differs from that in normal mouse strains and, based on this observation, it has been suggested that the strength of the different antigenic stimuli for B cells is in the order T_{ind} type 1 > T_{dep} > T_{ind} type 2. Of interest in this respect is the function of the Lyb3 molecule itself, a non-allelic cell surface receptor with a molecular weight of 68 kD. Treatment of B cells *in vitro* with anti-Lyb3 causes a 10-20-fold increase in the number of plaque-forming cells

to sheep erythrocytes (a T_{dep} antigen) in all strains tested. In fact, anti-Lyb3 is a polyclonal B cell activator, acting preferentially on IgG secretion as well as accelerating affinity maturation in the secondary immune response. This suggests that the Lyb3 molecule acts as a receptor for signals for maturation and proliferation. Since the Lyb5$^+$ population has low mIgM, relatively small amounts of anti-IgM are sufficient to crosslink the surface receptors and trigger the cells − an indication that low levels of antigen may also be sufficient to trigger the population. This population is less readily tolerized than the Lyb5$^-$ population. It is not certain how much this inability to tolerize the Lyb5$^+$ cells is intrinsic or due to their arising later in ontogeny, when the other elements of the immune system are more fully developed. The X-linked gene determining the development of this subset also controls the expression of a private class II MHC specificity (Ia-W39), which distinguishes an Ir gene.

Another difference between the Lyb5$^+$ and Lyb5$^-$ subsets occurs in the response to the T dependent antigens (T,G)-A--L and (H,G)-A--L *in vitro*. It appeared originally that the response to these antigens was MHC-restricted, when either Lyb5$^+$ or Lyb5$^-$ cells were the responders. Closer analysis of the response showed that in both cases T cell interaction with antigen-presenting cells was MHC-restricted, as was the interaction between Lyb5$^-$ and T_H cells, but Lyb5$^+$ cells do not require MHC-restricted interactions to proliferate. The action of T cells in inducing proliferation of Lyb5$^+$ cells can be substituted with soluble T cell factors alone.

Putting these various pieces of data together a picture emerges of an Lyb5$^+$ population less readily tolerized, more easily triggered and able to respond differently to T_{dep} and T_{ind} antigens. Furthermore, in some situations the Lyb5$^+$ population is responsible for autoantibody formation (experimental and spontaneous autoimmune haemolytic anaemia). It is notable that some of the antisera used to define the subpopulations of B cells in mice also react on a proportion of B cells in humans. Another finding which suggests that humans have analogous B cell subpopulations to the mouse is the fact that patients with Wiskott Aldrich syndrome (which includes immunodeficiency) are unable to respond to some type 2 T_{ind} antigens. More recent studies have produced human B cell-specific monoclonal antibodies which appear to differentiate B cell subsets, but the relationship of these to the subpopulations in mice is undetermined.

Interestingly, a small population of mouse B cells which express the Ly1 marker (normally associated with T cells) have also been shown to produce IgM autoantibodies, but the relation of this subset to the Lyb5$^+$ populations was not determined in these experiments.

B cells have also been classed into different populations according to their location in secondary lymphoid tissues. For example, B cells in splenic PALS (periarteriolar lymphoid sheaths) fall into two types. Marginal zone B cells recirculate slowly and are more sensitive to the drug cyclophosphamide than follicular B cells. In addition, the marginal zone cells express relatively little mIgD, and studies depleting the follicular B cells with anti-IgD indicate that the residual marginal zone cells can still respond well to type 2 T_{ind} antigens. Whether it is possible to equate this population with the Lyb5$^+$ subset in mice is doubtful, and it is still uncertain to what extent the differences between the types of lymphocyte seen in secondary lymphoid tissues are dependent on precommitment to particular differentiation pathways, or on the micro-environment of the tissue. An experiment which sheds light on this question involves the total lymphoid irradiation of recipient animals followed by repopulation with fetal haemopoietic cells. The marginal zones take longer to repopulate than the follicles, and it is thought that the marginal zone cells require a longer developmental period. This does not, however, determine finally whether they are a distinct population, or part of the main B cell differentiation sequence.

Expression of Immunoglobulin Genes

The initial steps involved in the formation of a recombined VDJ heavy chain gene and a VJ light chain gene have been summarized in Chapter 2. These rearrangements are necessary for the generation of the wide variety of immunoglobulin V regions seen in the B cell population. Generally these gene rearrangements only occur in B cells, but rearrangements are occasionally observed in T cells, which shows that rearrangement of the Ig genes does not necessarily commit a prelymphoid cell to the B cell lineage. It is interesting that T cell receptor genes are sometimes rearranged in B cells, but again the rate of rearrangement is much less than for the appropriate receptor. Although the Ig gene rearrangement is a necessary prerequisite for Ig formation, it is not the only factor controlling Ig expression, since it is possible to transfect non-lymphoid cell types with functionally re-arranged Ig genes and subsequently to find that they do not express the mRNA for the Ig gene. Even when transfecting Ig genes into lymphoid cells, it is found that their expression is much greater when the recipient cell is a myeloma than, for example, a thymoma. Therefore, regulatory mechanisms within the B cell are also required for expression of immunoglobulin genes.

Gene rearrangement takes place in an ordered sequence. In cells producing κ chains, the λ chain genes are in the germline configuration and the λ DNA is methylated and DNAse insensitive, indicating that it is functionally inactive. By contrast, in cells producing λ

chains the κ chain DNA contains non-functional gene rearrangements. This information, along with the finding of aberrant rearrangements of κ genes in some κ producers and λ genes in some λ producers may be explained by the hypothesis that the pre-B cell sequentially rearranges its two κ genes followed by its λ genes. Once a functional rearrangement has been produced, there is a block on further light chain gene rearrangements. It is thought that heavy chain gene rearrangement precedes that of light chain genes, since heavy chain rearrangements are seen in cells which lack any alterations in their light chain genes (Fig. 4.3).

Since many aberrant immunoglobulin mRNAs are produced in pre-B cells, this implies that it is necessary for the cell to actually synthesize a functional polypeptide to block further gene rearrangements. Presumably, cells which fail to produce a functional rearrangement of one light and one heavy chain are clonally deleted at an early stage of development. Sequential rearrangement of genes in this way provides an explanation for allelic exclusion, that is, the observation that any one B cell, at random, only expresses one heavy (H) chain and one light (L) chain - the others are either aberrantly rearranged, or in the germline configuration.

Another level of control of immunoglobulin genes is seen in the degree of methylation of the genes. Methylation of bases is noted in quiescent genes and appears to act as a long-term control mechanism, since the methylation develops over some time. This applies to many genes, not just those for immunoglobulins. When genes become demethylated, they also become sensitive to the action of DNAse. For example, V region genes are insensitive to DNAse until they start to rearrange. It is notable that in IgM-producing cells both maternal and paternal C_μ genes are demethylated, and class switching is accompanied by loss of methylation in the C gene region of both chromosomes, not just on the chromosome with the functional VDJ. This also indicates that methylation is probably not involved in determining which Ig genes are expressed.

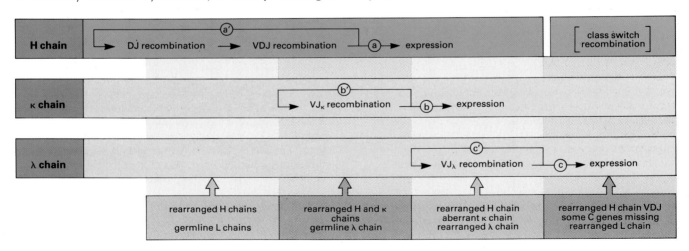

Fig. 4.3 DNA rearrangements during B cell development.

During B cell development, a number of recombinations occur within the genes for the heavy and light chains. The initial event is a DJ joining in the heavy chain, followed by linking of this unit to a V segment. The cell has two possible attempts (a and a') to produce a functional H chain gene. This is followed by VJ recombination in the κ genes (again, two attempts are possible). If a functional gene is produced, further recombination is prevented, otherwise the λ genes will be acted upon similarly until a functional L chain gene is produced, or the cell is aborted. At some time later, and after several cell cycles, the B cell may recombine its heavy chain C genes in an irreversible class switching event. If the DNA of the B cells is examined at each of the different stages, the condition of the H and L chain gene stacks will be as indicated in the lower panels.

Transcription and Expression of Ig Polypeptides

The level of expression of Ig polypeptides is determined primarily by the rate at which the mRNA is transcribed. The transcription initiation sites are signalled by the characteristic TATA box sequence lying approximately 25 base pairs (bp) 5' to the initiation site. This serves to orientate the RNA polymerase. Transcription initiation sequences on genes in the germline configuration are transcriptionally silent, although they may be expressed *in vitro* when injected into oocytes. This shows that the control of transcription in B cells is determined by gene segments remote from the initiation site.

Examination of the DNA sequences 5' to the leader peptide of light chains has identified a highly conserved transcription *promoter*. This transcription promoter consists of an octanucleotide lying between 90 and 160 base pairs upstream of the transcription initiation site. A second 15 base pair conserved sequence also occurs in this region. Interestingly, the inverse sequence of this octanucleotide is seen in the equivalent position upstream of one heavy chain transcription initiation site. Experimental deletion of the transcription promoter on κ genes transfected into a myeloma prevented expression of the gene.

There is also evidence for transcription *enhancer* regions amongst the Ig genes. These regions are usually on the same DNA strand as the genes they control but may be quite distant from them (>500bp), and in some cases they will still act in different orientations on the chromosome. These enhancers can be recognized by transferring DNA segments from the Ig gene region of B cells into cells which can demonstrate the presence of the enhancer.

mental data supporting this idea. For example, some B cell lines have deleted enhancer regions but still express Ig. Thus, assuming that these lines reflect normal B cell regulation, it is debated whether the enhancers are mandatory for Ig gene expression.

After transcription of the heavy chain gene mRNA, processing of the transcripts plays a part in determining which heavy chain isotype is expressed. Post-transcriptional regulation of Ig synthesis also occurs to a limited extent, after the mRNA is produced, although this is less important than the various DNA and RNA rearrangements. It is noted that expression of the heavy chains is determined by the presence of light chains. A number of cell lines produce heavy chains but do not express them, and in experiments where such cells are fused with myelomas capable of producing light chains the hybridoma cell is capable of producing Ig. It is thought that Ig heavy chains are rapidly degraded within the cell if they do not combine with light chains. This explains why myelomas secreting light chains are relatively common, while those secreting heavy chains are very rare. It also indicates an additional and final control mechanism producing coordinate synthesis of light and heavy chains. Although glycosylation is mandatory for the normal expression of some Ig isotypes (IgE, IgA and IgM), there is as yet no evidence that cells can glycosylate particular Ig peptides in different ways in different conditions, and so this step could not affect the gene expression in normal B cells. There is some evidence that the glycosylation of antibodies in B cells producing rheumatoid factors differs from the process in other B cells, but this could not be considered a normal control mechanism.

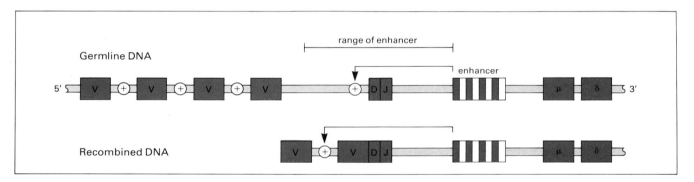

Fig. 4.4 Elements controlling H chain gene transcription. Three elements control transcription: a) a TATA box (not shown) immediately preceding each V gene, which signals the starting point for transcription, b) a transcription promoter (+) lying upstream of each V gene, and c) an enhancer region located between the J and C genes. Following the initial DJ recombination, sterile transcripts may be generated by the influence of the enhancer acting on a region between V and D, but after VDJ recombination the promoter preceding the newly recombined V segment now comes within range of the enhancer to generate active VDJ+C transcripts.

For example, the enhancer will activate transcription of a particular gene in the recipient cell. Conversely, the absence of enhancers may be inferred in deletion mutants. Both approaches have identified enhancer regions lying in the gene segment between the J and C genes, and their presence is suspected in both L and H chain genes. Upon VDJ recombination the transcription promoters 5' to the V region genes are brought within range of the transcription enhancers (2-3 kb) (Fig.4.4). While the presence of enhancer regions provides an explanation for the way in which the recombined V region (and not other V regions) is transcribed, there are some discrepancies in the experi-

Class Switching

Individual B cells only express antibody of one idiotype, but this may be represented on antibodies of different classes; a B cell's surface Ig receptors may be IgM alone, or IgM and another class, or either IgG, IgA or IgE alone. mIgD does not occur in isolation, but it is seen on a proportion of the cells expressing IgM. The earliest B cells in neonatal spleens express mIgM, but dual immunofluorescence studies have shown that IgM/IgA- or IgM/IgG-bearing cells develop shortly afterwards, both in normal and nude (athymic) mice, which shows that T cells are not required to initiate class switching. Some class switching occurs in germ-free animals, showing that antigen is also unnecessary.

Furthermore, some neonatal B cells can switch to IgG or IgA production without coexpressing IgD. IgD is the one class which lacks a 5' switching sequence, therefore IgD transcripts can only be produced together with IgM transcripts. This has led to the developmental scheme illustrated in Figure 4.5, in which the expression of IgD is an option on the main line of development.

Two possible mechanisms may underlie class switching: the mechanisms do not exclude each other, and it is possible that the second precedes the first or vice versa.

2. There is a gene rearrangement involving recombination between the switch regions preceding each of the C gene isotypes (except IgD), and consequent loss of the intervening genes (see Fig. 4.5).

Although both hypotheses account for class switching, they have different sequelae: a cell which switches class by altering its RNA processing (1) may subsequently switch back to its original class but, if DNA recombination has occurred (2), C genes have been lost and it cannot revert. If class switching involves gene deletion, the presence of dual isotype producers can only be explained by the long-term persistence of mRNA for IgM.

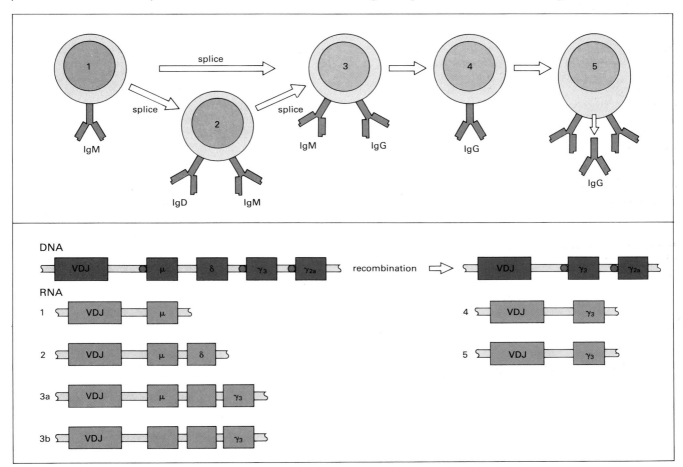

Fig. 4.5 Mechanisms for class switching in B cells. The upper part of the diagram shows the possible patterns of membrane Ig (mIg) expression which may occur during B cell ontogeny, and the lower part shows the heavy chain heteronuclear RNA transcripts which can produce the various combinations of heavy chains at each stage (1 - 5). Early B cells (1) express mIgM produced from a short transcript which probably only contains the VDJ and IgM C genes. These cells may then express IgM and IgD (2), or IgM and IgG (3a), here illustrated as γ_3, by differential splicing of the long RNA transcript. Cells may also switch to another class without necessarily losing the IgM and IgD genes (3b). If recombination occurs, however, this is associated with an irreversible class switch (4). At any stage the cell may produce secreted rather than membrane Ig by altering its RNA splicing mechanism, to generate mRNA lacking the membrane exons (5). Note that unlabelled boxes represent exons which are removed during RNA splicing.

1. Very large heteronuclear RNA transcripts are generated from the Ig gene region, which include the recombined VDJ segment and several H chain genes. This transcript may be spliced so that either the IgM or one of the other C genes is joined to the VDJ. This is certainly the mechanism by which IgM and IgD mRNA can be generated from a single transcript, but there is increasing evidence to support the view that even larger transcripts containing C_γ and C_α genes may also be produced.

Since there is evidence (summarized below) for both mechanisms, it is possible that differential transcription precedes gene recombination. It has been known that myelomas can switch isotype expression *in vitro*. Generally the switching occurs from a C gene higher up the gene stack (5') to one further down (e.g. μ to γ). Sublines of cells which have switched in this way may revert to the original isotype, and analysis of the frequency of revertants shows them to be at least as common as the original switch.

It may be debated whether myelomas have normal class switching mechanisms, but further support for differential transcription comes from studies in SJA/9 mice infected with nematodes. Using a FACS (Fluorescence Activated Cell Sorter), populations of B cells have been isolated from these animals which express both mIgM and mIgE. These cells do not have deletions in the heavy chain C genes, again indicating that deletion of genes is not necessary for class switching. Recent data have led to the tentative identification of very large transcripts of heteronuclear RNA containing several C genes, and if such transcripts could be isolated from dual producer B cells, this would provide conclusive evidence for the role of class switching mediated at the RNA level, even though the technical difficulties in locating these transcripts are great. Many hybridoma cells express more than one Ig isotype, and cells expressing up to seven isotypes have been detected although, in general, cells which express several isotypes are increasingly rare, with increasing numbers of expressed isotypes. It is hard to imagine that multiple isotype expression could be explained on the basis of gene recombination and persistence of long-lived mRNA for deleted genes.

Evidence for the role of gene recombination with the elimination of intervening sequences comes directly from Southern blot analyses of myeloma DNA, showing alterations in the C region DNA. Switching is directed by recombination between the S regions preceding the C genes, and there is evidence that the recombination can take place either on a single chromosome or, less commonly, it may involve crossing over between sister chromatids. Although it might be theoretically possible for a B cell with C gene deletions to revert isotype by using the non-rearranged chromosome, many myeloma lines have C gene deletions on both chromosomes and consequently may never revert their expression. With the evidence finely balanced for either mechanism, it is probable that both are applicable in different circumstances (see Fig. 4.5).

Signal for Isotype Switching

B cells producing IgG and IgA are detected early on in neonatal spleens, which indicates that class switching can occur before antigen stimulation and without T cell help. Nevertheless, the observation that immune responses to T_{dep} antigens usually induce IgG and/or IgA, whereas responses to T_{ind} antigens often do not, has led to the supposition that T cells are involved in the control of class switching. (Strictly speaking, even T_{ind} antigens may require some help from T cells to produce a response, although this is not usually an MHC-restricted interaction). The question then arises as to whether the T cells induce the switching themselves, or whether they are responsible for the selective expansion of B cells which have already switched. B cell isotype switching independent of T cells has been examined using LPS. This mitogen appears to act primarily on B cells in the mouse and induces switching. mIgM$^+$ cells are most responsive to LPS; this population turns over rapidly, and peaks in numbers around the time of birth. While LPS can induce switching to any of the other isotypes, the proportion of switched cells bearing each isotype varies greatly. The frequency of each isotype is IgG3>IgG2b>IgG1 and IgG2a>IgE & IgA. This is roughly the order of the C genes in the mouse C gene stack, with IgG3 being closest to IgM. Furthermore, this proportionality is the same in both athymic and normal animals. The switching induced by LPS is sometimes accompanied by gene deletion, indicating that gene recombination can occur in B cells without T cell intervention. Interestingly, a number of type 2 T_{ind} antigens also tend to produce a switch to IgG3. The switch from IgM to IgG production is associated with cell division, since the inclusion of inhibitors of cell division at levels which do not cause cell death and which permit some growth prevent LPS-induced class switching. These observations lead to the conclusion that class switching is programmed into the B cell during its differentiation, and with no additional stimuli the cell can switch to a new isotype. The frequency of occurrence of isotypes in this type of class switching depends partly on the proximity to the recombined VDJ gene (and thus on the transcription enhancer), and partly on particular DNA sequences which may favour some isotypes. This explains why the observed frequency of new isotypes does not correspond exactly to gene order.

Antigen can also influence switching; for example, mice raised in germ-free environments express a low but constant number of anti-PC B cells in their spleen which are predominately IgM. If these animals are then colonized with *Proteus morganii*, there is both an increase in the numbers of total anti-PC cells and an increase in the proportion of those expressing IgG and IgA. This may in turn be due to the effect of T cells.

Although T cells are not necessarily required to induce switching, they have a profound influence on the isotype expressed. For example, if B cells are cultured *in vitro* in the presence of T cell-conditioned medium (spent medium in which T cells have been grown), the production of IgG1 is favoured (cf. LPS which favours IgG3 and IgG2). Similarly, if mice are primed for the production of anti-DNP, the T_{dep} antigen DNP-Hy induces mostly IgG1, while the T_{ind} antigen DNP-ficoll does not. This difference is only seen in euthymic (normal) mice. Also with respect to T cell action, it is noted that significant numbers of IgA- and IgE-producing cells only arise *in vitro* when T cells are present. This leads to the possibility that particular T cells are able to help particular isotype producers. Evidence for this comes from experiments on Peyer's patch T cells. These cells cause a preferential expansion of IgA-producing cells in the presence of LPS, and this effect is particularly marked when the T cells are cocultured with Peyer's patch B cells as compared to splenic B cells. This shows that T cells have the ability to preferentially expand B cells producing a particular isotype. It may be significant that Peyer's patch T cells have Fc$_\alpha$ receptors.

Other T cell populations have been described which carry receptors for other Ig classes including IgG, IgE and IgM, and this might underlie a mechanism for differential activity on B cells producing different isotypes. The alternative explanation for preferential help involves isotype-specific T helper factors. Such factors have been described for the selective regulation of IgE synthesis, but even in this instance where the factors appear to be soluble MHC-restricted IgE binding proteins, they also share a common antigenic determinant with Fc$_\epsilon$ receptors. This suggests that a mechanism for selective isotype help (or suppression) involves either the presence of isotype-specific receptors on the T cell surface or the secretion of factors binding the particular isotype.

The question now arises as to whether a particular T cell can only help B cells of one isotype or antibody responses of all isotypes. Analysis of the helper potential of T cell lines shows that they can initiate the development of B cells producing different isotypes. The spectrum of isotypes generated in this instance is partly dependent on the source of the B cells, but there is also a characteristic profile for each T cell line. T cell clones also support development of several isotypes, with the spectrum of isotypes developing being similar to that of the parental T cell line but usually more restricted, that is, some isotypes are not expressed. Since both the source of B cells and the type of T cells influence the range of isotypes, a theory of class switching can be developed in which both populations play a role. Thus, B cells themselves can generate a range of isotypes which is partly dependent on the local environment. As noted above, Peyer's patch B cells tend to generate IgA on antigen challenge even in athymic mice. Given a particular B cell population, T cells can now modulate the isotype expression by selectively expanding particular sets of B cells. Furthermore, by increasing the rate of B cell division T cells can affect the rate of class switching by gene recombination. Calamé has suggested that T cells could act by releasing isotype-specific factors which selectively alter areas of chromatin in the heavy chain C genes. Although there is no evidence for this yet, it is notable that somatic mutation which accompanies affinity maturation of T dependent responses also becomes activated at the time of class switching. This explains how antibody affinity maturation is most marked in responses to T dependent antigens.

B CELL SURFACE MARKERS

Although mIg is the characteristic marker of functional B cells, they also express a variety of other surface proteins which receive signals from other parts of the immune system and allow them to make an antibody response. As noted above, surface Ig first appears on immature B cells which may undergo a number of class switching events: terminally differentiated plasma cells express very little surface Ig, although the production of secreted Ig may account for up to 30% of their total protein synthesis. Other surface proteins include receptors for IgG (Fc) and for C3b (CR1 and CR2), and class I and II MHC molecules. B cells are presumed to carry receptors for a number of lymphokines, including B cell growth and differentiation factors and IFN_γ, which make them able to respond to signals from T cells and antigen-presenting cells. The

function of the various B cell-stimulating factors in the antibody response is outlined in Chapters 10 and 11. The receptors for these factors are only partially characterized, but it can be inferred that their presence on the B cell surface modulates with the state of activation of the cell, since the ability to respond to the factors varies with time. In general, the expression of the various receptors increases on activated B cells and declines to virtually nil on plasma cells. The receptor for IL-2 (TAC) appears on a subpopulation of activated human B cells (20 - 30%), and a receptor for this lymphokine can also be induced on mouse B cells by LPS stimulation. A number of other molecules appear on subpopulations of B cells. These include Ly1 which occurs on a small minority of cells also expressing IgM but not IgD (see above), Qa-2 which is more usually associated with T cells, and the Mls determinant. It is debatable whether these proteins represent true differentiation markers like Lyb3, 5 and 7, or whether their presence reflects developmental stages within the cell cycle. As will be indicated in the following section, activation of B cells requires at least three separate signals to move a resting B cell into proliferation, differentiation and finally into an antibody-producing cell. Since each step requires sequential induction of additional receptors, the presence of populations of B cells expressing different sets of receptors does not imply separate differentiation pathways.

THE ACTIVATION OF B CELLS

The great majority of B cells are quiescent, that is, they are in the G_0 phase of the cell cycle. Activation of B cells involves a shift into the G_1 phase, prior to DNA synthesis (S), and the cells then proceed through the G_2 phase towards cell division. Three phases of B cell activation can be distinguished, each requiring separate signals: a) a signal which moves the cell from G_0 to G_1, b) a second signal which initiates DNA synthesis; once this phase is complete the cell is normally committed to division, and c) a group of factors causing the proliferating cells to mature into antibody-forming cells (Fig.4.6). Some of the evidence for this scheme is outlined below.

Anti-Ig and LPS have been used to dissect the first two steps in B cell activation. Anti-IgM (anti-μ), which cross-

Fig. 4.6 Stimulators of B cell activation. F(ab')$_2$ with anti-Ig specificity, Con A and LPS can all stimulate B cells and render them susceptible to signals for proliferation, but they differ in the degree to which they activate the cells, as reflected in a number of parameters indicated here.

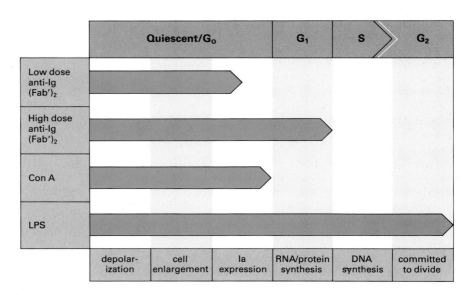

links the surface immunoglobulin on the great majority of B cells, causes the cells to decrease their membrane potential and increase in size, stimulates RNA synthesis, induces expression of Ia molecules on potentially responsive cells, and increases the sensitivity of the cells to a proliferative signal from LPS. The low doses of anti-μ used in these experiments do not by themselves cause cell division, although very high doses of anti-μ can do so. A number of other stimulators, such as Con A, have similar effects. It is now possible to push these cells into division by treatment with low doses of LPS or higher doses of anti-Ig. In this case, the anti-Ig must be $F(ab')_2$ anti-Ig, whereas the initial stimulation does not have this requirement. These data point to the requirement of separate signals for the shift from G_0 to G_1 and from G_1 to G_2.

How does this relate to B cell activation by T_{dep} and T_{ind} antigens? In one experiment, the type 1 T_{ind} antigen TNP-*brucella* could induce cell division of 80% of TNP-binding cells; that is, it was able to supply both signals, which indicates that crosslinking of receptors on the B cell may be enough to cause activation, particularly if accompanied by a polyclonal activation signal with mitogenic activity. This would be equivalent to LPS in the experiments mentioned above. A type 2 T_{ind} antigen was also able to induce division of 40% of potentially responsive cells, but the T_{dep} antigen TNP-SRBC was unable to induce cell division. This reinforces the idea that T_{dep} antigens require a second signal from T cells to proliferate. The first stage of T_{dep} antigen presentation is MHC-restricted, unlike the subsequent steps, and it explains the observation that the expression of Ia molecules which are required for T dependent MHC-restricted help appear on the B cells at a very early stage of activation preceding cell division. If, as proposed in this scheme, it is necessary to express Ia to be responsive to T cell activation, other signals may be required even before mIg-mediated B cell stimulation to induce Ia expression. One candidate for this function is BSF1, which does not have the ability by itself to induce cell division, but acts very early to induce Ia, or Ia and Ie expression. T cells can be induced to cooperate with B cells in an MHC unrestricted

fashion by crosslinking the cells with Con A. This indicates that the second activation signal from the T cell does not itself use the Ia on the B cell: only the first antigen/MHC signal requires Ia.

The T_{ind} antigens may either signal to the B cell directly via crosslinking of the surface Ig, or the cells may require an additional activation signal via an independent receptor. It has previously been mentioned that the Lyb3 molecule can act as a receptor for a B cell activating stimulus, and it has been noted that Lyb3+ cells can be activated by antigen and T cells in an MHC-unrestricted manner. This implies that the Lyb3 molecule is an alternative receptor to the mIg in receiving the initial activating stimulus (cf. Ti/T3 and T11 on human T cells), to push the cells into G_1.

Subsequent cell division and differentiation is directed by MHC-unrestricted factors, including the interleukins and B cell stimulating factors (BCGFII, BCDF and T cell replacing factor). These factors may be functionally divided into three types:
1. Those from antigen-presenting cells which are required for proliferation.
2. The T cell factors which also induce division.
3. The T cell factors which induce differentiation.
With respect to B cell division, it is necessary for both T cell factors and IL-1 from APCs to be present to induce continued proliferation. They act synergistically. The first cell division occurs within 24 hours of activation from G_0, and the B cell clone may then undergo several cycles of division, before falling back into a quiescent state, if IL-1 and T cell factors are limiting, or undergo terminal differentiation into an antibody-secreting cell. Cells which have returned to the resting state may be reactivated if their surface receptors become occupied with antigen. In keeping with this scheme it is noted that receptors for IL-1 and BSF1 appear on B cells at an early stage of activation, while receptors for IL-2 and transferrin (present on most dividing cells) appear later.

The late acting factors (third stage) include T cell replacing factor (TRF) which contains a mixture of BCGFII and BCDF. The possible role of IL-2 in stimulating B cell division has been hotly debated, but there is increasing

Fig. 4.7 Activation steps in the B cell cycle. B cells require several signals for activation. The initial signal is supplied by antigen, with T cell help for T_{dep} antigens, along with BSF1 which induces Ia. This moves the cell from its quiescent state into G_1, when it expresses lymphokine receptors. At this point it may be driven to proliferation by IL-1 and T cell factors including BCGFII. Subsequent differentiation of the proliferating cells requires the continued presence of T cell lymphokines to maintain the B cells in the cell cycle. T independent antigens appear to be able to drive the cell into G_1 without MHC-restricted help from T cells. The details of this scheme are not fully established, and the precise order of action may ultimately be found to vary slightly from that shown here.

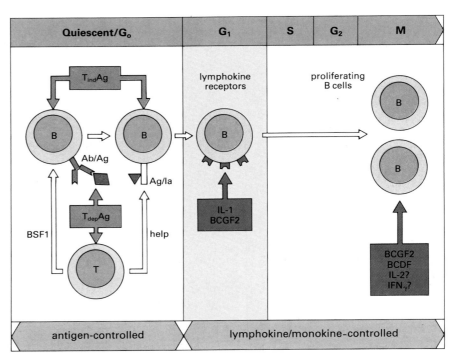

evidence that at least some B cells express the IL-2 receptor (TAC) and are susceptible to its actions. The function of IFN_γ in causing B cell differentiation is more doubtful, but the function of the B cell-stimulating factors as primary regulators of B cell differentiation is accepted. A synthesis of the various steps involved in B cell activation is shown in Figure 4.7. The various factors maintain cell division and induce differentiation into antibody-producing cells. Even polyclonal B cell activators such as LPS, although they can shift the cell through the first two stages of activation, are not as effective as T cells in causing terminal differentiation of the B cells with the associated class switching. The role of B cell growth factors in the development of the antibody response is further discussed in Chapters 10 and 11. B cell lines have been isolated at various stages of development. The most primitive lines lack even DJ rearrangements, but may develop them in culture. Early B cell lines respond to IL-3, while differentiated lines often require T cell growth factors for their maintenance. It is thought that many B cells may be programmed after stimulation to undergo terminal differentiation. If this is so, at which stage do B cells 'park' as memory cells?

MEMORY B CELLS

Since most antibody-producing cells in an animal are fully differentiated and have lost the majority of their surface antigen receptors, they are presumably unable to respond to further triggering, so it is thought that B cell memory resides in cells higher up the differentiation pathway. Memory cells are derived from B cells driven into proliferation by appropriate signals which have subsequently reverted to G_0 and are capable of responding again if the antigen returns.

A functional characteristic of memory cells is that they respond to a small antigenic stimulus and, having once been stimulated by antigen, they cannot be subsequently tolerized. It has been found that neonatal B cells which express high levels of mIgM are relatively easily tolerized by the use of anti-IgM, whereas adult B cells with relatively less mIgM are not. This is not due to an inability of neonatal B cells to proliferate, since they can be stimulated quite well with LPS. In contrast to mIgM, the levels of mIgD rise as B cells mature, and the most readily stimulated B cell population is that with high levels of mIgD and low levels of mIgM. Thus, adult B cells (cells with low mIgM and high mIgD) have the characteristics expected of memory cells. This has led to the supposition that mIgD might be involved in determining how readily a B cell is triggered and thus might be a marker for memory B cells. Indeed, removal of mIgD from B cells makes them more easily tolerized by T dependent antigens. Since IgM and IgD on a single cell share idiotypes and antigen-binding activities, it is unlikely that IgD is more efficient than IgM at binding antigen. Thus, if IgD is involved in the triggering of memory B cells, the mechanism must relate to the way in which mIgD links to components within the plasma membrane. Although it is attractive to assign this function to IgD (especially since other explanations of its function are unconvincing), it is equally possible that IgD is merely a marker of more mature cells which are more readily triggered, and that the association is coincidental. If, however, IgD is associated with readily triggered memory cells, this implies that the memory resides in a population of cells which

have not undergone recombinational class switching.

Other possible receptors involved in the development of memory are the C3b and C3d receptors (CR1 and CR2). These receptors develop on mature B cells, and it is noted that antigens in complement-fixing immune complexes are efficiently taken up within germinal centres of the lymph node, where B cells proliferate in a primary immune response. Complement (C3) is also involved in the development of the antibody response: C3 depletion inhibits the development of the normal secondary response to antigens. By implication, therefore, the receptors on the B cell for complement (C3) products facilitate the uptake of antigen-containing complexes and thus aid the development of the secondary immune response and B cell memory.

THE DEVELOPMENT OF T CELLS

Unlike B cells, the T cells in mammals differentiate in a discrete organ, the thymus. The early ontogeny of T cells is therefore more easily studied. In a series of experiments, Le Douarin and colleagues have demonstrated that the avian thymus has windows of receptivity for colonization by pre-T cells during embryonic development. After the thymus has been colonized by T cells, it becomes refractory to further cell immigration for a period. Thus, cells appear to colonize the thymus in waves. In chick/quail T cell chimaeras, the first window of receptivity when pre-T cells may enter the thymus occurs at six days of development. Subsequent windows occur at intervals of approximately six days. There is at least one more window, and perhaps several altogether. Similar studies performed on the bursa of Fabricius show that this organ also has windows of receptivity, the first being at approximately nine days. It is uncertain how this study in birds relates to mammalian thymic development, but it is certain that colonization of the thymus in the neonatal period is critically important for T cell development. Indeed, thymic function decreases so markedly with age that the organ appears superfluous in the adult. Adult thymectomy does not impair immune function. Possibly there is some peripheral development of T cells in the adult, from peripheral or bone marrow pre-T stem cells. This would explain why the thymus appears to be dispensable, whereas T cell function is essential throughout life. Differentiation of T cell subsets starts in the thymus (see below), and the thymus exerts an influence over subsequent T cell function via the activities of thymic hormones.

The Development of T Cells in the Thymus
Cells which enter the neonatal thymus do not appear to be committed to the T cell lineage, since their surface and cytoplasmic markers are essentially similar to pre-B cells and they lack any rearrangements of the T cell receptor genes. This means that the environment of the organ provides the signal for the differentiation pathway. Similar considerations apply to the bursa of Fabricius in birds, where much of the experimental work on lymphocyte development has been done. Within the thymus four separate regions can be distinguished. These are:
1. The subcapsular region which contains the most immature cells.
2. The cortex which contains the majority of the proliferating thymocytes.

Fig. 4.8 Markers of mouse thymocytes. The most immature mouse thymocytes are found in the subcapsular region whence they move into the cortex where there is considerable proliferation. Tdt (terminal deoxyribonucleotidyl transferase) is lost in cortical thymocytes, but the markers Thy1 and T200 appear at this stage. Ly1 also appears in the cortex. Initially this is coexpressed with Ly2, but there is a considerable increase in the levels of Ly1 as cells mature into medullary thymocytes. In the medulla cells expressing Ly1 alone are found, as well as cells coexpressing Ly1 and Ly2. A few cells may express Ly2 only.

Regions of the thymus	Subcapsular region	Cortex	Cortico-medullary junction	Medullary thymocytes
Cell numbers		proliferation	selective death	
Tdt				
Thy1				
T200				
Ly1 Ly2				Ly1$^+$ Ly1$^+$2$^+$ Ly2$^+$

3. The corticomedullary junction.
4. The medulla containing relatively few cells which express surface markers of mature T cells.

Even within the various regions, subpopulations of thymocytes can be distinguished based on surface markers (Fig. 4.8). The development during the passage through the thymus involves considerable proliferation and cell death. It is supposed that the differentiation process involves education to recognize external antigen plus MHC, as well as the elimination of anti-self MHC-reactive cells, and cells responding to self MHC plus a self antigen. It is unlikely that the enormous level of cell death within the thymus can be accounted for entirely in terms of elimination of self-reactive cells, and it is more likely that pre-T cells which fail to generate a functional receptor account for much of this loss during transit in the thymus. It has also been supposed that cortical thymocytes pass into the medulla before they leave the thymus, but a number of cortical thymocytes express the surface antigen recognized by the monoclonal antibody MEL-14. This antibody recognizes a receptor involved in homing of T cells to peripheral lymphoid organs, and is characteristic of mature T cells. Therefore, it is possible that both cortical and medullary thymocytes are sufficiently mature to exit for peripheral lymphoid tissues.

In humans, cortical thymocytes express T4 and T8 surface markers, but lose one of these molecules in the final stages of thymic development, so that they emerge as mature helper cells expressing T4 (CD4) or cytotoxic/suppressor cells expressing T8 (CD8) only. Human cortical thymocytes may also be distinguished from all other T cells, since they express the developmental marker T6 (CD1).

One important step in thymic T cell development is the interaction between developing thymocytes and the stromal cells of the thymus. In particular, the interaction with cells expressing MHC class II molecules appears to be most important. For example, treatment of neonatal mice with anti-Ia antibody prevents development of helper T cells. It is also noted that Ia molecules are absent from embryonic nude mouse prethymic cells. There are three separate cell types which express Ia within the thymus. These are:

1. Epithelial reticular cells which extend throughout the cortex and medulla, and which express class II MHC molecules very strongly. These cells also express class I molecules. These constitute the main stromal cell type within the cortex, but are less common in the medulla where a minor set have relatively little Ia.
2. Interdigitating reticular cells, similar to those seen in the T cell areas of secondary lymphoid tissues. They are seen in the medulla and express high levels of Ia.
3. Macrophages are also present and, as elsewhere, their expression of Ia molecules is variable.

There has been some controversy over the possible role of a population of stromal cells isolated from the thymus which appear to partly internalize the developing T cells, termed thymic 'nurse' cells. There has been some doubt as to their separate identity and role in antigen presentation. The evidence is weighed in favour of their existence, but their function in education has only been inferred from their surface markers. Examination of neonatal thymus shows the cortical thymocytes to be very closely apposed to Ia-bearing epithelial reticular cells.

Expression of the T Cell Receptor
The genes for the Ti portion of the T cell receptor are expressed early on in thymic development, in a definite sequence. The first transcripts to be expressed are for the apparently non-functional Tiγ chain. This chain, which should not be confused with the γ chain of T3, does not produce significant quantities of receptor peptide and lacks glycosylation sites. Therefore, the reason for its early expression in thymocytes is obscure. β chain transcripts are seen shortly afterwards, at approximately day 17 of development in mouse thymus, and α chain transcripts appear shortly thereafter. Presumably expression of the Ti is dependent on translation of the mouse equivalent of human T3, which determines expression of the receptor as a whole. There is now direct evidence that such an equivalent molecule exists. The expressed protein is therefore an α/β dimer, which appears on approximately half of the thymocyte population. The level of receptor is relatively low on neonatal thymocytes: approximately 5,000 receptors per cell, compared with the 20/40,000 seen on mature T cells.

Gene rearrangements in the T$_\beta$ chain of thymocytes occur from day 14 of thymic development. As with immunoglobulins, the initial recombination is a DJ joining which may generate sterile RNA transcripts. This is followed by VDJ recombination, so that virtually all of the initial population of thymocytes have recombined by day

Fig. 4.9 The rearrangement of Ti β chain genes. Gene rearrangements in the β chain of mouse Ti can be mapped by preparing hybridoma T cells from mouse thymus at different ages. They can then be quantified by looking for alterations in the restriction enzyme digests of the genes encoding the T_β chain. Liver cells (control) have no rearrangements of T_β; in fetal thymus DJ recombinations appear, which peak at day 16 and are followed by a wave of further rearrangements (e.g. VDJ recombination), so that the majority of cells in the day 17 mouse thymus have rearranged their T_β chains. The incidence of unrearranged chains in the adult thymus is very low.

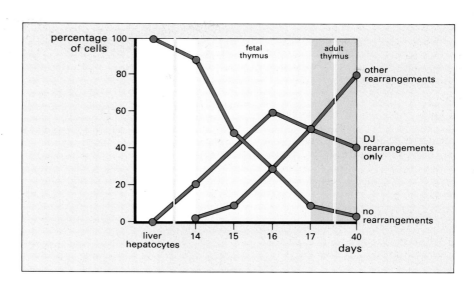

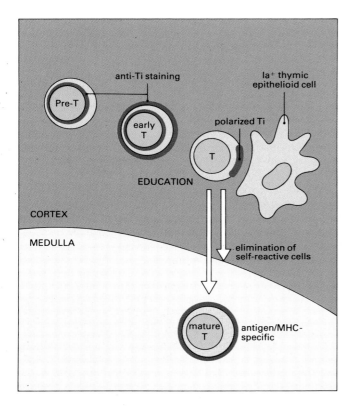

Fig. 4.10 Expression of the T cell receptor. Using antibodies specific for the T cell receptor on thymic sections, it is found that the receptor (brown) is initially expressed on early thymic T cells where it is seen in the perinuclear region. On more mature cells the receptor molecules are still present in the cytoplasm, but they also start to appear on the cell membrane. Developing cortical T cells undergo a process of education in close proximity to Ia-bearing thymic epithelial cells. T cells which are seen closely apposed to epithelial cells have their surface receptors polarized towards the epithelial cell. Exactly what occurs during this process is unknown, but it may involve education to recognize antigen only in association with the animal's own Ia haplotype, or self tolerance may develop at this stage. Considerable numbers of cells are eliminated during transit through the thymus, and the self-reactive cells may fall into this group. Mature medullary thymocytes express virtually all of their Ti on the cell membrane, as do peripheral T cells.

17, and so the great majority of adult thymocytes also have rearranged T_β genes (Fig.4.9). Interestingly, a number of thymocytes also develop rearrangements in the Ig heavy chain genes, albeit at a very slow rate. It is thought that this is a coincidental side effect of activation of the recombinational mechanisms which are primarily directed at the T cell receptor genes, but which act in an identical way on the Ig genes, if they are available.

Antibodies are now available which recognize families of expressed Ti,V_β chains – equivalent to the V gene subgroups of immunoglobulins. Using an antibody which recognizes a family of V_β genes expressed on approximately 20% of T cells, Marrack and her colleagues have been able to show that the genes for the T cell receptor are allelically excluded (cf. immunoglobulins). They examined T cells of F1 animals where one parent had this V gene family and the other lacked it. Only 10% of the T cells from these F1 animals expressed the V gene family, but the levels on those T cells were equivalent to the levels on the first parental strain. In effect, in the F1 mouse half the T cells express the maternal and half the paternal allele, but if the gene is expressed this is at normal levels, which is to say that the genes are allelically excluded.

The location of the T cell receptor on thymocytes is instructive. This is initially intracytoplasmic, around the nucleus of the developing cortical cell. The receptor then appears on the surface of the cell. Thymocytes which are closely apposed to epithelial reticular cells have their receptors sharply polarized on the membrane towards the epithelial cell. This has led to the idea that the educational process involving thymocyte/reticular cell interaction occurs by the recognition of Ia plus an unidentified factor on the reticular cell by the newly generated T cell receptor (Fig.4.10). These studies lead to the conclusion that the environment of the thymus is at least as important as the thymocytes in the development of the T cell repertoire.

Factors Influencing Post-Thymic Development

The role of the thymus in T cell development is fully established, but there is also evidence that the thymus can produce peptides which influence T cell development in the periphery. For example, it was noted that thymectomized mice which became pregnant started to show development of peripheral lymphoid tissues and some restoration of immune system function, indicating that molecules crossing the placenta from the fetal mice could

Factor	Occurrence	Size	Charge	Comment	Main effects
Thymosin Fraction 5 (>30 peptides)	isolated from calf thymus present in serum and spleen extracts	1000-15000 D $\alpha_1 = 3108$ D $\alpha_7 = 2200$ D $\beta_3 = 5500$ D	α pI <5 β pI 5-7 γ pI >7	$\alpha_1, \alpha_3 \beta_3, \beta_4$ and β_2 are active $\beta_1 \equiv$ Ubiquitin β_3 and β_4 have homology	α_1 (most active fraction) increases mouse T cell mitogen response; increases numbers of Ly123$^+$ cells; enhances MIF production; α_7 induces suppressors and T cell markers
Thymopoietin (2 peptides)	isolated from bovine thymus present in plasma	5560 D (49 amino acids)	?	Thymopoietin I and II differ by 2 amino acids; peptide of residues 32-36 (TP5) is active; no homology with thymosin α_1	induces T cell markers on nude mouse bone marrow and spleen
Thymulin: Facteur Thymique Serique (FTS)	isolated from mouse or pig serum; present in thymus	867 D (9 amino acids)	pI = 7.5	active form contains zinc (FTS - Zn)	induces cells bearing T cell markers in thymectomized animals
Thymic Humoral Factor (THF)	thymus extracts	3000 D (30 amino acids)	pI = 5.8		promotes thymocyte proliferation and differentiation; enhances T cell mitogen response

Fig. 4.11 Thymic hormones. The factors listed are the better characterized thymic hormones. These molecules have either been isolated from the thymus and/or shown to depend on it for their production. They have been assayed by numerous protocols, and their effects include inducing the differentiation of T cells. Although their effects are diverse, they generally appear to act at an early stage of T cell development rather than during the response to antigen.

influence the maternal peripheral immune system. Subsequently, it was shown that thymic grafts isolated within millipore chambers could also partly restore deficient immune responses. The factors responsible are called thymic hormones. In spite of the nomenclature, they are not like conventional hormones in that they cannot functionally replace the thymus *in toto*, and some of the molecules responsible for 'thymic hormone' activity may also be generated in other tissues.

A considerable number of such factors have been described, of which the best characterized are thymosin, thymopoietin, thymulin and thymic humoral factor. These peptides have either been isolated from the thymus or, in the case of thymulin, they were originally identified in serum and have subsequently been identified in the thymus using specific antibodies. Thymosin fraction 5 extracted from calf thymus contains at least 30 separate peptides, mostly structurally distinct, of which the most active are α_1, α_7, β_3 and β_4. Activities which have been ascribed to it include the induction of T cell markers on bone marrow cells, enhancement of MIF production and, in other systems, induction of suppressor cells. The evidence indicates that different thymosin peptides can act at different stages of development but, since many of the thymosin preparations used also contained interleukins and other lymphokines, the results are hard to interpret. One scheme for the role of thymosin states that α_1 at high doses, and β_3 and β_4 induce prethymocytes, and α_1 subsequently favours the differentiation of T helper cells, whereas α_7 acts within the thymus promoting the development of Ly123$^+$ cells and ultimately promotes the development of T suppressor cells. Thymosin α_1 also causes IFN$_\gamma$ production from mature T cells, and can thus influence late events in the immune response.

Thymopoietin consists of two structurally related peptides, with some similarities at the active site to β_2 microglobulin, IgG, and so on. The activity of thymopoietin resides in a pentapeptide (TP5) corresponding to amino acids 32-36 of thymopoietin II. The molecule is found in serum but is absent from patients with DiGeorge syndrome (thymic aplasia) and, like thymosin, it produces a variety of effects including the ability to induce T cell markers on bone marrow and splenocytes from nude mice.

Thymulin was originally identified in serum and termed Facteur Thymique Serique (FTS). It disappears from serum shortly after thymectomy, and can be identified on a proportion of thymic epithelial cells. Furthermore, it was subsequently identified as one of the components of thymosin fraction 5. The molecule is a nonapeptide which is only active when linked to zinc. There are specific receptors on peripheral T cells for thymulin, but these are not present on B and null cells.

Although the receptors have been identified on mature T cells, it appears that thymulin acts relatively early on in T cell development, since it accelerates loss of Tdt from early T cells and induces Ly123 cells in the mouse and Leu2a-reactive (=T8) cells in humans. It has been suggested that thymulin promotes the differentiation of cells capable of secreting IL-3. These then induce IL-2 producing T helper cells. As with all these experiments, a differentiation factor acting at an early stage of T cell development can exert numerous diverse effects on the immune response as a whole, acting through different T cell subpopulations.

The thymic humoral factor was originally assayed by its faculty of restoring the ability of splenocytes from neonatally thymectomized mice to mount a graft-versus-host reaction. It also promotes thymocyte maturation and differentiation (thymic hormones, see Fig. 4.11).

The peptide ubiquitin (UB), which was originally identified in thymosin (β_1) and thymopoietin preparations, is a 74 amino acid peptide and was at one time thought to be a thymic hormone. It is debatable whether it has any intrinsic T cell stimulatory activity, or merely accentuates responses to other immunologically active molecules. Furthermore, it has been identified in a variety of other animal and plant tissues, and is no longer considered a *bona fide* lymphocyte differentiation factor.

There are three possible roles for these thymic peptides:

1. They may be involved in intrathymic differentiation, modulating the proportions of each T cell subpopulation.
2. They may be required to maintain the peripheral pool of differentiated T cells.
3. Some of them appear to mimic the actions of the interleukins and other lymphokines involved in the response to antigen/MHC.

The nature of the interaction between the thymic epithelium and developing thymocytes is not known. It is noted that many of the peptides, for example, thymulin and thymosin factor 5, act on cells expressing receptors for the lectin PNA (which is a marker of immature thymocytes) and appear to accelerate their development as judged by loss of this receptor and of Tdt (i.e. function 1).

In respect of the second function, it must be stated that this feature was the first pointer to the existence of these peptides. Although the crucial role of the thymus in neonatal T cell development is fully accepted, the thymus involutes with age but the individual maintains a population of post-thymic T cell precursors in the periphery throughout life. This population of cells shows considerable capacity for further expansion, and in the mouse it expresses an Ly123 phenotype and lacks immune functions. In addition, numerical arguments hold that the neonatal colonization of peripheral lymphoid organs by newly differentiated thymocytes cannot be sufficient to maintain the peripheral T cell population indefinitely. Therefore, the post-thymic T cell precursors must be important in supplying mature T cells throughout life. These extrathymic cells may either arise from bone marrow stem cells independently of thymic development, or they may be T cells which have previously passed through the thymus and are not fully differentiated, retaining the capacity to divide repeatedly. In view of the

implied importance of the interaction between thymic epithelium and thymocytes in the development of the T cell repertoire, the first theory for their origin seems less likely. Thus, one role for the thymic hormones is to maintain an active population of precursor lymphocytes within the periphery, which can divide throughout life.

With respect to the role of these peptides in the response to antigens, it is notable that *in vitro* cultures of T cells are maintained and respond to antigen without thymic hormones, whereas lymphokines such as IL-2 are essential for the maintenance of all T cell lines. In all cases the roles of these peptides in specific immune responses can be ascribed either directly or indirectly to the selective expansion of precursor cell populations. The functions of the lymphokines in antigen-specific T cell expansion are described in the following section regarding the cell cycle, and also in Chapters 10, 11 and 12 in relation to the immune response.

ACTIVATION OF T CELLS

As with B cells, T cell activation takes place in sequential stages. For example, an optimal dose of the mitogen PHA induces T cell division if the cells are cultured for up to 18 hours, but if they are cultured for a shorter period, they undergo a temporary increase in size and then fall back into the resting state. Nevertheless, following this brief stimulation they are pushed into G_1 and become sensitive to the action of other stimulatory factors, including IL-2 (Fig. 4.12). This suggests a similar control of the cell cycle to that seen in B cells, with an antigen/MHC-specific step driving the T cells into G_1, accompanied by expression of IL-2 receptors; in the second phase the cells are committed to divide in the presence of IL-2 and other cytokines. However, the situation with T cells is more complicated than for B cells, since IL-2 which is required for T cell proliferation is also produced by the T cells themselves. The action of IL-2 in T cell proliferation is dependent on three factors: a) the concentration of IL-2 present, b) the density

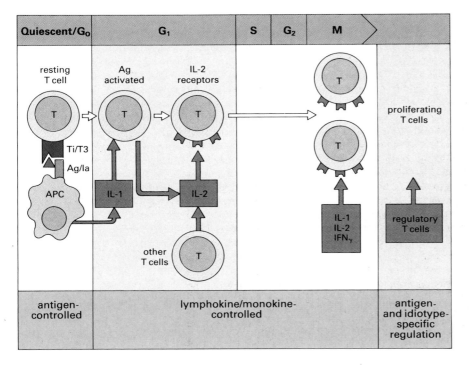

Fig. 4.12 T cell activation. Resting T cells (T_H) are stimulated by a signal of antigen/MHC from antigen-presenting cells expressing Ia. This pushes the T cell from G_0 into G_1; at this stage the cells start to express receptors for IL-2. IL-1 from antigen-presenting cells also increases IL-2 receptor expression. These T cells may now receive a proliferation signal of IL-2 derived either from themselves, if they can produce IL-2, or from other T cell populations. T cells stimulated to divide are subject to regulation by other lymphokines, including IL-1 and IFN, as well as being susceptible to immunoregulation by other T cell populations. After division, the levels of IL-2 receptor are decreased on the cell surface, and a continued stimulation by IL-2 is required if the cells are to continue proliferating.

of IL-2 receptors on the cell, and c) the length of time available for the IL-2 to interact with the cells. Thus, the control of proliferation by IL-2 depends on a critical cumulative dose being received by the cell. This explains why it is necessary for T cells to be in contact with IL-2 for several hours, even though the IL-2 receptors of the cells reach equilibrium binding within 15 minutes. IL-2 receptors appear on T cells following antigen/MHC activation but preceding DNA synthesis (S phase), and receptor density gradually increases until a critical density is reached. The cells may then receive a sufficient cumulative dose of IL-2 (if present) to initiate DNA replication and division. The quantity of IL-2 receptor on the cells following division declines unless the cells are restimulated. Thus, activated cells may relapse into G_0. This group of T cells, which have been stimulated to divide but have reverted to G_0, are thought to be the memory T cell population. Since IL-2 is consumed by cells during their replicative cycle, a continuous source is required to maintain division.

While this theory explains how proliferation of activated T cells is controlled, it is more difficult to understand where the initial IL-2 comes from, since IL-2 is only generated by cells which are already in G_1. Either the initial antigen stimulus is sufficiently strong to initiate IL-2 production in the responding population, or IL-2 comes from another cell population. In the first hypothesis, a triggered population is pushed to a 'flip/flop' condition where it either generates enough IL-2 to drive its own division (as occurs if mitogen is present for a long period), or it flops back into G_0 (as occurs for short mitogen stimulations). Note in this case how mitogen-mediated proliferation of T cells is IL-2 dependent. There is also evidence for other cell populations being able to generate IL-2, for example, the thymulin-sensitive peripheral T cells. It is likely *in vivo* that IL-2 is supplied to the responding cell population both from external sources and by the responding population itself. In addition, the responding population also requires signals from antigen-presenting cells (see Fig. 4.12).

Although IL-1 is not required for the initial stimulation of T cells into G_1, expression of IL-2 receptors is augmented by IL-1, and at least one T cell clone has been reported that absolutely requires IL-1 for the expression of the IL-2 receptor. Physiologically, IL-1 will usually be supplied to the T cell by the antigen-presenting cells at the same time as antigen/MHC interactions. At present then, it appears that IL-1 is not essential for all cells, but it may modulate developing T cell responses. The critical role of the antigen/Ia signal in stimulation of T cells is set out in the following chapters.

T CELL DIFFERENTIATION MARKERS

It is generally accepted that the two main lymphocyte subpopulations, T_H and T_C/T_S, result from distinct differentiation pathways which are distinguished by Ly1/Ly23 in the mouse and by T4/T8 in the human. The more recently discovered molecule L3T4 on mouse T cells appears to be a functional equivalent of T4 and therefore is also a marker of helper cells. In some experiments, the surface phenotype of mouse T cells appears to modulate to express the other subpopulation Ly marker when stimulated *in vitro*. It is therefore possible that the Ly markers are not stable indicators of a single cell population, although virtually all experiments assume that they are. Attempts

have also been made to equate other cell surface markers with different functional subsets of T cells. These markers include the Qa locus antigens, lectin-binding sites and MHC class II molecules. It had been hoped that these molecules would provide ways of uniquely identifying functional T cell subsets, although this assumption has never been proven. To give two examples: (1) The T suppressor cell in mice is $Ly2^+$ and acts on antigen-specific helper cells or B cells, but it is thought to be induced by an $Ly1^+$ cell expressing Qa1. (2) The helper cell in mice is $Ly1^+$, and in some circumstances is acted on by an $Ly1^+$ contrasuppressor which reacts with anti-I-J antisera. Experiments which purport to equate the action of a particular subpopulation with a particular cell phenotype by depleting the responding population of cells with that phenotype can sometimes be faulted, since they do not take account of successive chains of regulation of the sort mentioned above.

T cell interactions between different subsets may take place at two levels, which correspond to the two main stages of T cell proliferation and development. These are:
1. In the initial proliferation of virgin T cells.
2. At the stage of antigen-induced proliferation.
The interactions of different subpopulations in an immune response are discussed in Chapter 10, but *in vivo* and in long-term *in vitro* experiments the former type of interactions may be important. It has been stated that $Ly1^+$ and $Ly23^+$ cells in the mouse develop from $Ly123^+$ thymocytes and post-thymic precursors: similarly in humans T4 and T8 positive cells develop from T4/T8 positive thymocytes. Therefore, the proportion of the different phenotypes which develop can be varied by modulating the proportion of cells directed into each differentiation pathway from the common precursor. In mice there is much evidence that peripheral $Ly1^+$ and $Ly23^+$ cells can feed back onto post-thymic $Ly123^+$ precursors, thereby indirectly influencing the control of immune reactions. This may be seen as a possible complement to the actions of the thymic hormones, IL-3 and other cytokines which feed forwards to modulate the functions of the mature T cell populations.

SUMMARY

Lymphocytes undergo two main phases of proliferation during their development. The first is associated with development in the primary lymphoid organs, before the cells colonize the periphery, and the second may occur if the cells come into contact with an appropriate antigenic stimulus. During the first phase, T cells differentiate in the thymus from immature T cells expressing markers characteristic of both helper and suppressor cells, into mature T cell subpopulations expressing only one of these surface phenotypes. B cell development takes place in the fetal liver and bone marrow, and is therefore less accessible for study. Nevertheless, there do appear to be different functional subsets of B cells, which may be distinguished by their surface markers or anatomical locations. It is not entirely certain, however, that these different B cell subsets do not represent different stages in B cell ontogeny.

The development of T and B cells is associated with rearrangements of genes for their antigen receptors, in a defined sequence: $H/\kappa/\lambda$ in B cells, $\gamma/\beta/\alpha$ in T cells. Many rearrangements are non-functional, therefore only a proportion of cells produce functional rearrangements and others are eliminated. The process of T cell maturation involves an education step, in which the T cells interact with thymic epithelium expressing Ia molecules. Whether this step determines antigen/MHC reactivity or results in the elimination of self-reactive clones is uncertain. Possibly both processes (or neither) may occur during this phase of development in the thymic cortex. The thymus can also influence T cell development in the periphery by secreting factors (thymic hormones) which affect T cell function and differentiation.

The second phase of proliferation occurs if lymphocytes receive an appropriate antigenic stimulus. Resting lymphocytes require two signals to initiate proliferation. The first signal is antigen-specific, and is transduced via the antigen receptor. This drives the cells from G_0 to G_1. At this stage they become susceptible to the actions of lymphokines — BCGFII, BCDF and so on for B cells, IL-2 and IL-3 for T cells. IL-1 also modulates proliferation of both populations. These lymphokines and monokines drive the cells from G_1 into the S phase, and several cycles of proliferation may ensue. If the proliferation factors are absent or at low levels, antigen-activated cells may relapse into G_0. The population of cells which have undergone several rounds of division and subsequently reverted to the resting state are thought to constitute the memory population. The process of B cell maturation also requires factors which induce terminal differentiation into antibody-secreting cells. This process is associated with class switching, which sometimes involves further recombination of the antibody genes. Class switching proceeds from IgM to C genes further down (3') the IgH C gene stack. Mutational mechanisms are activated at this time, which affect the whole Ig gene region and permit slight modifications of the original Ig genes. This process, when it is accompanied by antigen selection, underlies antibody affinity maturation.

FURTHER READING

Bach J.F. (1983) *Thymulin (FTS-Zn)*. Clin. Immunol. Allergy **3**, 133.

Calamé K. (1985) *Mechanisms that regulate immunoglobulin gene expression*. Ann. Revs. Immunol. **3**, 159.

Cebra J.J., Komisar J.L. & Schweitzer P.A. (1984) *C_H isotype switching during normal B-lymphocyte development*. Ann. Revs. Immunol. **2**, 493.

Goldstein A.L., Low T.L.K., Zatz M.M., Hall N.R. & Naylor P.H. (1983) *Thymosin*. Clin. Immunol. Allergy **3**, 119.

Hayakawa K., Hardy R.R., Honda M., Herzenberg L.A., Steinberg A.D. & Herzenberg L.A. (sic) (1984) *Ly-1 B Cells: Functionally distinct lymphocytes that secrete IgM autoantibodies*. Proc. Nat. Acad. Sci. **81**, 2494.

Howard M. & Paul W.E. (1983) *Regulation of B cell growth and differentiation by soluble factors*. Ann. Revs. Immunol. **1**, 30.

Huber B.T. (1982) *B cell differentiation antigens as probes for functional B cell subsets*. Immunol. Revs. **64**, 57.

Incefy G.S. (1983) *The role of thymic hormones on human lymphocytes*. Clin. Immunol. Allergy **3**, 95.

Kishimoto T. (1985) *Factors affecting B cell growth and differentiation*. Ann. Revs. Immunol. **3**, 133.

Klaus G.G.B. & Hawrylowicz M. (1984) *Cell cycle control in B lymphocyte stimulation*. Immunol. Today **3**, 15.

MacLennan I.C.M., Gray D., Kumararante D.S. & Bazin H. (1982) *The lymphocytes of the splenic marginal zones: a distinct B cell lineage*. Immunol. Today **3**, 305.

Mather E.L., Nelson K.J., Haimovich J. & Perry R. (1984) *Mode of regulation of immunoglobulin mu and delta expression varies during B lymphocyte maturation*. Cell **36**, 329.

Melchers F. & Anderson J. (1984) *B cell activation: Three steps and their variations*. Cell **37**, 715.

Moller G. (Ed.) (1980) *The effects of anti-immunoglobulin sera on B lymphocyte function*. Immunol. Revs. **52**, 3.

Mond J.J. (1982) *Use of T lymphocyte regulated type 2 antigens for the analysis of responsiveness of Lyb5$^+$ and Lyb5$^-$ B lymphocytes to T lymphocyte-derived factors*. Immunol. Revs. **64**, 99.

Mosier D.E. & Subbarao B. (1982) *Thymus-independent antigens: complexity of B cell activation revealed*. Immunol. Today **3**, 217.

Samelson L.E., Lindsten T., Fowlkes B., Elsen P., Terhorst C., Davis M., Germain R. & Schwartz R. (1985) *Expression of genes of the T cell antigen receptor complex in precursor thymocytes*. Nature **315**, 765.

Shimuzu A. & Honjo T. (1984) *Immunoglobulin class switching*. Cell **36**, 801.

Singer A., Asano Y., Shigeta M., Hathcock K.S., Ahmed A., Fathman C.G. & Hodes R.J. (1982) *Distinct B cell subpopulations differ in their genetic requirement for activation of T helper cells*. Immunol. Revs. **64**, 137.

Smith K. (1984) *Interleukin-2*. Ann. Revs. Immunol. **2**, 319.

Stutman O. (1983) *Role of thymic hormones in T cell differentiation*. Clin. in Immunol. Allergy **3**, 9.

Tucker P. (1985) *Transcriptional regulation of IgM and IgD*. Immunol. Today **6**, 181.

Wall R. (1983) *Biosynthesis and regulation of immunoglobulins* Ann. Revs. Immunol. **1**, 393.

5 Class I and II Molecules of the Major Histocompatibility Complex

The ability to distinguish 'self' from 'non-self' is a protective characteristic of virtually all multicellular organisms, ensuring that defence mechanisms are directed towards invading microorganisms and other foreign molecules without causing damage to host tissues. The fundamental features are highly polymorphic cell-surface recognition structures and mechanisms for the destruction of non-self. The existence of self/non-self discrimination in mammals was first demonstrated by the ability of mice to reject grafts of foreign tissues, such as skin or tumours. This ability to reject non-self tissues was subsequently mapped to a region (termed H-2) on chromosome 17, which became known as the major histocompatibility complex (MHC). The cell surface structures involved in rejection were initially characterized by using alloantibodies, produced in one inbred strain of mice immunized with cells of other strains differing only at the MHC. Subsequently, with the use of specific antibodies to molecules encoded by small regions of the MHC and using techniques borrowed from protein chemistry and molecular biology, the characteristics of MHC genes and their products have been analysed in considerable detail. Similar techniques have also been used to characterize the human MHC, known as the Human Leucocyte Antigen (HLA) system which is located on chromosome 6. The similarities between the mouse and human major histocompatibility complexes suggest that other species will also be found to have MHC regions with broadly similar gene products and functions. Recent studies involving a number of species, particularly the rat, have substantiated this view.

Three classes of molecules, denoted I, II and III, have been identified in the MHC of both mouse and man (Fig. 5.1). At least three separate class I loci (termed H-2K, -D and -L in the mouse and HLA-A, -B and -C in man) encoding classical transplantation antigens have been demonstrated. Other class I genes in the mouse map to the right of the MHC in regions known as Qa-2,3 and Tla. Products of these loci differ in tissue distribution and probably also in function. For example, certain Qa antigens can be expressed by distinct T lymphocyte subpopulations. A human equivalent of the Qa-2,3/Tla genes probably also exists but has not yet been characterized. Class II genes, encoded in the I-A and I-E regions of the mouse MHC and the HLA-D region of man, are identical to the immune response (Ir) genes known to control murine responses to different antigens. Class I products are primarily recognized by cytotoxic T cells, whereas class II gene products (often called Ia antigens) are primarily involved in the activation of T helper cells, although there are exceptions to this general rule. The class III genes encode several components of the complement system. Since there is no evidence for functional or structural similarities between these products and the class I and II molecules, it is perhaps better to consider these genes to be closely linked to the MHC rather than a part of it. The MHC could then be more neatly defined as a cluster of loci involved in triggering T lymphocytes. The major feature of the MHC is the extreme polymorphism of some of the class I and II genes. For example, more than 50 different alleles have been demonstrated at both the H-2K and -D class I loci of mice.

Fig. 5.1 Organization of the murine and human MHC. The location and major loci of the class I (brown), class II (pink) and class III (grey) regions are shown. The Qa-2,3 and Tla regions of the mouse Tla complex have more recently been shown to contain class I genes and are thus now considered part of the MHC. The class III genes primarily encode complement components (e.g. C4 and Slp in mouse; C4, C2 and Bf in human), and although they are located within the H-2 and HLA complexes, they ought not be considered as MHC genes.

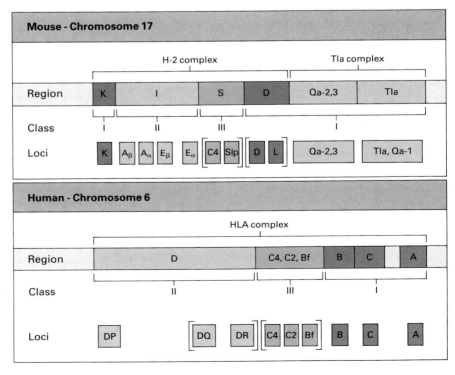

Class I molecules are somewhat more polymorphic than class II molecules, although the Qa-2,3 and Tla region class I genes exhibit little polymorphism. The generation and molecular basis of MHC polymorphism will be discussed in subsequent sections of this chapter.

STRUCTURE OF CLASS I AND II MOLECULES

Class I Molecules

Class I molecules are comprised of a glycosylated polypeptide chain of 45 kD (heavy chain) in close, non-covalent association with β_2 microglobulin (β_2m), a 12 kD polypeptide which is also found non-associated in serum. Amino acid sequence analyses of both human and murine class I molecules have demonstrated that the heavy chain is divided into five distinct regions: three extracellular domains, a transmembrane region, and a cytoplasmic domain (Fig.5.2).

The three extracellular domains, designated α_1 (N-terminal), α_2 and α_3, can be cleaved from cell surfaces with the enzyme papain. These domains, each of about 90 amino acids, bear a striking resemblance to immunoglobulin (Ig) domains. The α_2 and α_3 domains both have intrachain disulphide bonds enclosing loops of 63 and 86 amino acids respectively, and the α_3 domain also appears to fold like an Ig constant region. Both human and mouse heavy chains have an N-glycosylated asparagine residue (86) in the α_1 domain. Murine heavy chains are also N-glycosylated at residue 176 in α_2, and some (D^b, K^d, L^d) have additional carbohydrate side chains at residue 256 in α_3. Each carbohydrate side chain consists of 12-15 invariant sugar residues. In addition to the major papain cleavage site between α_3 and the transmembrane region, there is also a minor cleavage site between the second and third domains.

The transmembrane region consists of about 25 hydrophobic uncharged residues, which assume an α-helical conformation and traverse the cell membrane. There is a cluster of about five basic amino acids (arginine and lysine), immediately C-terminal to the transmembrane region. Such highly charged regions are typical of membrane-bound proteins (for example, glycophorin and cytochrome b6), and they probably help to anchor the polypeptide chain in the membrane by interacting with the negatively charged phospholipid headgroups of the inner membrane.

The hydrophilic cytoplasmic domain is about 30 (human) to 40 (mouse) residues long and consists of approximately 50% polar amino acids, particularly serine. Some of these serine residues may be phosphorylated. For example, the HLA-A2 heavy chain is phosphorylated by a cyclic AMP-dependent protein kinase at two serine residues in the cytoplasmic domain. Such phosphorylation has been postulated to be involved in transmitting signals from the MHC molecule to appropriate intracytoplasmic mediators. This region of the heavy chain also has free cysteine residues which could become involved in disulphide binding to other heavy chains, or cytoplasmic proteins. However, a cloned, truncated H-2L^d gene lacking exons coding for the cytoplasmic region has recently been shown to be expressed in the membrane and to function normally, implying that interactions between cytoplasmic proteins and class I molecules are not required for function. The lack of conservation in the

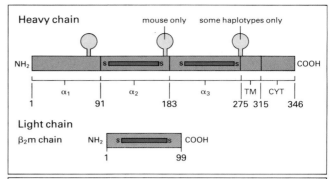

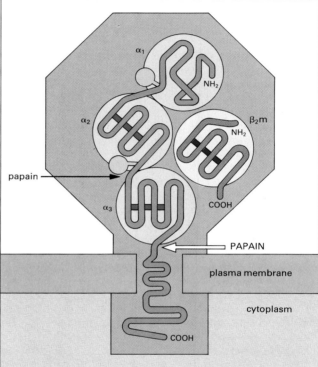

Fig.5.2 Structure of MHC class I molecules. The general features of class I molecules are illustrated here by the murine H-2K^b molecule. The heavy chain, encoded by the MHC, is divided into five regions: three extracellular globular domains (α_1, α_2 and α_3), a hydrophobic transmembrane (TM) segment, and a short, hydrophilic cytoplasmic domain (CYT). The amino acid residues at the boundaries of these domains are numbered (upper diagram). The non-MHC encoded β_2 microglobulin (β_2m) light chain associates non-covalently with the heavy chain, particularly through interactions with the α_3 domain. Carbohydrate attachments (grey) are found primarily in the α_1 and α_2 domains in mice and the α_1 domain in humans, although additional glycosylation occurs in α_3 in some murine haplotypes. Intrachain disulphide bonds (red bars) in α_2, α_3 and β_2m stabilize the structure of the molecule. The conformation adopted by the non-disulphide-bonded α_1 domain is not known. The major (large arrow) and minor (small arrow) papain cleavage sites are also shown.

membrane and cytoplasmic regions among different class I molecules would also support this view.

The class I light chain β_2m forms a single Ig-like domain, by disulphide bonding of its two cysteine residues. It also has strong sequence homology with Ig constant regions and is thought to associate with the class I heavy chain primarily through interaction with the α_3 domain, in the same way as inter-domain Ig interactions. β_2m is encoded outside the MHC on human chromosome 15 and on mouse chromosome 2. It is a non-polymorphic protein in humans, dimorphic in mice (a single amino acid change at position 85), with a high degree of sequence homology among species implying evolutionary conservation. The function of β_2m appears to be to stabilize the class I molecule. It may also be involved in transporting heavy chains to the membrane, but this is not yet certain. Although β_2m is essential for the structural integrity of class I molecules, it is still unclear whether or not it contributes directly to the functions of class I molecules.

Class II Molecules

The products of class II genes (I-A and I-E in the mouse, DR, DQ and DP in humans) are heterodimers comprising heavy (α) and light (β) glycoprotein chains. The α chains have molecular weights of 30-34kD and the β chains range from 26-29kD, depending on the locus involved. For example, at least 20 different mouse I-A region haplotypes exist, and all have α chains of 34-35kD and β chains of 26kD. However, E_α chains of the k and r haplotypes are 34kD, whereas those of the p or d haplotypes are 31kD. All E_β chains appear to be 28-29kD. Amino acid sequences deduced from class II cDNA clones have complemented direct sequencing data to give the current view of the structure of α and β chains. On the basis of sequence and susceptibility to proteolysis, each chain has been shown to consist of four domains: two extracellular domains of approximately 90 amino acids each, α_1 and α_2 or β_1 and β_2, and a transmembrane region of about 30 residues followed by a short cytoplasmic domain (Fig.5.3).

The two N-terminal domains, α_1 and β_1, show no sequence homology with Ig, whereas the α_2 and β_2 domains, like α_3 and β_2m of class I molecules, have the characteristics of a single Ig domain. The class II α_2 and β_2 domains are most homologous to the $C_\gamma3$ and $C_\mu4$ Ig domains, and are as similar to Ig as the various Ig C domains are to each other. The β_1 domain has cysteine residues at positions 15 and 79, which are disulphide-linked to give a 64 amino acid loop. The three-dimensional structure of the α_1 domain is at present unknown, but as it lacks cysteine residues it cannot form disulphide bonds. Both α_2 and β_2 domains have disulphide loops enclosing 56 amino acids. Class II molecules are N-glycosylated at asparagine residues in α_1, α_2 and β_1. The carbohydrate side chains are mostly of a complex type involving mannose, galactose, fucose and glucosamine units. Heterogeneity in carbohydrate attachments accounts for much of the difference in molecular weight of class II molecules. Differential glycosylation of identical class II molecules may also occur between cell types. It is conceivable that they could lead to both qualitative and quantitative variations in the capacity of class II bearing cells to present antigens to T cells (see Chapter 6).

The extracellular domains are connected to the trans-membrane region by a short hydrophilic region, rich in glutamic acid and proline (α chain) or serine (β chain). The transmembrane regions of the α and β chains are thought to form α-helices packed together and, like the class I heavy chains, they have a cluster of positively charged residues anchoring the chains in the membrane. The hydrophilic cytoplasmic regions are of variable, but generally short, length (10-15 residues).

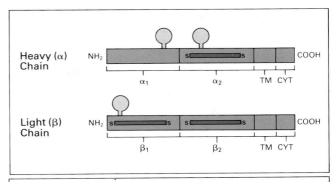

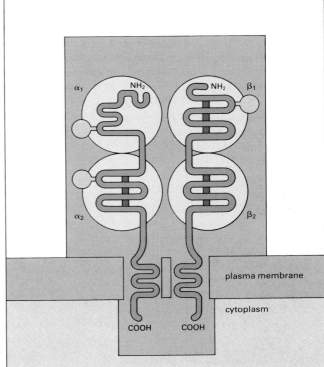

Fig.5.3 Structure of MHC class II molecules. The general features of class II molecules are illustrated by prototypic α (heavy) and β (light) chains, as some variation exists in the precise length of the various regions. Each chain is divided into four major regions: two extracellular globular regions (α_1, β_1, α_2, β_2), a short hydrophobic transmembrane region, (TM) and a short hydrophilic cytoplasmic region (CYT). Carbohydrate attachments (grey) account for much of the molecular weight differences between the α and β chains. The conformation of the disulphide-bonded β_1 and the non-disulphide-bonded α_1 domains is unknown. The α_2 and β_2 domains have a strong sequence homology with immunoglobulin constant regions, and thus probably adopt a β-sheet conformation.

Structural Correlates of I-J

The I-J subregion of the H-2 complex was originally defined serologically and mapped between I-A and I-E by using antisera raised in I-J disparate strains, such as the apparent intra-I-region recombinant mouse strains B10.A(3R) and B10.A(5R), which carry and express identical class II genes. Such antisera recognize polymorphic determinants expressed on suppressor T cells (and the recently described contrasuppressor cells) and soluble secretory products of these cells. Thus, it was thought that

I-J represented part of the antigen receptor of T suppressor cells. Molecular analysis of the region between I-A and I-E has indicated that the putative I-J region would have to map to a 1 kb length of DNA entirely within the intron separating the β_1 and β_2 exons of the E_β gene. This evidence, coupled with the observation that cloned DNA from the putative I-J region fails to hybridize to RNA from I-J$^+$ suppressor T cell lines, implies that the I-J locus is not encoded within the I region. It now seems probable that I-J molecules are encoded by a non-H-2 gene and expression of this gene is somehow regulated by I-region genes. Although the I-J gene has not yet been identified, recent evidence indicates that I-J^k expression requires complementation of at least two genes: one on chromosome 4, called the Jt gene, and another on chromosome 17, perhaps the E_β gene. Other genes on chromosome 12 may also influence the expression of I-J. The binding of monoclonal anti-I-J^k antibodies to cell surface I-J^k determinants is blocked by treatment of the cell with α-mannosidase, implying that the I-J determinant involves a glycoprotein structure.

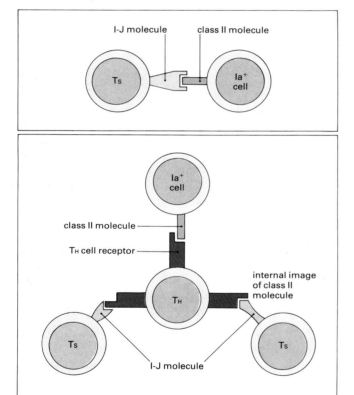

Fig.5.4 Two hypothetical models to explain the nature of I-J molecules. Both of these models depict I-J molecules as receptors on some T cell subsets (Ts in this Figure), which are either directly or indirectly selected for by class II molecules (but encoded outside of the MHC). The simplest model (upper diagram) shows the I-J receptors directly recognizing class II molecules. In the other model (lower diagram), I-J receptors may recognize part of a conventional T cell receptor (α/β complex) on a T helper cell (or possibly Tc cell), which is itself specific for a class II molecule. In this model, a subset of the I-J receptors might mimic the self class II molecule, and so represent an 'internal image' of the class II molecule. It is postulated that these I-J receptor molecules are distinct from the α and β chains of conventional T cell receptors found on T$_H$ and Tc cells.

Perhaps the most attractive hypothesis to date is that I-J molecules are T cell receptors whose selection is influenced by I-region genes. Such receptors could be either anti-self class II, or they could recognize (or be recognized by) other T cell receptors for self class II molecules. A subset of such receptors might even mimic self class II molecules: 'internal images' of class II molecules (see Chapter 13), (Fig.5.4). Therefore, class II molecules would dictate the receptor structures on I-J bearing T cells, thus accounting for the pseudomapping of I-J to the I-region of the MHC. These I-J$^+$ T cell receptors seem to be expressed in T cell subsets (for example, suppressor, contrasuppressor), which regulate T helper activity and are probably distinct from the α and β subunits of T$_H$ cell receptors, since these cells are routinely I-J$^-$. Preliminary biochemical analysis suggests that I-J molecules are 25kD compared with the 40-45kD for the T$_H$ receptor polypeptides.

Testing of this model will require the isolation of I-J structural genes, as well as an understanding of the roles played by I-region and non-H-2 genes in regulating the expression and polymorphism of I-J molecules. For the present time, it seems that I-J is best regarded as an idiotype of the T cell receptor of certain T cell subclasses. Certainly, whatever the localization of I-J determinants, they are intimately involved in the exchange of information amongst T cell subsets.

THE IMMUNOGLOBULIN SUPERGENE FAMILY

The homology in sequence and domain structure between class I and II molecules and immunoglobulins has also been demonstrated in many other gene products known to be involved in vertebrate immune responses. These include the Thy-1 polypeptide, the T cell antigen receptor and T cell γ-chain (see Chapter 3), the poly-Ig receptor for IgA and IgM, and the T8 molecule (Fig.5.5). The genes encoding these products may, therefore, have a common evolutionary origin and are collectively known as the 'immunoglobulin supergene family' after the first genes to be analysed. A supergene family is a set of multigene families (for example, heavy Ig chains) and single copy genes (for example, Thy-1), which are related by sequence but not necessarily by function.

The domain structure common to all the products of the immunoglobulin supergene family consists of sequences of approximately 100 amino acids folded into two sheets of anti-parallel β strands which are stabilized by a conserved disulphide bridge between cysteine residues approximately 65 amino acids apart. Each member of the family has one or more of these conserved domains. The exon-intron organization of the genes in this family usually corresponds to the domain organization of their products.

It is thought that the primordial gene of the Ig supergene family encoded a cell surface protein and would, therefore, have had a leader sequence, a domain structure and a transmembrane region. Evolutionary processes subsequently led to the development of V and C domain structures and, following further divergence, they have ultimately produced the variety of cell surface molecules known to be important in triggering cells involved in the immune response. Whether all such molecules are members of the Ig supergene family and all family members are involved in immune responses is not yet known.

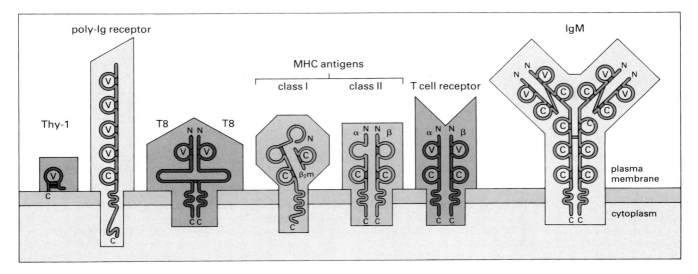

Fig.5.5 Products of the immunoglobulin (Ig) supergene family. Immunoglobulin-related molecules of immunological relevance are depicted on the surface of a cell. Regions related to Ig domains are depicted by circles with similarities to a variable (V) or constant (C) domain indicated. Disulphide bonds are shown in dark red (for the poly-Ig receptor these have been predicted from the amino acid sequence but are not established). IgM is shown as a typical surface Ig molecule. The conformation of non-Ig-like regions in the MHC and T8 molecules is unknown.

CLASS I AND II GENES

Our current understanding of MHC genes has come through application of the methods of molecular genetics. For simplicity, this section will describe the organization and structure of murine and human genes separately, followed by a discussion of the nature of polymorphism of class I and II genes.

Murine Class I Genes

Class I genes in the mouse fall into two main categories: the classical transplantation antigens encoded within the K and D regions of the H-2 complex, and genes in the Qa-2,3 and Tla regions to the right of H-2 some of which encode class I molecules expressed in a tissue-specific manner. The postulated function of Qa-2,3 and Tla genes will be expanded upon later. More than 50 alleles have so far been identified at both the H-2K and -D loci, whereas the Qa-2,3/Tla genes are much less polymorphic. The advent of molecular genetic methods has led to the isolation and characterization of many class I genes. However, because of a lack of amino acid sequence data, only a few of these genes have been correlated with known, serologically detectable, class I molecules. Sequencing of different class I genes has revealed an exon-intron organization similar to antibody genes (Fig.5.6 overpage). Each gene is divided into eight exons precisely matching the domain structure of the class I molecule (see Fig.5.2). A leader sequence encoded by the first exon is followed by exons 2, 3 and 4 which encode the α_1, α_2 and α_3 domains respectively. The fifth exon codes for the hydrophobic transmembrane segment, and the remaining three exons encode the cytoplasmic domain and a 3' untranslated region. The β_2m gene, which is a single copy gene coordinately regulated with class I genes, consists of four exons with most of the coding region (amino acids 3-95 of the total of 99) present in the second exon (see Fig.5.6).

The use of cosmid vectors to clone large DNA fragments has enabled the complexity and linkage relationships of class I genes to be studied. Using this approach the BALB/c mouse (H-2^d) has been shown to have at least 33 class I genes, most of which are located in the Qa-2,3/Tla region (see Fig.5.7). Similarly, the B10 mouse (H-2^b) has a minimum of 26 class I genes: 10 in the Qa-2,3 region (Q1-10), 13 in the Tla region (T1-13), 2 in the K region (H-2K^b and K1) and the H-2D^b gene. Thus, although the number of class I genes appears to vary from one strain to the next, most of the genes are found in the Qa-2,3/Tla region. The function of such large clusters of class I genes in this region is open to question. It has been proposed that they are important in the generation of polymorphism of class I molecules. Whether or not most of these genes are normally expressed, or whether their products serve as restricting elements in antigen recognition by T cells, is still unknown. Both BALB/c and B10 mice have two genes (K and K1) at the K region, but only one of these (K) appears to be expressed. Mice of the b and k haplotypes, as well as the BALB/c mutant strains dm1 and dm2, fail to express H-2L gene products. This has recently been shown to be due to a deletion of the entire, or a large portion of, the 5' region of the L gene. The localization of murine class I genes in relation to class II genes differs from that seen in the major histocompatibility complexes of other species. In mice, the H-2K locus is centromeric to the class II genes, and the H-2D, L, Qa-2,3 and Tla loci are telomeric, whereas in other species all class I genes are telomeric to class II genes. The similarity between H-2K and Qa genes has led to the suggestion that this anomaly might have arisen from a translocation of a Q6 and Q7-like gene pair from the Qa-2,3 locus to give rise to the H-2K gene in its present position.

The identification of serologically defined class I genes has been achieved by transfection experiments. Mouse L cells lacking thymidine kinase were cotransfected with class I genes and the herpesvirus thymidine kinase gene. Over 90% of cells found to express the thymidine kinase gene also expressed the introduced class I molecule (detected with monoclonal antibodies). All serologically defined BALB/c class I genes have now been identified in this way, with the exception of Qa-1 for which no mono-

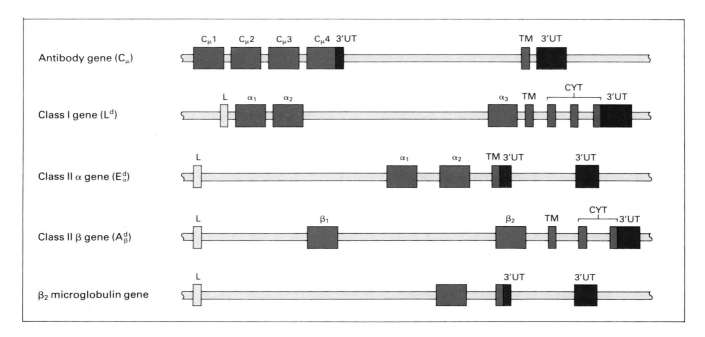

Fig. 5.6 Schematic representation of the exon-intron organization of antibody, class I, class II and β_2 microglobulin genes. The organization of typical murine genes is illustrated. Exons which correspond closely to the domain structure of the coded peptide chain are shown as boxes, with translated exons in red and 3′ untranslated (3′UT) regions in maroon. The intervening introns are shown in pink and their lengths are approximately to scale. L = exons encoding leader or signal peptides; TM = transmembrane exons; CYT = exons encoding cytoplasmic regions.

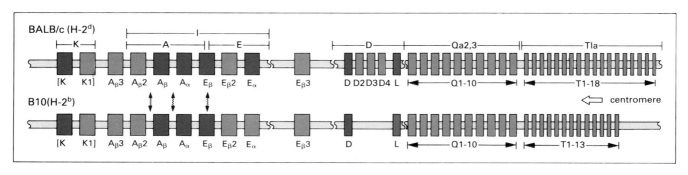

Fig. 5.7 Murine class I and II genes. Genes of the H-2^d and H-2^b haplotypes are illustrated. Genes known to be transcribed and translated to produce a functional MHC molecule are shown in red. The other genes (dark pink) are either known pseudogenes or their functional usage is uncertain. Note that the H-2^b haplotype (represented here by the B10 mouse strain) lacks a functional E$_\alpha$ gene, and therefore cannot produce cell surface I-E molecules (although it still produces cytoplasmic E$_\beta$ chains). The H-2^b strain also lacks a functional H-2L gene. The additional genes (D2, D3 and D4) in the D region of the BALB/c (H-2^d) mouse are thought to have arisen by gene duplication. Postulated regions of hypermutation (hot spots) in the I-region are here indicated by the vertical arrows.

clonal antibody is yet available. For example, in BALB/c mice, transfected Q6, 7, 8 and 9 genes could all be used to produce serologically detectable Qa-2 antigens. However, which of these genes (if any) are normally used by lymphocytes to produce Qa-2 products is still not known. The transfection approach, coupled with genetic methods to produce recombinant MHC molecules (exon shuffling), has also been very useful in defining the regions of class I molecules which are recognized by cytotoxic T cells. The results from such experiments will be elaborated in Chapter 7.

Murine Class II Genes

The α and β chains of murine class II molecules are encoded by separate genes located in the I region of the H-2 complex (see Fig. 5.1). The use of recombinant inbred mice in mapping immune responsiveness subdivided the I region into five subregions: A, B, J, E and C. However, only the I-A and I-E regions have been biochemically defined. Molecular genetic methods have been unable to establish the existence of separate B, J and C loci, suggesting that their initial characterization was an illusion created by the complex interactions involved in controlling immune responses.

A substantial portion of the I region has been characterized by probing cosmid libraries of mouse DNA with human class II cDNA clones, and by using chromosome walking procedures. There appears to be no more than two α genes and six β genes, and of these only A$_\alpha$, A$_\beta$, E$_\alpha$ and E$_\beta$ appear to be expressed to produce two functional class II molecules: I-A and I-E. The A$_\beta$3 gene has a seven base pair deletion which makes it non-functional.

Whether or not the other genes ($A_\beta2$, $E_\beta2$ and $E_\beta3$) are functional is not known.

Some mice (b, s, f and q haplotypes) fail to express I-E class II products. The b and s strains fail to make E_α chains because of a deletion of approximately 650 base pairs in the promoter region. However, they express normal cytoplasmic levels of E_β chains which can be utilized in hybrid I-E molecules in F1 hybrids between b or s haplotypes and strains expressing E_α. Mice of the f and q haplotypes fail to make both E_α and E_β chains. The E_α chain defect appears to reside at the level of RNA splicing, whereas the E_β defect has not yet been clarified.

The $A_\beta2$, A_β, A_α and the 5' end of E_β are located in the I-A subregion, whereas the 3' end of E_β, $E_\beta2$ and E_α are in the I-E subregion. The $A_\beta3$ gene maps telomeric to the H-2K region (for the b haplotype), and the $E_\beta3$ gene maps telomeric to E_α near the S region (Fig.5.7).

The intron-exon organization has now been elucidated for a number of murine class II genes and, like class I genes, it correlates very closely with the domain structure of the class II product (see Fig.5.6). Both α and β genes have separate exons encoding the leader sequence and the first and second domains. However, the E_α gene uses a single exon to code for the transmembrane and cytoplasmic regions, and has a fourth intron in the 3' untranslated region.

Human Class I Genes

Three different loci, HLA-B, -C and -A, encode the expressed human class I molecules (Fig.5.8).

Human Class II Genes

Human class II genes are located in the D region of the HLA system. This D region appears to be more complex than the murine I region. Current evidence suggests that at least six α and eight β chain genes are encoded within the D region. These are organized in three different families of genes called DR, DQ and DP, with the exception of one α (DZ_α) and one β chain gene (DO_β) whose map positions are uncertain, but which do not fit into one of the three families (see Fig.5.8). The DR family consists of a single α gene (DR_α) and three β genes ($DR_\beta1$, $DR_\beta2$, $DR_\beta3$), whereas the DQ and DP families have two α and two β genes each. These genes are called $DQ_\alpha1$, $DQ_\alpha2$, $DQ_\beta1$, $DQ_\beta2$ and $DP_\alpha1$, $DP_\alpha2$, $DP_\beta1$, $DP_\beta2$. The DR, DQ and DP α chains associate primarily with the β chains of their own family. It is not yet known which α and β chains give rise to which serologically detectable class II molecules. It is also not clear which genes are expressed and whether or not the expression is the same for all haplotypes. Nucleotide sequence determination suggests that the $DP_\alpha2$, $DP_\beta2$ and DO_β genes are pseudogenes and, thus, not expressed. The DZ_α gene appears to be intact, but since it produces abnormally large mRNA molecules, it is not known whether these molecules can be translated and their products expressed at the cell surface.

The order of genes within the DR and DQ families is unknown, but the DP gene family has been cloned in overlapping cosmids and shown to have the order $DP_\alpha1$, $DP_\beta1$, $DP_\alpha2$, $DP_\beta2$.

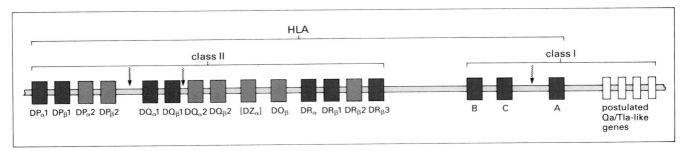

Fig.5.8 Human class I and II genes. HLA genes known to encode a functional class I or II molecule are shown in red. The remaining genes (dark pink) are either pseudogenes (e.g. $DP_\alpha2$, $DP_\beta2$, DO_β), or their functional usage is uncertain. The human equivalent of the murine Qa/Tla genes (open boxes) has been postulated but not yet found. Regions of possible hypermutation (hot spots) are indicated by arrows. (Previously used nomenclatures for the class II genes are as follows: DQ = DC, DS, LB, MB; DP = SB; $DQ_\alpha2 = DX_\alpha$; $DQ_\beta2 = DX_\beta$; $DP_\alpha2 = SX_\alpha$; $DP_\beta2 = SX_\beta$).

The A and B loci exhibit the most extensive polymorphism as determined by their serologically detectable products. For example, the B locus has nearly 50 recognized specificities, whereas the C locus only has about ten different alleles. These class I loci are analogous to the murine H-2K, D and L loci. Although human equivalents of the Qa-2,3/Tla loci have been suggested, their existence awaits demonstration.

Human class I molecules are structurally very similar to their murine counterparts, therefore it is not surprising that their intron-exon organization is also virtually the same. The only apparent difference is that human class I genes have only two cytoplasmic region exons instead of the three in the mouse. Functional studies of human class I genes have recently been aided by their successful transfection and expression in mouse L cells. This has also shown that mouse β_2m can associate with human class I heavy chains to produce a functional molecule.

The orientation (direction of transcription) of the α genes is reversed compared with that of the β genes, an observation also made with murine α and β genes. Both genetic and biochemical analyses have shown that DR genes are the human counterpart for mouse I-E genes (E_α and $E_\beta2$) and DQ genes are equivalent to murine I-A genes (A_α, A_β and E_β). No murine analogue of DP has yet been detected, although some evidence suggests that the non-functional $A_\beta3$ gene may be analogous to DP_β.

The intron-exon organization of human class II genes is very similar to that of mouse class II genes, with distinct exons encoding the major portions of the different domains of the expressed product. For example, a DQ_β gene has five exons. The first exon encodes a 5' leader sequence, a signal peptide (32 amino acids), and the first four amino acids of the β_1 domain. The second and third exons encode the β_1 and β_2 domains respectively, and the fourth exon codes for the transmembrane region and the first six amino acids of the cytoplasmic region. Finally, the fifth exon encodes the remaining amino acids of the cytoplasmic region and a 3' untranslated sequence.

ALLOANTIGENICITY

As mentioned previously, most class I and II molecules (with the exception of Qa-2,3/Tla antigens) are highly polymorphic structures. This polymorphism was originally defined through the use of alloantisera, alloreactive lymphocyte populations and, more recently, monoclonal antibodies. The list of different HLA specificities has grown very large (Fig.5.9). Unfortunately, in most cases the location of the epitopes recognized by the antibodies or T cells used to define these specificities is still unknown. In this section, the molecular basis of the observed polymorphism will be discussed. Mechanisms involved in generating and maintaining this variability at the genetic level will be described later.

DR		DQ	DP	B		C	A
DR1	Dw1	DQw1	DPw1	Bw4	Bw47	Cw1	A1
DR2	Dw2	DQw2	DPw2	B5	Bw48	Cw2	A2
DR3	Dw3	DQw3	DPw3	Bw6	B49	Cw3	A3
DR4	Dw4		DPw4	B7	Bw50	Cw4	A9
DR5	Dw5		DPw5	B8	B51	Cw5	A10
DRw6	Dw6		DPw6	B12	Bw52	Cw6	A11
DR7	Dw7			B13	Bw53	Cw7	Aw19
DRw8	Dw8			B14	Bw54	Cw8	A23
DRw9	Dw9			B15	Bw55		A24
DRw10	Dw10			B16	Bw56		A25
DRw11	Dw11			B17	Bw57		A26
DRw12	Dw12			B18	Bw58		A28
DRw13	Dw13			B21	Bw59		A29
DRw14	Dw14			Bw22	Bw60		A30
DRw52	Dw15			B27	Bw61		A31
DRw53	Dw16			B35	Bw62		A32
	Dw17			B37	Bw63		Aw33
	Dw18			B38	Bw64		Aw34
	Dw19			B39	Bw65		Aw36
				B40	Bw67		Aw43
				Bw41	Bw70		Aw66
				Bw42	Bw71		Aw68
				B44	Bw72		Aw69
				B45	Bw73		
				Bw46			

Fig.5.9 Currently recognized HLA alloantigenic specificities. Distinct antigenic specificities detected at each HLA subregion are listed. HLA-A, -B, -C and -DR (D-related) are detected serologically, whereas HLA-D specificities are detected in a mixed lymphocyte reaction. Many of the specificities are not yet sufficiently well characterized, and these are given the 'w' (workshop) designation.

Class I Molecules
Amino acid sequence analysis and tryptic peptide mapping have shown that H-2K and -D, and HLA-A and -B molecules are highly polymorphic, whereas H-2L and HLA-C molecules appear less so. The amino acid sequence variability in class I antigens is clustered in three main (hypervariable) regions of the α_1 and α_2 domains (residues 62-83, 95-121, 135-177 in the mouse; 68-80, around 110 and around 175 in humans). The α_3 domain appears to be much more conserved. The most conserved region is the second disulphide loop. Clearly, this third domain needs to be conserved in order that it can correctly associate with

β_2m to produce a functional class I molecule. No characteristic sequences have been identified which could classify a gene as being a product of a particular locus. That is, there is no evidence for 'K-ness' or 'A-ness' and so on.

Regions of variability often coincide roughly with the positions at which mutations occur in the H-2K locus of the mouse. Such mutations, detected by parent to offspring skin-grafting, have been found most frequently in the H-2K^b locus and these are known as the 'bm' series of mutants (Fig.5.10). A number of these mutants differ in only one amino acid resulting from a single nucleic acid base substitution (for example, bm5). In other cases, two amino acid changes are involved, and some of these required two base changes (for example, bm1). Similar mutations also seem to occur in human class I molecules (see Fig.5.10). For instance, variant HLA-A2 molecules have been detected, either with allospecific T cells or by using HLA-A2-restricted cytotoxic T cells specific for influenza virus. Two of these mutations (DR1 and M7 in Fig.5.10) resulted from a single amino acid change and appear to be analogous to the bm mutations. These mutants have been very useful for studying the molecular basis of functional and serological polymorphism. Mutant class I molecules are not normally discriminated by standard serological reagents, but as they were originally detected by graft rejection, they are clearly functionally different. However, monoclonal antibodies have since been produced which can recognize bm mutant molecules. Formaldehyde fixation will destroy the serological determinants on H-2K^b, but it has no effect on determinants recognized by cytotoxic T cells. Thus, since graft rejection is a T cell-mediated phenomenon, it would seem that class I epitopes recognized by antibodies are not necessarily the same as those seen by T cells. Studies with cloned cytotoxic T cells and DNA-transfected target cells have directly demonstrated that more than one distinct epitope on the same class I molecule can be recognized by T cells.

The association of β_2m with the heavy chain alters both the three-dimensional conformation of the class I molecule and the ability of antibodies to bind to epitopes on the heavy chain. These observations imply that some antibodies recognize conformational determinants (see Chapter 8) on class I molecules. It is thought that the clustered regions of variability in the α_1 and α_2 domains are largely responsible for the differences in antigenic structure. Although it is not yet clear whether the regions of variability represent actual epitopes, it has recently been claimed that residues 61-83 (highly variable in human class I molecules) of the HLA-B7 heavy chain specify an alloreactive site.

Class II Molecules
A high degree of polymorphism is also seen in class II molecules. Studies with tunicamycin and glycosidases have shown that carbohydrate attachments do not contribute to this polymorphism. Two-dimensional gel electrophoresis studies and β chain cDNA probing of restriction fragments of human class II molecules have shown that most polymorphism occurs in DR and DQ β chains, while DP β chains are largely non-polymorphic. Of the α chains, only DQ$_\alpha$ is polymorphic, DR$_\alpha$ chains being virtually invariant. As with class I molecules, allelic variations are not random but occur clustered in particular regions of the molecule; for example, around amino acid 50 in the DQ$_\alpha$ chain. Similarly, the DQ$_\beta$ chain has three major clusters of amino acid variability at residues 52-58, 70-77 and 84-90

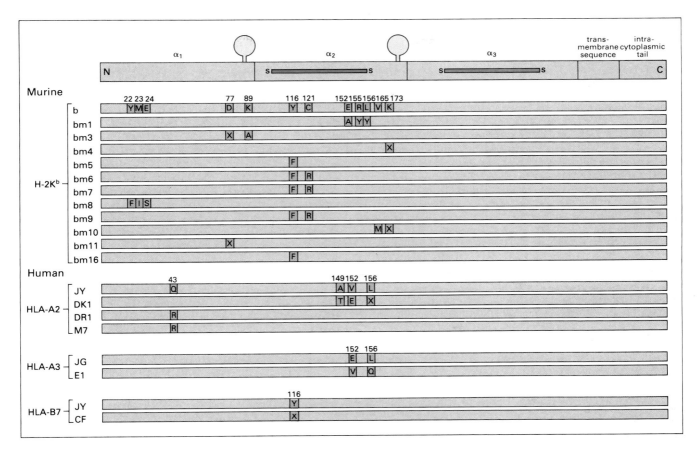

Fig.5.10 Mouse and human MHC class I mutants.
Mutations in the murine H-2K^b locus (bm series) were identified by skin grafting between a very large number of mice of an H-2^b strain. Similar mutants, also occurring naturally in humans, have been distinguished by their differential reactivity with cytotoxic T cell populations. For example, serologically identical HLA-A2 molecules can be subdivided into four subtypes by this approach. In both the murine and human mutants, amino acid differences are clustered in the α$_1$ and α$_2$ domains, with particular sites

being especially mutable. In this diagram amino acid differences between the mutant and the corresponding prototypic sequence (b, JY, JG) are represented in one letter code (defined below) at the position numbered in the prototype: (A = alanine, C = cysteine, D = aspartic acid, E = glutamic acid, F = phenylalanine, G = glycine, H = histidine, I = isoleucine, K = lysine, L = leucine, M = methionine, N = asparagine, P = proline, Q = glutamine, R = arginine, S = serine, T = threonine, V = valine, W = tryptophan, Y = tyrosine, X = unknown amino acid replacement).

of the β$_1$ (N-terminal) domain. The polymorphism of DR$_β$ chains is also located in three hypervariable regions in the N-terminal region.

In the mouse, only I-E α chains are non-polymorphic. Like DQ molecules, I-A α and β chains have non-random amino acid variability. In I-A α chains there are three clusters of hypervariable residues at positions 11-15, 48-60 and 69-77, whereas I-A β chains have extensive polymorphism which appears to be more scattered throughout the N-terminal domain. The variation between E$_β$ alleles also occurs in the first domain. Most of the allelic amino acid substitutions in these genes are non-conservative, and thus, might be expected to significantly alter the secondary structure within certain regions of the first domain. It therefore seems that, whereas interlocus (isotypic) variation occurs in all four extracellular domains of class II dimers, allelic variation in both mouse and human molecules is localized in the N-terminal α$_1$ and β$_1$ domains. It has been suggested that the three-dimensional folding of the α and β chains may allow juxtaposition of the hypervariable regions to form a site which can interact with antigen or the T cell receptor in a similar way to the formation of antigen-binding sites in immunoglobulin

molecules. Alternatively, regions of sequence variability might produce many local changes in surface topography of the molecules. This would produce new epitopes and also influence binding to antigen and T cell receptors (see Chapters 6 and 8). Unfortunately, there is no information on the folding of class II molecules to support or refute these hypotheses.

The B6.C-H-2^{bm12} (bm12) mutant mouse has not only been useful in demonstrating that class II molecules are Ir gene products, but has also provided much useful information on the basis of structural and functional polymorphism. Peptide mapping and nucleotide sequencing have shown that the mutation involves three productive nucleotide differences (i.e. producing an amino acid change) in a region of 14 nucleotides in the second exon of the I-A$_β$ gene. Two of the three are non-conservative, which lead to changes in structure and different associations with the I-A α chain. Studies with alloreactive T cell clones have indicated that at least two different epitopes on the I-A β chain can be recognized by T cells, one of which is altered by the bm12 mutation and the other is not. The role of class II epitopes in antigen presentation to T cells will be discussed in the next chapter.

THE GENETIC BASIS OF POLYMORPHISM

The mechanisms involved in generating the polymorphism of class I and II molecules, as well as their relative importance, is still the subject of hot debate. Clearly, random point mutations could contribute to the generation of allelic products, particularly if fixed in the population by phenotypic selection pressure. However, different class I and II alleles differ at multiple residues, unlike other allelic proteins, such as immunoglobulins and globins, which generally differ at single residues. Some of the allelic polymorphism is seen as clusters of highly polymorphic sequences interspersed with conserved regions. For example, the frequently occurring H-2K^b mutants (bm series) generally have two or more relatively closely spaced amino acid substitutions. In addition, the same variants are seen repeatedly in independently derived mutants. Furthermore, non-allelic genes can share polymorphic sequences which differentiate alleles. Thus, it seems that mechanisms other than simple random point mutations are involved in generating the observed polymorphism.

The mechanism postulated to account for the generation of multiple nucleotide substitutions in class I and II alleles has been termed 'gene conversion' or 'copy substitution' (to distinguish it from the classical meiotic gene conversion originally described for certain fungi). Donor gene sequences present elsewhere in the genome (probably other class I and II genes) are thought to be copied and substituted in a non-reciprocal fashion onto recipient genes. Although the precise mechanism is unclear, it would probably be mediated through homologous flanking regions in the two genes, and could occur following the resolution of heteroduplex hybrid DNA formed as a recombination intermediate. It has been proposed that the major function of class I genes mapping to the Qa-2,3/Tla region of the mouse MHC is to act as donor genes for such conversion events which generate diversity of class I molecules in the H-2 region. For example, a donor gene Q10 mapping to Qa-2,3 has been identified as generating the H-2K^b mutant bm1. Similarly, the mutant bm6 appears to have incorporated a Q4 gene segment. Nucleotide sequence comparisons of E$_\beta$^{b} and the A$_\beta$^{bm12} chain from the bm12 mutant have been taken as evidence that the bm12 mutation was produced by the transfer of a stretch of 14-44 nucleotides from the exon encoding the E$_\beta$^{b} first domain to the equivalent region in A$_\beta$^{b}. In contrast to class II β genes, A$_\alpha$ genes have shown no evidence for gene conversion, even though they have a similar clustering of regions of allelic polymorphism. These observations, together with the lower mutation rate of the D^b gene compared to the K^b gene, suggest that gene conversion does not occur with the same frequency in all class I and II genes.

There appears to be a 'hot spot' for recombination within a 2 kilobase region of the intron between the first and second exons (including part of the second exon) of the E$_\beta$ gene. A similar region may also exist between DP and DR/DQ, in the human D region. Recent data also indicate that other hot spots occur in I-A and DQ, as well as between HLA-C and -A. Analysis of overlapping cosmid clones of BALB/c and AKR mouse I regions has indicated that the 'hot spot' in E$_\beta$ forms a sharp boundary of polymorphism. The A$_\beta$2, A$_\beta$, A$_\alpha$ and E$_\beta$ genes are extremely polymorphic, whereas E$_\beta$2 and E$_\alpha$ are non-polymorphic. In microorganisms, 'hot spots' often occur in regions with short palindromic sequences, which allow single DNA strands to form short loops. The repair of unpaired regions of these loops can lead to multiple nucleotide substitutions. Such a mechanism might also operate in the H-2K^b gene which has palindromic sequences in the region containing multiple nucleotide substitutions in bm mutants.

Other mechanisms, such as gene duplication and deletion and differential RNA splicing, could also contribute to the generation of diversity among class I and II molecules. For example, because of the close similarity of DR$_\beta$1 and DR$_\beta$3 genes, it has been proposed that they arose as a result of a recent gene duplication event. The possible combinations of α and β chains in the offspring of parents mismatched at class II MHC loci will also serve to expand the diversity of class II molecules. For example, it has been shown that APCs from F1 mice can express novel antigenic and functional class II domains.

At present, the relative contribution of the mechanisms suggested above to the diversification of the MHC remains to be determined. Clearly, the exertion of selection pressure on the different mutations generated has also played a very important role.

BIOSYNTHESIS

Class I Molecules

There is very little information available on the nature of the primary RNA transcripts of heavy chain genes, but it is known that the mature mRNA molecules have about 1640 bases. The primary translation products of both heavy chain and β$_2$m mRNA have N-terminal extensions containing a signal sequence which directs the nascent polypeptide chains to the endoplasmic reticulum. Following insertion of the heavy chain into the membrane of the endoplasmic reticulum, the signal sequence is enzymatically removed. Glycosylation occurs concomitantly with translation. Studies with tunicamycin, which blocks N-linked glycosylation, have demonstrated that the carbohydrate moieties are not required for membrane insertion or for transport to the membrane. Transport may require β$_2$m because the Daudi cell line, which does not synthesize β$_2$m, fails to express HLA-A and -B antigens, even though class I molecules and their mRNA are present in normal amounts in the cytoplasm. Association of the heavy chain with β$_2$m in the endoplasmic reticulum is complete within five to ten minutes after completion of the heavy chain. If association does not take place within this time, a conformational change occurs which renders the heavy chain unable to associate with β$_2$m. Following association, transport to the surface occurs in membrane-bound vesicles formed from the endoplasmic reticulum, which are called 'coated vesicles'. This takes 25-60 minutes, during which time the oligosaccharide side chains are modified such as to render them insensitive to endoglycosidase H, but sensitive to endoglycosidase D. Phosphorylation and addition of a fatty acid side chain to a free cysteine in the cytoplasmic tail also occur post-synthetically. The addition of the acyl moiety is also thought to be important for transport. The differential RNA splicing which can occur in the cytoplasmic domains may be important for generating different effector functions.

An unusual category of class I mRNA molecules has recently been described, which has codons for hydrophilic amino acids as well as a termination codon in the exon normally encoding the transmembrane region. These mRNA molecules appear to be expressed in liver cells only, and it is thought that they direct the synthesis of soluble class I molecules. An example of this phenomenon is the Q10 gene of the Qa-2,3 region of B10 mice, which is a highly conserved (non-polymorphic) gene only transcribed in the liver. Mouse L cells transfected with the Q10 gene, coupled to a metallothionein I promoter, have been shown to secrete class I polypeptides with a molecular weight of 38kD; this is somewhat smaller than membrane-inserted class I molecules. Class I molecules have also been immunoprecipitated from serum and have a similar molecular weight, although it is not known whether they were secreted or merely shed from cell surfaces. The function of such secreted class I molecules is unknown, but they could conceivably play an immunoregulatory role.

Class II Molecules

The biosynthetic pathways of class II α and β chains are similar to those of other membrane proteins, such as glycophorin, surface Ig and class I molecules. Biosynthetically, immature class II molecules are associated with a third glycoprotein chain, called the invariant (γ) chain because of its lack of allelic polymorphism between different strains of mice. The γ chain is a methionine-rich, basic polypeptide of 31 kD in molecular weight which is N-glycosylated at two positions. It exists, in part, as disulphide-bonded dimers and also associates non-covalently with a number of other poorly characterized molecules. The γ chain is produced in excess and interacts non-covalently with α and β chains before they associate. Unbound γ chains remain in the endoplasmic reticulum, while the $\alpha\beta\gamma$ complex is transported to the cell membrane. The γ chain has a transmembrane region and becomes inserted into the cell membrane, but is no longer associated with the mature class II molecules. The dissociation of the γ chain appears to occur during passage of the $\alpha\beta\gamma$ complex through an as yet unidentified acidic compartment within the cell. Although it seems likely that the γ chain is involved in intracellular transport and/or assembly of class II molecules, large amounts are probably not required, since transfected L cells (which produce very little γ chain) can express the class II product normally. Some evidence suggests that the human γ chain may be required to allow glycosylation of DR_α chains. The synthesis of α, β and γ chains is coordinately regulated even though the γ chain gene is not MHC-linked, being found on chromosome 18 in the mouse and on 5 in humans. Recent evidence suggests that at least three distinct molecular variants of γ chain are produced by human cells. Whether or not these γ chains associate preferentially with different class II molecules is unclear.

Antigenic determinants on class II molecules change during synthesis. Unassociated α and β chains have a different antigenic structure, but even after association some antigenic determinants are subsequently lost or gained. Studies with tunicamycin have shown that N-linked carbohydrates are not required for these conformational changes. The α and β chains must associate in order for either to be expressed on the cell surface.

In contrast to class I molecules which are constitutively expressed by virtually all nucleated cells, the expression of class II molecules is more restricted and highly susceptible to regulatory control mechanisms. The regulation of class II expression affects a cell's ability to present antigen to T lymphocytes (see Chapter 6). Gamma interferon (IFN_γ) and other T cell products (see Chapter 11) can induce and amplify the expression of class II molecules (as well as class I molecules), whereas PGE_2, glucocorticoids, α-fetoprotein and bacterial endotoxin lipopolysaccharide (LPS) can reduce expression. LPS may, in fact, act by stimulating PGE_2 production by macrophages. Recent experiments have shown that, following transfection of an $E_\beta{}^b$ gene, macrophages will only express the class II product after treatment with IFN_γ, suggesting that DNA sequences associated with class II genes may play a regulatory role in cell-type specific regulation. A separate study has since identified a cell-type specific transcriptional enhancer element in the DNA associated with the mouse $E_\beta{}^d$ gene, which might account for such regulation. Both class I and II molecules are internalized and recycled during constitutive endocytosis, a phenomenon which might allow fragments of processed foreign antigens to associate with MHC molecules prior to their coexpression on the cell membrane (see Chapter 6).

TISSUE DISTRIBUTION OF CLASS I AND II MOLECULES

Class I antigens were thought to be expressed on the surface of all nucleated cells, as well as on the erythrocytes of some species, even though the level of expression could vary from one cell to the next. For example, cells of the immune system express particularly high levels of class I antigens. However, recent studies have suggested that class I antigens are not ubiquitously distributed. Using a sensitive immunoperoxidase staining technique on human tissues, class I antigens were only weakly detectable on most endocrine cells (with the exception of the adrenal gland), and not found at all on corneal endothelium, the exocrine region of the pancreas, acinar cells of the parotid gland, central nervous system neurons, or the villous trophoblast. Capillary endothelium, interstitial dendritic cells, fibroblasts and lymphatics of all tissues express class I antigens.

Class II antigens are generally thought to be expressed predominantly on B cells and antigen-presenting cells (see Chapter 6). However, it is becoming apparent that other cell types can also express class II antigens, under either physiological or pathological conditions. Endothelial cells and lymphatics in most tissues normally express class II molecules, and activation of human T cells also leads to class II expression. In addition, epithelial cells in a number of different organs, such as the small intestine, trachea, tongue, tonsils, epiglottis, proximal renal tubules, urethra and epididymis, may carry class II antigens. Interestingly, capillaries in the human brain and placenta do not appear to express class II antigens: this is an observation which might relate to the fact that both of these tissues are relatively immunologically privileged. A number of tissues have been shown to bear class II antigens under pathological conditions. For example, thyroid epithelial cells of some patients with Graves' disease and Hashimoto's thyroiditis express class II molecules. In addition, class II expression is seen on β cells in the pancreatic islets of Langerhans of patients and BB rats with insulin-dependent diabetes. As yet, very little is known about the relative expression of the different class II loci or *in vivo* functions of these molecules on tissues of non-lymphoid origin. It is reasonable to speculate that these class II antigen-bearing cells could present foreign antigen to T cells. Indeed, class II-positive thyroid epithelial cells have recently been shown to present peptide antigens to cloned human T helper cells.

A summary of the distribution of class I and II molecules on various human tissues and cell types is given in Figure 5.11; the evidence was obtained by using an immunoperoxidase staining method.

SUMMARY

Class I and II molecules of the MHC are highly polymorphic cell surface recognition structures, which enable the immune system to distinguish self from non-self and to respond appropriately. Class I molecules consist of a membrane-bound glycoprotein chain, encoded within the MHC, in non-covalent association with $\beta_2 m$, which is

Tissues	Class I	Class II
Cells of the Immune System		
B cells	strongly positive	strongly positive
T cells (activated cells only)	strongly positive	variable
Macrophages	strongly positive	variable
Dendritic cells	strongly positive	strongly positive
Nervous System		
Peripheral	strongly positive	negative
Central	negative	negative
Dura	strongly positive	strongly positive
Cardiovascular System		
Myocardium	weakly positive	negative
Intercalated discs	strongly positive	negative
Respiratory System		
Epiglottis	strongly positive	strongly positive
Trachea	strongly positive	strongly positive
Urogenital System		
Kidney glomeruli	strongly positive	strongly positive
Kidney tubules	strongly positive	variable
Liver		
Sinusoidal lining cells	strongly positive	strongly positive
Hepatocytes	variable	negative
Endothelium		
Capillaries (*except brain and placenta)	strongly positive	strongly positive
Larger vessels	strongly positive	variable

Tissues	Class I	Class II
Cells of the Endocrine System		
Thyroid	weakly positive	variable
Pituitary	weakly positive	negative
Pancreatic Islets of Langerhans	weakly positive	variable
Adrenal	strongly positive	negative
Gastrointestinal Tract (epithelium)		
Tongue	strongly positive	negative
Oesophagus	strongly positive	negative
Stomach	weakly positive	negative
Small Intestine	strongly positive	strongly positive
Colon	strongly positive	negative
Miscellaneous		
Breast (epithelial and glandular tissues)	strongly positive	strongly positive
Exocrine pancreas	negative	negative
Parotid acinar epithelium	negative	negative
Parotid ductal epithelium	strongly positive	negative
Muscle	weakly positive	negative
Cornea-squamous epithelium	strongly positive	negative
Cornea-endothelium	negative	negative
Langerhans cells	strongly positive	strongly positive
Lymphatics	strongly positive	strongly positive
Fibroblasts	strongly positive	negative
Placenta-villous trophoblast	negative	negative
Placenta-epidermis	weakly positive	negative

strongly positive	weakly positive	variable, depending on activation state	positive under some pathological conditions	negative

Fig.5.11 Distribution of MHC class I and II antigens on human tissue. The distribution of class I and II antigens in various tissues and on different cell types shown here is based on data obtained using a sensitive immunoperoxidase staining method. Since immunological mediators (e.g. IFN$_\gamma$) released during an immune response can modulate the expression of both class I and II molecules, the levels of these antigens expressed may vary quite considerably. This table should, therefore, be considered only as a general guide. Based on data from Daar *et al.*, 1984.

encoded on a different chromosome. Class I products are primarily involved in the recognition of antigen by cytotoxic T cells. Class II molecules are membrane-bound heterodimers of heavy (α) and light (β) glycoprotein chains, both encoded within the MHC, which are primarily involved in the activation of T helper cells. The polymorphism of both class I and II molecules is primarily located at the N terminus and is often localized in hypervariable regions. Disulphide bonding in class I and II molecules gives rise to domain structures, some of which have close homology to immunoglobulin constant domains. Such homologies also exist for a number of other molecules involved in immune responses, and together they are known as members of the immunoglobulin supergene family.

Class I genes can be divided into two categories: those encoding classical transplantation antigens (mouse H-2K, D, L, and human HLA-A, -B, -C genes) and others (Qa-2,3/Tla genes in the mouse) mapping adjacent to, but outside, the MHC. Although the majority of class I genes in the mouse map to the Qa-2,3/Tla region, which of these

are expressed and what role they play is still not clear. One possibility is that they provide a pool of genetic information which is used in the generation of polymorphism of class I molecules. There are considerably fewer class II genes than class I genes. In the mouse I-A and I-E regions there are two α and six β chain genes, but only four of these (A_α, E_α, A_β, E_β) appear to be expressed. In the human HLA-D region the situation is more complex, with six α and eight β chain genes most of which fall into three families termed DR, DQ, and DP. As in the mouse, not all of these genes are expressed.

The polymorphism of class I and II genes appears to be generated by a combination of the genetic mechanisms of recombination, gene conversion and gene expansion and contraction. Although the function of this polymorphism is not known, it seems likely that it gives an entire species the potential to present any antigenic structure it may encounter, and thus improve its chance of survival. The role of class I and II molecules in presenting antigens to cytotoxic and helper T cells will be discussed in subsequent chapters.

FURTHER READING

Bach F.H. (1985) *The HLA class II genes and products: the HLA-D region.* Immunology Today **6**, 89.

Bach F.H. (1984) *Structural and functional studies of HLA class II antigens.* Scand. J. Immunol. **20**, 1487.

Bodmer W.F., Albert E., Bodmer J.G. Dausset J., Kissmeyer-Nielson F. Mayr W., Payne R., Van Rood J.J., Trika Z. & Walford R.L. (1984) *Nomenclature for factors of the HLA System 1984.* Immunogenetics **20**, 593.

Bodmer J. & Bodmer W. (1984). *Histocompatibility 1984.* Immunology Today **5**, 251.

Boss J.M. & Strominger J.L. (1984) *Cloning and sequence analysis of the human major histocompatibility complex gene DC-3$_\beta$.* P.N.A.S. **81**, 5199.

Burnside S.S., Hunt P., Ozato K. & Sears D.W. (1984) *A molecular hybrid of the H-2D^d and H-2L^d genes expressed in the dm1 mutant.* P.N.A.S. **81**, 5204.

Daar A.S. Fuggle S.V. Fabre J.W. Ting A. & Morris P.J. (1984) *The detailed distribution of HLA-A,B,C, antigens in normal human organs.* Transplantation **38**, 287; 293.

Dausset J. & Cohen D. (1984) *Molecular genetics of the HLA system, new tools for the study of HLA and disease.* Clin. Immunol. Allergy **43**, 581.

Devlin J.J. Lew A.M. Flavell R.A. & Coligan J.E. (1985) *Secretion of a soluble class I molecule encoded by the Q10 gene of the C57BL/10 mouse.* EMBO J. **4**, 369.

Erlich H., Stetler D., Sheng-Dong R. & Saiki R. (1984) *Analysis by molecular cloning of the human class II genes.* Fed. Proc. **43**, 3025.

Gillies S.D. Folsom V. & Tonegawa S. (1984) *Cell type specific enhancer element associated with a mouse MHC gene, E$_\beta$.* Nature **310**, 594.

Gould B. & Strominger J. (1984) *HLA-A2 antigen phosphorylation in vitro by cyclic AMP-dependent protein kinase. Sites of phosphorylation and segmentation in class I major histocompatibility complex gene structure.* J. Biol. Chem. **259**, 13504.

Hood L., Kronenberg M. & Hunkapiller T. (1985) *T cell antigen receptors and the immunoglobulin supergene family.* Cell **40**, 225.

Hood L., Steinmetz M. & Malissen B. (1983) *Genes of the major histocompatibility complex of the mouse.* Ann. Rev. Immunol. **1**, 529.

Hurley C.K., Giles R.C. & Capra J.D. (1983) *The human MHC, evidence for multiple HLA-D-region genes.* Immunology Today **4**, 219.

Kappes D. J. Arnot D. Okada K. & Strominger J.L. (1984) *Structure and polymorphism of the HLA Class II SB light chain genes.* EMBO J. **3**, 2985.

Kaufman J.F., Auffray C., Korman A.J., Shackleford D.A. & Strominger J. (1984) *The class II molecules of the human and murine major histocompatibility complex.* Cell **1**, 13.

Klein J., (1984) *Gene conversion in MHC genes.* Transplantation **38**, 327.

Klein J., Figueroa F. & Nagy Z.A. (1983) *Genetics of the major histocompatibility complex: the final act.* Ann. Rev. Immunol. **1**, 119.

Kobori J.A., Winoto A., McNicholas J. & Hood L. (1984) *Molecular characteristics of the recombinant region of the six murine major histocompatibility complex (MHC) I-region recombinants.* J. Mol. Cell Immunol. **1**, 125.

Lafuse W.P. & David C.S. (1984) *Ia antigens. Genes, molecules and function.* Transplantation **38**, 443.

McDevitt H.O., Mathis D.J., Beroist C., Karter M.R. & Williams V.E. (1984) *Structure, regulatory polymorphisms and allelic hypervariability regions in murine I-A.* Fed. Proc. **43**, 3012.

McIntyre K.R. & Seidman J.G. (1984) *Nucleotide sequence of mutant I-Aβ^{bm12} gene is evidence for genetic exchange between mouse immune response genes.* Nature, **308**, 551.

McLaughlin-Taylor E., Woodward J.G., McMillan M. & Frelinger J.A. (1984) *Distinct epitopes are recognized by cytolytic T lymphocyte clones on the same class I molecule: direct demonstration using DNA-transfected targets and long-term cytolytic T cell clones.* Eur. J. Immunol. **14**, 969.

Melief C. (1983) *Remodelling the H-2 map.* Immunology Today **4**, 57.

Mengle-Gaw L. & McDevitt H.O. (1985) *Genetics and expression of mouse Ia antigens.* Ann. Rev. Immunol. **3**, 367.

Mengle-Gaw L., Conner S., McDevitt H.O. & Fathman C.G. (1984) *Gene conversion between murine class II major histocompatibility complex loci. Functional and molecular evidence from the bm12 mutant.* J. Exp. Med. **160**, 1184.

Murphy D.B. (1985) *Commentary on the genetic basis for control of I-J determinants.* J. Immunol. **135**, 1543.

Murre C. Reiss C.S. Bernaben C. Chen L.B. Burakoff S.J. & Seidman J.C. (1984) *Construction, expression and recognition of an H-2 molecule lacking its carboxyl terminus.* Nature, **307**, 432.

Pease L.R. (1985) *Diversity in H-2 genes encoding antigen-presenting molecules is generated by interactions between members of the major histocompatibility complex gene family.* Transplantation **39**, 227.

Ploegh H.L., Orr H.T. & Strominger J.L. (1981) *Major histocompatibility antigens, the human (HLA-A,-B,-C) and murine (H-2K, H-2D) class I molecules.* Cell **24**, 287.

Ritzel G., McCarthy S.A., Fotedar A. & Singh B. (1984) *Gene conversion may be responsible for the generation of the alloreactive repertoire.* Immunology Today **5**, 343.

Sachs D.H. (1984) *The major histocompatibility complex.* In Fundamental Immunology (page 347). Paul W.E. Ed. Raven Press, N.Y.

Servenius B., Gustafsson K., Widmark E., Emmoth E., Andersson G., Larhaumar D., Rask L. & Peterson P.A. (1984) *Molecular map of the human HLA-SB (HLA-DP) region and sequence of an SBα (DPα) pseudogene.* EMBO. J. **3**, 3209.

Travers P., Blundell T.L., Sternberg M.J.E. & Bodmer W.F. (1984) *Structural and evolutionary analysis of HLA-D region products.* Nature **310**, 235.

Weiss E.H., Golden L., Fahrner K., Mellor A.L., Devlin J.J., Bullman H., Tiddens H., Budd H. & Flavell R.A. (1984) *Organization and evolution of the class I gene family in the major histocompatibility complex of the C57BL/10 mouse.* Nature **310**, 650.

Williams A.F. (1984) *The immunoglobulin superfamily takes shape.* Nature **308**, 12.

IMMUNE RECOGNITION

6 Antigen Processing and Presentation

It has long been known that, whilst B cells can recognize soluble antigens directly, most T cells require the presence of an accessory cell population in order to be activated by antigens. The classical studies of Rosenthal and Shevach were the first to demonstrate that this accessory cell population serves to present the antigen in a manner requiring histocompatibility between the presenting cell and the responding T cell. We now know that T cells need to interact both with antigen and with self MHC molecules. Class I molecules are required for antigen presentation to most cytotoxic T cells, whereas helper T cells recognize antigen in association with self class II molecules (Ia). In this chapter the mechanisms and cells involved in presenting antigenic determinants to class II-restricted T cells will be discussed. Similar mechanisms may well be utilized by cytotoxic T cells restricted to class I molecules, but this concept will be covered in the next chapter.

The following sections deal with the proposed mechanisms whereby antigens are processed (if necessary) into a form which can associate with Ia antigens at the surface of antigen-presenting cells (APCs), where it can be recognized by the T cell receptor of responding cells. With the exception of antigen-specific B cells, these mechanisms are probably common to all antigen-presenting cell types discussed. However, different antigen-presenting cells may vary in their ability to provide the additional activation requirements of some T cells. Finally, the possible roles of different antigen-presenting cells *in vivo* will be discussed briefly.

ANTIGEN PROCESSING

The studies of Gell and Benacerraf in 1959 were the first to show that, whilst B cells primarily recognize determinants found on native molecules, T cells can recognize both native and denatured forms of the antigen. This observation was subsequently confirmed by many different workers using a variety of protein antigens. However, it was only in 1980 that Chesnut and his colleagues demonstrated that the T cells responding to native antigen were the same cells which responded to the denatured antigen. Further research produced a considerable body of evidence indicating that many antigens (particularly protein and bacterial antigens) required some form of 'processing' prior to presentation to T cells (see Fig.6.1). This processing involves binding of antigen to the surface of the antigen-presenting cell (APC) followed by active catabolic events which convert the antigen to a form which is recognizable, in association with class II molecules, by TH cells.

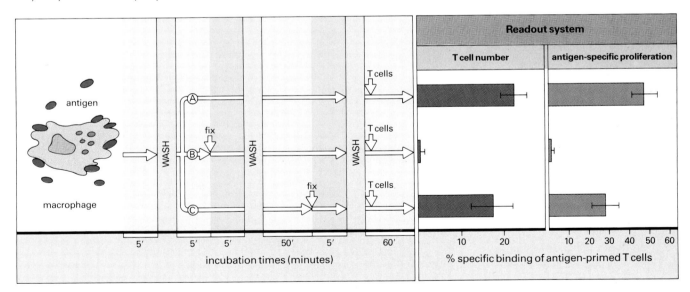

Fig.6.1 Antigen presentation by fixed macrophages. Macrophages were incubated with antigen (*L. monocytogenes*) for 5 minutes and, following extensive washing, they were treated in three different ways (A-C) before addition of antigen-primed T cells. Macrophages in A were left untreated. In B and C, cells were fixed with paraformaldehyde after 5/60 minutes incubation at 37°C respectively. T cells were then spun onto all the antigen-pulsed macrophages and incubated for an hour. After this time, non-adherent cells were removed, counted and tested for antigen-specific responses (in this case results from proliferation assays are shown). The specific binding of T cells to the antigen-pulsed macrophages in A-C was then determined from the decrease in T cell number and reduction in proliferative responses. This experiment demonstrated that T cells recognize antigen at the surface membrane of the macrophage, but only after a lag period of antigen handling by these APCs. Modified from Ziegler and Unanue, 1981.

Antigen Binding

With the exception of antigen-specific B cells (see later), binding of soluble antigen to antigen-presenting cells occurs via non-specific, non-covalent interactions with poorly characterized structures at the cell surface. Antigen in immune complexes can also bind specifically through receptors for Fc and C3 (see Chapter 15). The degree of non-specific binding appears to be proportional both to the size of the molecule and to the antigen concentration. A defect in the APC's ability to bind antigen will produce a block to the presentation of antigen. For example, alveolar macrophages are unable to present the bacterial antigens of *Listeria monocytogenes* because they lack a bacterial binding protein. However, if the bacteria are first opsonized with specific antibodies, alveolar macrophages can then both bind and present the bacterial antigens.

Metabolic Events

The first evidence that an active processing step was required before antigen could be presented to TH cells came from the studies of Ziegler and Unanue: *L. monocytogenes* was used as a particulate antigen in presentation experiments involving murine macrophages and polyclonal T cell populations. They found that there was a lag period between binding of the antigen to the macrophages and detection of antigen recognition by the T cells (see Fig. 6.1). Furthermore, T cells could still recognize antigen-pulsed macrophages which had been rendered metabolically inactive by fixation with paraformaldehyde. This implied that the T cells actually recognize antigen at the surface of the antigen-presenting cell, rather than non-specifically bind to the antigen-presenting cell and subsequently trigger it to produce an immunogenic moiety from a cytoplasmic compartment. However, antigen recognition by T cells only occurred when the cells were fixed after a lag period of 45-60 minutes (depending on antigen concentration and temperature). Similar results were obtained by Chesnut and colleagues in their studios of presentation of soluble protein antigens to antigen-specific, class II-restricted T cell hybridomas. These observations indicated that, following antigen binding, a short period of time (the lag period) was required for the antigen-presenting cell to process the antigen and express it at the cell surface in the form recognized by the T cell.

Attention was then focussed on the nature of the processing events which occur following antigen binding. Experiments designed to follow the fate of radiolabelled antigen in APCs had suggested that at least two pools of immunologically relevant antigenic material exist in the APC: one exposed on the surface where it can be recognized by T cells, the other sequestered within the cell. Antigenic material from the sequestered pool could subsequently be transported to the cell surface for presentation, or actively exported to the extracellular milieu where it could be utilized by other APCs. Since the antigenic material in both pools was primarily in a fragmented form, it was suggested that the sequestered pool was being processed by the APC and that proteolysis was involved in the processing step. Evidence in support of this suggestion has come from a number of experiments. Chloroquine and ammonia, which localize in lysosomes, have been shown to block the degradation of proteins in

Fig.6.2 Chloroquine inhibits antigen presentation to T cells.
Murine splenic macrophages were used as APCs in a proliferation assay using a T cell line specific for the bacterium *Corynebacterium parvum* (CP). APCs were pulsed with CP (+) or medium only (−) for two hours at 37°C. Where indicated, optimal concentrations of chloroquine (0.3-0.5mM) were added for the duration of the antigen-pulsing period, and removed during the washing period. After five days of cultivation, proliferative responses of the T cell line were measured by the

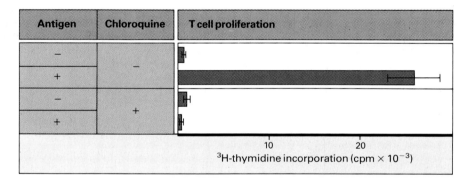

Antigen	Chloroquine	T cell proliferation
−	−	
+	−	
−	+	
+	+	

^{3}H-thymidine incorporation (cpm × 10^{-3})

incorporation of ^{3}H-thymidine. In the absence of chloroquine, the T cells responded well to CP. This response was completely abolished by the chloroquine treatment. Based on data from Guidos *et al.*, 1984.

Fig.6.3 Effect of the enzyme inhibitor, ZPADK, on antigen presentation to T cells. Guinea-pig peritoneal APCs were incubated with the cysteine proteinase inhibitor ZPADK (100/μm) or control in the presence of antigen (DNP-PLL or GA) at 37°C for two hours. After washing, the cells were fixed with paraformaldehyde and used to stimulate primed lymph node T cells in a proliferation assay. The response of the T cells was measured as the net incorporation of ^{3}H-thymidine above that using APCs not exposed to antigen. The results show that inhibiting cysteine proteinase activity

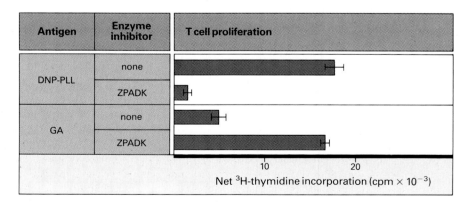

Antigen	Enzyme inhibitor	T cell proliferation
DNP-PLL	none	
	ZPADK	
GA	none	
	ZPADK	

Net ^{3}H-thymidine incorporation (cpm × 10^{-3})

with ZPADK markedly reduced the processing of DNP-PLL but enhanced processing of GA.

ZPADK=benzyloxycarbonyl-phenyl-alanyl-alanine-diazomethyl-ketone. Based on data of Buus & Wederlin, 1986.

lysosomes by raising the lysosomal pH. Macrophages treated with chloroquine were found to be incapable of presenting protein or bacterial antigens (Fig.6.2) and, in some cases, this inhibitory effect was correlated with a block in antigen degradation. That chloroquine was blocking the processing step and not inhibiting the recognition of antigen by the T cell was apparent from the observation that this agent had no effect if used after a one hour incubation to allow processing to occur. Such observations were interpreted to mean that antigen processing involves proteolysis in lysosomes. However, chloroquine can have other effects on cells such as decreasing membrane recycling and inhibiting the intracellular removal of iron from transferrin. In the latter case, lysosomes are not involved but the process is blocked because it requires an acid environment. Some studies have shown that antigen presentation by dendritic cells is also blocked by chloroquine, even though these cells are non-phagocytic *in vitro* and have a very poor lysosomal system. It has been suggested that dendritic cells can process antigens at the cell surface through the use of membrane ectoproteases, although this has not been directly demonstrated.

Studies with specific enzyme inhibitors have also implicated proteinases as being important in antigen processing. One study by Buus and Wederlin has clearly shown that cysteine proteinases are involved in processing the simple polypeptide antigen dinitrophenyl poly-L-lysine (DNP-PLL) which contains only Lys-Lys peptide bonds (Fig.6.3). It seems clear that proteolysis is important for the production of antigenic moieties recognized by

some T cells. Polymers of D-amino acids are not susceptible to degradation by proteinases, and are also non-immunogenic. However, rapid and extensive proteolysis could also account for the poor immunogenicity of some antigens. As shown in Figure 6.3, the presentation of the random copolymer of L-glutamic acid and L-alanine (GA) is markedly enhanced by inhibiting the action of cysteine proteinases. Since GA has four types of peptide bond (G-G, G-A, A-G and A-A), it is probably also susceptible to cleavage by a number of enzymes of other classes (serine, aspartic or metallo-proteinases). One of these may be important for producing antigenic fragments of GA. Clearly, protein antigens are much more heterogeneous than these synthetic polypeptides with respect to their enzyme susceptibilities, and one might expect that different enzymes can produce different antigenic fragments. Whether such antigenic fragments are recognized will depend primarily on the ability of the fragments to associate appropriately with MHC class II molecules, although the T cell receptor repertoire may also play a role. Differences in antigen-presenting capabilities of different types of APC could also be partly accounted for by differences in their levels of appropriate proteinases.

Perhaps the first direct evidence that the processed antigenic moiety recognized by T cells is a proteolytic fragment of the antigen came from studies of ovalbumin (OVA)-specific, H-2^d-restricted T cell hybridomas, by Shimonkevitz and colleagues in 1983. These cells all recognized OVA presented by untreated APCs, but failed to respond when the APCs were rendered metabolically inert by fixation (Fig.6.4). If, however, OVA peptides

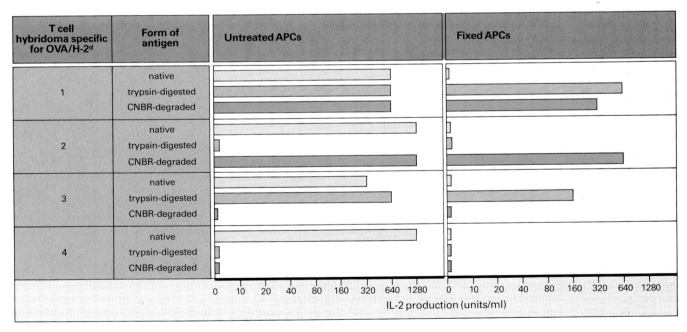

T cell hybridoma specific for OVA/H-2^d	Form of antigen	Untreated APCs	Fixed APCs
1	native		
	trypsin-digested		
	CNBR-degraded		
2	native		
	trypsin-digested		
	CNBR-degraded		
3	native		
	trypsin-digested		
	CNBR-degraded		
4	native		
	trypsin-digested		
	CNBR-degraded		

IL-2 production (units/ml)

Fig.6.4 Effect of APC fixation on the reactivity of chicken ovalbumin (OVA)-specific T cell hybridomas with native and degraded antigen. APCs were fixed or untreated before testing for their ability to present different forms of the antigen to a variety of T cell hybridomas, all restricted to H-2^d class II molecules. The response of the hybridomas was assessed by measuring IL-2 released into the culture medium. Representative hybridomas are shown to illustrate the four patterns of reactivity (1-4) which were observed with native, trypsin-digested and cyanogen bromide (CNBR)-degraded OVA. These four hybridomas all

had different epitopic specificities as assessed by their reactivity with OVA species variants. In all cases, fixed APCs were unable to present native OVA. However, most hybridomas (1-3) could respond to a degraded form of the antigen whether the APCs were fixed or not. Thus, previous antigen degradation had completely bypassed the active processing events normally required of the APC. In some cases (2 and 3) only one of the degraded forms of OVA were stimulatory. Thus, different modes of antigen degradation can either preserve or destroy different epitopes. Based on data from Shimonkevitz *et al.*, 1983.

(prepared either by digestion with the enzyme trypsin or by cleavage at methionine residues with cyanogen bromide) were used as the stimulating antigen, the majority of the hybridomas could respond whether the APCs were fixed or not. This cell-free proteolysis had completely replaced the active metabolic events involved in antigen processing by APCs. Clearly different cleavage procedures can produce different antigenic determinants which can be recognized by T cells (compare hybridomas 2 and 3 in Figure 6.4). The balance of the available processing pathways in the antigen-presenting cell is therefore likely to influence which of the potential epitopes are expressed at the cell surface in adequate amounts to stimulate T cells. A number of similar observations on protein fragments recognized by T cells have since been made with normal T cell populations (monoclonal and polyclonal), and with a variety of antigens. A T cell hybridoma which recognizes cytochrome c in association with I-E^k molecules can recognize the C-terminal peptide consisting of residues 66-104 without the need for antigen processing (i.e. with fixed or chloroquine-treated antigen-presenting cells). However, it requires processing events before it can recognize the slightly larger peptide 60-104. In this case, a lysine residue at position 99 is the major amino acid which contacts the T cell receptor and this forms an ionic bond with glutamic acid at position 61. Processing events would thus seem to be required in the region of residues 60-65 in order to disrupt this ionic interaction and leave lysine 99 free to interact with the T cell receptor.

However, not all T cells require that their antigen is fragmented before it can be recognized. In some cases, antigen denaturation (unfolding) is all that appears necessary for the antigen to be presented by fixed or chloroquine-treated APCs. (It is quite likely that the untreated APC actually produces an unfolded form of the antigenic region of the protein by proteolysis, since this is a lot easier under physiological conditions than unfolding an intact protein, particularly one with intramolecular disulphide bonds such as hen egg lysozyme). Smaller peptide antigens, such as the hormones insulin and angiotensin, can be recognized in an intact form by some T cells. Of course, other T

cells may also exist which do recognize processed forms of these same antigens.

Klein and his colleagues have argued that processing events are not essential steps in antigen presentation to T cells. They prepared liposomes with MHC class II molecules inserted into the lipid bilayer and then covalently coupled them with a variety of protein antigens. They found these liposomes to be capable of stimulating T cell clones or hybridomas in the complete absence of APCs. Other studies have investigated the processing requirements for activation of T cell clones which can be stimulated by soluble antigen in association with syngeneic class II molecules, and also by allogeneic class II molecules. In these experiments, only presentation of soluble antigen was affected by treating the APCs with chloroquine. Therefore, class II molecules which are present in the cell membrane apparently do not require any processing, even though they are intact protein molecules. The most attractive explanation for the differences in processing requirements of various antigens is that antigen needs to be present at the cell surface in a stable form so as to be recognized by specific T cells. The fact that many T cells recognize processed antigen in the form of fragmented or unfolded molecules probably reflects the nature of the APCs, in that most soluble proteins are either rapidly endocytosed or just do not spend sufficient time being bound to the cell membrane. A relatively stable membrane-bound form of the antigen is required so that it can interact appropriately with the MHC class II molecule and the T cell receptor (see following section).

ANTIGEN PRESENTATION

Early observations led to two major and contrasting hypotheses seeking to explain antigen recognition by T cells (Fig. 6.5). The 'dual receptor hypothesis' suggested that T cells possessed distinct receptors for binding antigen (appropriately processed, if necessary) and MHC molecules. The 'associative recognition hypothesis', on the

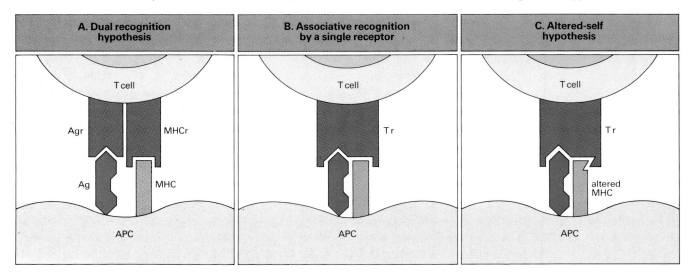

Fig.6.5 Hypotheses on T cell recognition of antigen. The dual recognition hypothesis (A) proposed separate T cell membrane receptors for antigen (Agr) and self MHC (MHCr). The associative recognition hypothesis (B), however, suggested that a single receptor recognized a combination of antigen and MHC. A modification of this hypothesis (C) proposed that antigen alters the self-MHC molecule which is then recognized by the T cell either alone or (as shown here) in combination with antigen.

Fig.6.6 Two alternative models to explain the recognition of antigen and MHC by a single T receptor. In A, the antigen and class II MHC molecule are shown to interact to produce a complex ligand which binds to a single site on the T cell receptor. The different sites of interaction between the three components involved are shown. The antigenic epitope contacts the T cell receptor paratope, and the histotope of the class II molecule contacts the T cell receptor restitope (restriction site interaction-tope). Antigen and the class II molecule interact via their agretope (antigen recognition-tope) and desetope (determinant selection-tope) respectively. The alternative model (B) suggests that no physical interaction occurs between the antigen and the

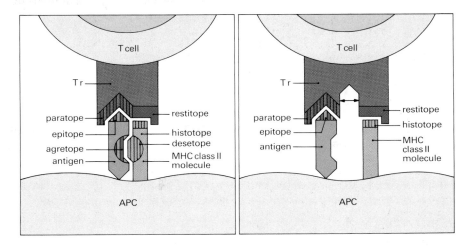

MHC molecule, which bind to discrete sites on the receptor molecule. Instead, an allosteric interaction (represented by the arrows) mediated by the T cell

receptor is suggested to account for the apparent interaction between antigen and the class II molecule. Modified from Schwartz, 1985.

Fig.6.7 Two models explaining the roles of the α and β chain of the T cell receptor in interacting with the antigen and MHC. In A, the α and β chains associate to form a single combining site which interacts with antigen and both chains of the class II molecule. In model B, a single antigen-binding site is formed by clonian-clonian interactions between one chain of the T cell receptor (β in this case) and one chain of the class II molecule. The other T cell receptor chain (α) might interact with the class II molecule to further stabilize the T cell-APC interaction.Based on data of Schwartz, 1985.

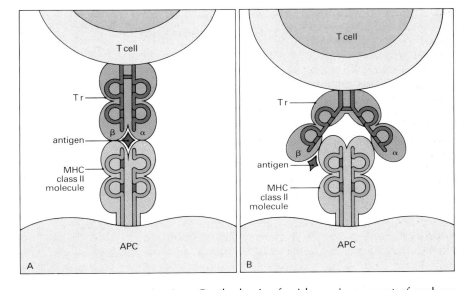

other hand, invoked the idea that the antigen in some way associates with an MHC molecule (perhaps during or after processing events), and that this is subsequently recognized by a single T cell receptor. The 'altered self hypothesis' modifies this second suggestion further, to propose that the self MHC molecule on the antigen-presenting cell is structurally altered following interaction with antigen, and that the single T cell receptor recognizes both antigen and altered self or possibly just altered self. At the present time, the evidence points strongly to the conclusion that T cells have a single receptor which is responsible for both antigen and MHC specificities (see Chapter 3). However, how such a single receptor interacts with antigen and MHC molecules is still hotly debated. Furthermore, it is still not clear whether class I- and II- restricted recognition of antigens follows the same or different rules. In this section the major models which have been proposed to explain antigen presentation to T_H cells will be outlined first, and the critical evidence for ar against them will then be discussed.

The Models
Perhaps most of the debate has centred around the problem of whether or not antigen (following processing if necessary) interacts with the MHC molecule during T cell

activation. On the basis of evidence in support of such an interaction (see below), Schwartz proposed in 1983 that regions on the antigen and class II molecule, distinct from those interacting with the T cell receptor, might physically interact in order to produce a single macromolecular ligand which binds to the T cell receptor (Fig.6.6). The region on the antigen which interacts with the MHC molecule was termed 'agretope' (antigen recognition -tope), and the complementary site on the MHC molecule was called 'desetope' (determinant selection -tope). An alternative possibility to explain the data available at that time was that the T cell receptor bound first to one component (either the antigen or the MHC molecule), and that this induced a conformational change in the receptor (an 'allosteric' effect) such that it could then interact specifically with the other component (the MHC molecule or antigen); thus, any direct physical interaction between antigen and MHC molecule is avoided (see Fig.6.6).

If antigen physically interacts with the MHC molecule to form a complex macromolecular ligand which contacts a single combining site on the T cell receptor, one must ask what roles are played by the α and β chains of the T cell receptor and class II molecule. Two alternative models are depicted in Figure 6.7. The simpler and more favoured model (A) suggests that the variable regions of the α and β chains of the T cell receptor interact to form a ligand-binding site similar to that formed by heavy and light chains of immunoglobulin (Ig). This ligand-binding site would then contact both chains of the class II molecule, with the antigen interacting with both molecules in the combining pocket so formed. An alternative model (B) proposes that a domain-domain interaction takes place between one chain of the T cell receptor and one chain of the class II molecule (since both types of molecule have domain structures similar to those of immunoglobulin; see Chapter 5). This interaction then forms the binding site for antigen, with both molecules contributing to specificity (see Fig.6.7). If the α and β chains of the T cell receptor are both pleiomorphic, this second model might predict that a single T cell could have specificity for two different antigens since both could form domain-domain interactions with a chain of the class II molecule. Alternatively, the other chain of the T cell receptor may simply interact with the class II molecule to further stabilize the interaction between T cell and antigen-presenting cell. To distinguish between these two models it would be necessary to ascertain whether or not the α and β chains of both T cell receptor and class II molecule influence the specificity of the T cell. However, this may still not answer the question, since one could still envisage slightly modified forms of model (A) (see Fig.6.7),

where antigen does not directly interact with all four components.

Other models have been proposed on the basis of evidence arguing against a direct binding of antigen to the MHC molecule. Parham, followed by Grey and colleagues, suggested that interaction between the antigen (after processing if necessary) and the MHC molecule only occurs after each has separately contacted the T cell receptor. This then causes the antigen and MHC molecule to come into close contact leading to an apparently specific interaction. According to this model, enforced interaction may be positive so that stabilization of binding occurs, leading to activation of the T cell (as seen with self Ia and specific antigen). On the other hand, the interaction could also be negative, perhaps due to steric hindrance or electrostatic repulsive forces, such that destabilization and dissociation of the complex occurs, in which case the T cell is not activated (for example, with a related but inactive antigen). This model is depicted in Figure 6.8. Since it is unlikely that antigen and the MHC molecule contact the T cell receptor simultaneously, it is suggested that the T cell receptor first interacts with the class II molecule and then antigen diffuses in the membrane of the APC to contact the receptor. However, it is still possible that antigen binds to the receptor first, followed by diffusion of the MHC molecule into the binding site. In this model, related

Fig.6.8 Proposed mechanism of T cell recognition of antigen/MHC, based on the hypothesis that antigen and the class II molecule only interact after each is contacted by the T cell receptor. If this interaction is positive, or even merely permissive, then the T cell will be triggered (A). If, however, repulsive forces result in a negative interaction, such as with a related (but inactive) antigen or an allogeneic class II molecule, then the interaction will be destabilized and no triggering will occur (B and C). In D, the observed alloreactivity of many antigen/MHC-specific T cells is explained by postulating that the allogeneic class II molecule can interact with both the antigen and MHC binding sites on the T cell receptor.

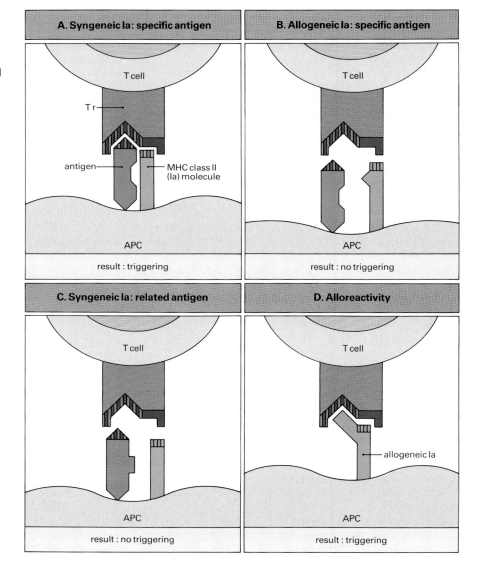

antigens may share an epitope with the specific antigen but not activate the T cell because it negatively interacts with the MHC molecule. In the model of Schwartz, discussed above, this would be explained by saying that the related antigen lacked an agretope for binding to the class II molecule (see Fig.6.6).

An alternative, more speculative, model suggested by Pernis and Axel proposes that the T cell receptor γ chain gene product plays a role in the recognition of the MHC molecule. In this model, an αβ heterodimer is responsible for binding antigen, and a heterodimer composed of an identical β chain and γ chain binds the self MHC molecule. It is proposed that these two heterodimers might associate in the membrane of the T cell to form a tetramer, in some ways similar to Ig, but with two distinct binding sites. Current evidence suggesting that the γ chain is only expressed in immature T cells and at low levels makes this a rather unlikely model.

At the present time it seems probable that the α and β chains of the T cell receptor recognize a complex ligand formed by an association of antigen and Ia. However, whether this ligand is formed independently (as in the model of Schwartz, Fig.6.6) or only in the presence of the T cell receptor (Parham's hypothesis) is still open to question. The available evidence pertaining to this question will now be discussed.

Interactions between Antigen, Class II Molecules and T Cell Receptors

Some of the first convincing evidence for an interaction between antigen and class II molecules during T cell activation came from Schwartz and his colleagues, using pigeon cytochrome c-specific T cell clones and hybridomas from B10.A mice. These T cells were also able to respond well to moth cytochrome c. It was found that the pattern of antigen cross-reactivity of these cells changed when the class II molecule was altered. For example, some clones could be stimulated with cytochrome c presented by either B10.A ($E_\beta^k:E_\alpha^k$) or B10.S(9R) ($E_\beta^s:E_\alpha^k$) APCs. When B10.A antigen-presenting cells were used, moth cytochrome c was more potent at stimulating the T cells than pigeon cytochrome c. However, with B10.S(9R) antigen-presenting cells the potency order was reversed (Fig.6.9). Since the T cell receptor is the same in both cases, these observations strongly suggested that class II molecules can influence the antigen specificity of the response, and led to the hypothesis that distinct subsites on antigens (agretopes) are responsible for binding to, or interacting with, MHC molecules. The evidence supporting the existence of agretopes on protein antigens is covered in more detail in Chapter 8.

An alternative line of evidence has come from antigen competition studies where non-stimulatory related antigens have been shown to block recognition of the specific antigen, perhaps by competing for binding sites on class II molecules. For example, Rock and Benacerraf studied T cell hybridomas specific for random polymers composed of glutamic acid, alanine and tyrosine (GAT) in association with I-A^d class II molecules. By pulsing the APCs with antigen before addition to the T cell hybridomas, they showed that the related antigen GT (a polymer of glutamic acid and tyrosine) which did not stimulate the T cells was able to block the response to GAT, if added during the pulsing period. This effect was specific as other T cell hybridomas specific for GAT-pulsed H-2^b APCs, or specific for different antigens, were unaffected. Furthermore, F1 APCs from H-2^b x H-2^d mice pulsed with GAT and GT simultaneously could present GAT only to the H-2^b-restricted T cells, and not to H-2^d-restricted T cells. Separate evidence that GT and GAT compete for a site on I-A^d class II molecules came from experiments with I-A^d-specific alloreactive T cell hybridomas (from H-2^b mice). The activation of a minority of these T cell hybridomas with I-A^d APCs could be inhibited with both GT and GAT implying that the alloreactive site on I-A^d recognized by these T cells is the same (or in close proximity to) a site with an affinity for GAT and GT.

One of the objections to the postulated binding of antigens to class II molecules during T cell activation has been that a small number of distinct Ia molecules could not have specific binding properties for the myriad of antigens which can be recognized by T cells. However, a number of recent experiments have indicated that there are multiple sites on class II molecules which are involved in T cell activation, either by interacting with antigen or with the T cell receptor. One study by Unanues' group utilized chemical modification procedures to demonstrate that two distinct determinants can be generated by a small (20 amino acids) lysozyme peptide in association with the I-A^k molecule. Molecular genetic techniques, such as site-directed mutagenesis and DNA-mediated gene transfer, have also been used to investigate the involvement of various regions of class II molecules in T cell activation. For example, Lechler and colleagues studied the contributions of A$_\alpha$ and A$_\beta$ chain polymorphisms to antigen-specific T cell activation. They created recombinant A$_\beta$ genes by exchanging all or half of the β$_1$ domain among A$_\beta$ genes of the b, d and k halotypes. These were then transfected, along with matched or mismatched A$_\alpha$ genes, into L cells which were subsequently used in antigen presentation experiments with a panel of T cell hybridomas of different antigen and Ia specificities. The results indicated that

Fig.6.9 The apparent antigenic specificity of a cytochrome c-specific T cell clone is dependent on the form of class II molecule. Cloned cells were tested in a proliferation assay using two different APC populations. With B10.A APCs, moth cytochrome c was clearly a more potent stimulator than the pigeon antigen, but this potency order was reversed when B10.S (9R) APCs were used. Since the T cell receptor is identical, this is strong evidence for antigen/Ia interaction (agretopes). From Matis et al., 1983.

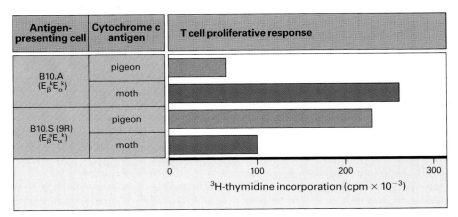

Antigen-presenting cell	Cytochrome c antigen	T cell proliferative response
B10.A ($E_\beta^k E_\alpha^k$)	pigeon	
	moth	
B10.S (9R) ($E_\beta^s E_\alpha^k$)	pigeon	
	moth	

^{3}H-thymidine incorporation (cpm × 10^{-3})

0   100   200   300

conformational determinants unique to a specific combination of α and β chains are important in I-A-restricted, antigen-specific T cell activation, and that multiple sites exist on a single class II molecule. Both halves of the N-terminal $A_\beta 1$ domain appeared to be important, whereas the $A_\beta 2$ domain did not seem to be involved. Allen and his colleagues used a panel of APCs with mutations in either A_α^k or A_β^k to present HEL and HEL fragments to ten different HEL-specific T cell hybridomas. The response patterns revealed that at least eight different determinants were formed by the association of HEL peptides with the I-A^k molecule. Thus, a simple globular protein can produce many T cell receptor ligands by the association of its processed fragments with a single Ia molecule.

Several investigators have shown that T cell activation can be achieved by utilizing planar lipid membranes or liposomes, in which class II molecules have been inserted, to present antigen. In most cases, antigen processing requirements were bypassed by using a small peptide form of the specific antigen, although one group of investigators directly coupled intact protein antigens to Ia-containing liposomes, and these were able to stimulate specific T cell clones and hybridomas. Such experiments indicate that the correct class II molecule and a relatively stable membrane form of antigen are the minimal requirements for T cell activation. Processing of antigen to fragments is probably required in many cases precisely because this produces a more stable binding of antigenic determinants at the cell membrane. Also implicit from these experiments is that it is unlikely that a processed antigen remains stable in the membrane of an APC by binding to proteins other than the class II molecule; this does not necessarily mean that the antigenic peptide binds to the class II molecule. A similar study by Coeshott and Grey failed to obtain antigen-specific stimulation with I-A^d-containing liposomes, although fusion of these liposomes with Ia-negative cells endowed them with antigen-presenting ability. These Ia-containing liposomes were also completely unable to block the specific activation of I-A^d-restricted, ovalbumin-specific T cell hybridomas, indicating that there is no separate high affinity Ia-binding site on the T cell receptor. Grey and his colleagues have also consistently failed to find evidence for binding of antigenic peptides to Ia molecules either by direct binding studies or antigen competition studies such as those described above. They have proposed that, if an antigen/Ia complex is important in T cell activation, it only occurs in the presence of the T cell

receptor. Direct evidence in support of this proposal has come recently from Watts and colleagues. They utilized a T cell hybridoma specific for a 17 residue peptide of ovalbumin in association with I-A^d-bearing antigen-presenting cells. The peptide can also be presented to this hybridoma by I-A^d-containing phospholipid planar membranes. They modified the peptide by coupling it to fluorescein (FL) and the I-A^d molecule by coupling it to another fluorescent probe, Texas red, and showed that antigen presentation still occurred. Using this system, the fluorescein on the peptide was excited by the appropriate wavelength of light, and the increase in fluorescence of the Texas red probe (normally excited at a different wavelength) on the I-A^d molecule was recorded. Transfer of energy from the excited fluorescein to Texas red occurs only when two molecules are within 40Å of one another. Such an effect was only noted in the presence of the specific T cell hybridoma, not other T cell hybridomas, and could be blocked by anti-I-A^d antibodies and by unlabelled peptide. This experiment argues against a direct interaction between antigen and Ia, except when juxtaposed by the T cell receptor.

Further evidence in favour of a physical interaction between antigen and class II molecules has come from the studies of Ashwell and Schwartz on a cytochrome c-specific T cell clone. This clone responds to a small peptide of moth cytochrome c in association with either $E_\beta^k : E_\alpha^k$ or $E_\beta^b : E_\alpha^k$. The moth peptide was 13-fold more potent with $E_\beta^k : E_\alpha^k$ than with $E_\beta^b : E_\alpha^k$ on the APC. Using a technique for estimating the avidity of the T cell receptor for its ligand (assumed in these experiments to be a complex between antigen and Ia), it was concluded that the avidity of the T cell receptor was the same for the moth peptide with both Ia molecules, and that the potency difference results from differences in the affinity of the peptide for the two Ia molecules. These observations do not discriminate between models proposing direct binding of antigen to Ia and those which claim that association only occurs in the presence of the T cell receptor. The data would also be consistent with one form of the 'altered self' model of T cell activation, where antigen itself is not directly recognized by the T cell receptor but induces a conformational change in the Ia molecule which then binds to the receptor. However, this particular model may be inappropriate as there is evidence that antigen can bind to the T cell receptor in the absence of MHC molecules under some circumstances. For example, Siliciano and colleagues showed

Fig.6.10 Binding of a lysozyme peptide (residues 46-61) to isolated I-A^k molecules. The peptide was labelled with the fluorescent compound 7-fluoro-4-nitro benzo-2-oxo-1, 3-diazole (NBD-F), and this molecule was shown to retain activity in stimulating an I-A^k-restricted, lysozyme-specific T cell hybridoma. Binding of labelled peptide to detergent-solubilized I-A^k and I-A^d molecules was measured by assaying fluorescence intensity after equilibrium dialysis. Binding of the labelled peptide was seen with I-A^k but not with I-A^d or the unrelated membrane molecule, glycophorin. This interaction appeared to be specific, since binding of fluorescent peptide could be blocked with the unlabelled peptide but not with a synthetic peptide analogue. Based on data of Babbitt et al., 1986.

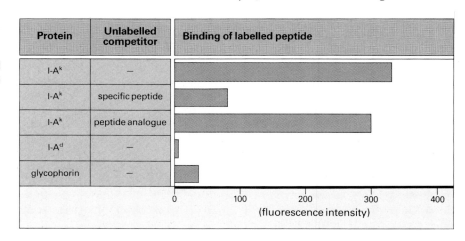

Protein	Unlabelled competitor	Binding of labelled peptide
I-A^k	—	
I-A^k	specific peptide	
I-A^k	peptide analogue	
I-A^d	—	
glycophorin	—	

0   100   200   300   400
(fluorescence intensity)

that class I-restricted, FL-specific, cytotoxic T cell clones could specifically bind multivalent forms of FL (for example, FL coupled to dextran or ficoll), and be activated to secrete lymphokines. Similar observations have also been made with class II-restricted arsonate-specific clones. These results imply that some T cell receptors have at least a low affinity for antigen.

More direct evidence for antigen binding to MHC molecules has come from studies showing that antigen-pulsed APCs release into the culture supernatant a moiety which can directly bind to specific T cells, and which appears to contain both antigen and Ia determinants. In one case, the antigen and MHC moieties appeared to be tightly linked. However, these experiments still await further biochemical analysis before the nature of the active component released from APCs is known. The first direct demonstration of antigen binding to MHC molecules came very recently from Babbitt and colleagues, using a fluorescently labelled peptide of lysozyme which stimulates T cells when in association with I-A^k molecules. Using detergent-solubilized Ia molecules, it was found that the labelled peptide bound at least ten times as well to I-A^k molecules as to I-A^d molecules or the unrelated membrane glycoprotein, glycophorin (Fig.6.10). Furthermore, binding could be blocked with an excess of unlabelled peptide, although not by a similar amount of a related, but non-stimulatory, analogue. Whether or not this observation can be repeated with other antigens remains to be seen. The observed association constant (5×10^{-5} M^{-1}) was moderately high and comparable to hapten binding by some antibodies. It may be that, in other cases, the affinity will be lower and therefore more difficult to demonstrate. Such a situation could have led to some of the results discussed above, where binding of antigen to Ia was only apparent in the presence of the T cell receptor because receptor binding stabilized the interaction.

In conclusion, therefore, the weight of evidence suggests that the T cell receptor recognizes a ligand consisting of antigen (often in a processed form) in association with an MHC molecule, but it is still open to argument whether this association is an active binding or merely a permissive interaction imposed on the two components by the constraints applied by the T cell receptor.

ANTIGEN-PRESENTING CELL TYPES

Originally, the role of presenting antigen to T cells was ascribed solely to the macrophage. However, in recent years it has become apparent that a variety of other cells can also present antigen to T cells. Any cell which expresses class II molecules should be able to present appropriately processed antigen to a T cell which has receptors of high enough affinity to be stimulated by antigen/Ia on its own. The ability to trigger T cells with additional requirements for activation (see later) will depend on whether the cell can cater to these needs. In this section, the presentation of antigen by cell types other than the conventional macrophage will be discussed.

Dendritic Cells
Lymphoid dendritic cells (DC) are bone marrow-derived non-phagocytic cells characterized by their irregular shape, constitutive expression of class II molecules at high levels, and a paucity of endocytic vesicles and lysosomes.

These cells are only present in relatively low numbers (less than 1%) in most lymphoid cell preparations, yet they have been shown to be very potent antigen-presenting cells in a variety of situations. It has been claimed that they are the most important cell type for presenting antigen to virgin T cells, but this has not yet been fully substantiated. Direct comparisons have been made between splenic dendritic cells and macrophages in mice, and between peripheral blood monocytes and dendritic cells in humans. There seems to be considerable overlap in the antigen-presenting capacity of these two cell types, although macrophages, because of their phagocytic activity, may be better equipped to process and present particulate antigens, such as bacteria. The presentation of protein antigens by both cell types involves processing of the antigen. Since DCs are very inefficient at endocytosis and have a poor lysosomal system, it has been suggested that processing can occur at the DC cell membrane, perhaps by membrane ectoproteases. Although it has not been directly demonstrated, DCs may also present antigen which has been processed and released by other cells.

B Cells
Both normal and neoplastic Ia-positive B cells have been shown to have the ability to present antigen to T cells. This presentation by non-specific B cell populations appears to follow similar rules to presentation by macrophages. However, recent evidence has clearly shown that antigen-specific B cells can present their antigen to T cells in a very efficient manner. This idea was first put forward by Benacerraf in 1978, but its validity has only been substantiated by experiments over the past few years. It is now known that the antigen-specific Ig molecules on the surface of B cells can serve as a means for the cell to specifically take up and concentrate the antigen. This antigen can then be processed and subsequently reexpressed at the cell surface in association with class II molecules where it is available to stimulate antigen-specific T cells. Because of the specificity and concentrating effect endowed by the Ig molecule, specific B cell presentation can occur at antigen concentrations much lower (as much as 1000-fold) than those required for presentation by macrophages and dendritic cells. This has been shown for both soluble and particulate antigens. Some evidence suggests that the B cells have to be activated before they can present antigen to most T cells. This might reflect the need for IL-1 by the T cells tested (see below), since activation has been shown to be required for B cells to make IL-1 (in a surface-bound form). Alternatively, antigen processing may occur much more efficiently in activated B cells. In fact, activation of B cells by lipopolysaccharide (LPS) has been shown to enhance binding and uptake of antigen.

Some T cell clones have been shown to be completely incapable of responding to B cell APCs. In one instance at least, the alloreactivity of an antigen/Ia-reactive T cell clone was also absent when B cells were used as APCs, arguing against differences in processing between macrophages and B cells in this case. Differential glycosylation of Ia molecules on B cells and macrophages might influence recognition by such T cells (see Chapter 5). Nevertheless, differences in antigen processing may well account for some of the differences between B cells and macrophages as APCs. It has been suggested that when antigen binds to the surface Ig molecule of a specific B cell, it is taken up into the cell as an immune complex, and it is this complex which is then subjected to processing events such as proteolysis.

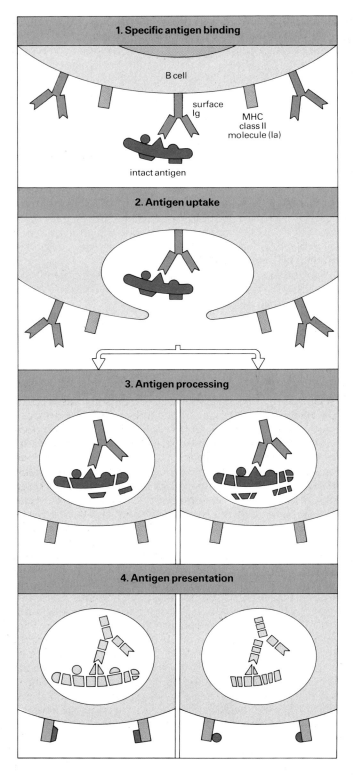

Fig.6.11 Proposed mechanism of antigen presentation by specific B cells. Specific antigen binding occurs through the surface Ig molecules (1). This complex is then taken into a cellular compartment for processing (shown here as a cytoplasmic vacuole, but processing might occur at the cell surface) (2). It is suggested that the Ig molecule specificity can influence which of the potential T cell epitopes become associated with Ia at the surface of the cell. Potential T cell epitopes in close proximity to the epitope recognized by the Ig molecule could either be protected from processing events and thus not expressed (3 and 4, left panel), or in some way positively selected (3 and 4, right panel).

The epitopic specificity of the B cell could thus influence the epitopes of a protein antigen which are presented to T cells, if the presence of bound Ig either enhanced or impeded presentation of some T cell epitopes on the antigen (perhaps those adjacent to the B cell epitope). This concept is illustrated in Figure 6.11. Since antigen presentation by B cells, rather than the old idea of antigen bridging, is probably the basis of cognate helper interactions between T and B cells, it can be seen that the specificity repertoires of the two cell types can influence one another.

Other Antigen-Presenting Cells
A wide variety of cell types have now been shown to have some antigen-presenting capacity provided they express, or can be induced to express, class II molecules. This is not surprising, since some T cells appear to have only the minimal requirement of antigen/Ia for their activation. Included in the list are skin Langerhans cells, liver Kupffer cells, astrocytes in the brain, human natural killer cells, endothelial cells, articular chondrocytes, thyroid epithelial cells and human dermal fibroblasts. In some cases, these cells have been shown to be incapable of presenting antigen to, and of activating, resting T cells, but will present to previously activated cells (for example, T cell clones).

It seems that different APC types have different presenting abilities depending on the requirements of the responding T cell. For example, splenic and bone marrow macrophages were shown to be capable of triggering an apocytochrome c-specific T cell clone to proliferate and to secrete the lymphokines IL-2 and macrophage activating factor (MAF). However, a B lymphoma cell line could trigger the same clone to release MAF, but was unable to stimulate IL-2 release or proliferation. This was not due to differences in antigen processing events or levels of Ia expression; it may reflect the lack of stabilizing interactions between the lymphoma cells and the T cell clone (see below). Ramila and Erb have shown that T cells grown in long-term culture can become more selective in their APC requirements. For example, T cell lines grown with macrophages as APCs were found to be unable to respond to B lymphoma cells and *vice versa*. Finally, in some species (for example, humans, guinea-pigs and rats) activated T cells express class II molecules and may be able to present soluble antigens to other T cells. In experiments by Lamb and colleagues, the outcome of such presentation by T cells may be the delivery of tolerogenic signals rather than activation.

MODULATION OF APC FUNCTION

It has been seen in previous sections that the minimal requirement for T cell activation is probably a composite ligand comprising antigen (processed if necessary) in association with polymorphic regions of MHC molecules. Clearly, the level of activation of any particular T cell will be dependent upon the affinity of its receptor for this complex ligand, and upon the concentration of the ligand available to interact with the receptor. In the latter case, changes in the level of either MHC molecules or antigen will alter the degree of activation. The level of antigen available can be influenced by the efficiency of processing events in the APC and the stability of the antigen at the cell surface. The level of MHC molecules can be influenced in a number of ways (see Chapter 5).

Fig.6.12 Role of IL-1 in activation of T cells. The activation of a conalbumin/ I-A^k-specific T cell clone is shown as assessed by IL-2 release, proliferation and expression of IL-2 receptors. An anti-clonotypic monoclonal antibody specific for this cell stimulated a large release of IL-2, but failed to trigger proliferation because it was unable to stimulate the expression of IL-2 receptors. However, if APCs or IL-1 were added together with the monoclonal antibody, the T cell clone was activated as well as, or even better than, with antigen and APCs. IL-1 alone was ineffective, demonstrating that it plays an accessory role in T cell activation, perhaps by promoting the expression of IL-2 receptors. Based on data from Kaye J. *et al.*, 1984.

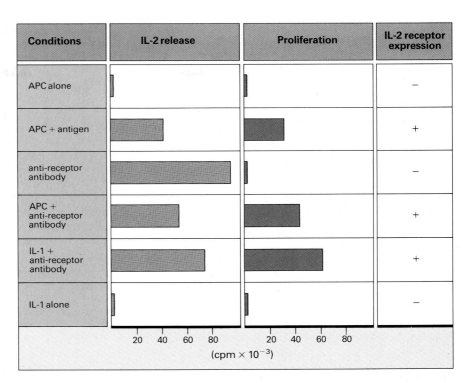

Conditions	IL-2 release	Proliferation	IL-2 receptor expression
APC alone			−
APC + antigen			+
anti-receptor antibody			−
APC + anti-receptor antibody			+
IL-1 + anti-receptor antibody			+
IL-1 alone			−

(cpm × 10^{-3})

However, many T cells appear to have additional requirements before they can be activated. Some cells may be activated to give some responses by antigen/Ia alone, but they require further stimuli or stabilization before their full range of activities can be manifested. These additional requirements will be covered in this section.

Interleukin-1 (IL-1)

Considerable evidence indicates that IL-1 (see Chapter 11) is necessary for the optimal activation of some T cells. A number of studies have suggested that resting or memory T cells require IL-1, but recently activated T cells (for example, T cell lines and clones) do not have this requirement. One study utilized transformed human B cells as APCs, and showed them to be incapable of presenting the antigen tetanus toxoid (TT) to purified resting T cells, unless IL-1 was provided. Yet the same B cells could present TT to activated T cells without added IL-1. If monocytes were used as APC, activation occurred because these cells could secrete IL-1. However, in the presence of antibody to IL-1, monocytes could only stimulate previously activated T cells. It had been suggested that B cells were unable to make IL-1, but Unanue and colleagues have demonstrated that B cells can produce membrane-bound IL-1. However, unlike the production of IL-1 by macrophages, this required triggering of B cells as well as the presence of T cell lymphokines. Surface membrane IL-1 may also be found in an active form on fixed APCs.

Another study investigated the role of IL-1 in the activation of cloned antigen-specific T cells by using WEHI-5B lymphoma cells as APCs. Recombinant IL-1 was found to significantly enhance the antigen-specific proliferation of cloned T cells, but it had little effect on IL-2 release by the same T cells. Antibody to IL-1 was able to block the enhancement, but it had no effect on the response driven in the absence of exogenous IL-1. Under conditions of suboptimal triggering with antigen, IL-1 led to an enhanced expression of IL-2 receptors which probably accounted for the increased proliferation observed. Thus,

it seems that IL-1 can have pleiotropic effects on T cell activation. The requirement for IL-1 by resting T cells could be because they have a higher threshold for stimulatory signals than previously activated T cells. Kaye and colleagues have studied the activation requirements of a T cell clone specific for conalbumin in association with I-A^k. An anti-clonotypic antibody which specifically binds to the receptor of this T cell could be shown to stimulate these cells in the complete absence of APCs, provided a source of IL-1 was also added to the cultures. Further analysis revealed that, in the absence of IL-1, the antibody could stimulate an abundant release of IL-2, but proliferation of the cells did not ensue because IL-2 receptors were not induced on the cell surface (Fig.6.12). When IL-1 or APCs which could make IL-1 were also added, IL-2 receptors were induced and the cells then proliferated. These observations strongly support the idea that the pleiotropic effects of IL-1 are at least partly mediated through its promoting the expression of IL-2 receptors. Experiments by Durum and colleagues have suggested that class II molecules on APCs may be involved in transducing signals which result in the release of IL-1. Monoclonal anti-I-A antibodies were found to block the release of IL-1 by macrophages triggered by signals such as LPS, concanavalin A, or even activated T cells.

Cell Surface Molecules

Obviously, cell surface class II molecules are the prime requirement for antigen presentation to TH cells. The level of expression of these molecules can be regulated in a variety of ways (see Chapter 5), and this will clearly influence the efficiency of an antigen-presenting cell. A number of studies, including those using L cells transfected with class II molecules, have indicated that a proportional relationship exists between antigen and Ia levels. That is, a relative deficiency in Ia levels can be overcome by an increase in antigen concentration and *vice versa*. There also appears to be a certain threshold level of antigen/Ia association which must be surpassed before activation occurs. Studies with anti-clonotypic antibodies such as those described above (see Fig.6.12) have shown that crosslinking of T cell receptors is required. This can occur very efficiently at the surface of an APC, provided it expresses adequate levels of processed antigen and class II molecules. The fluidity of the cell membrane may allow these molecules to move within the membrane in order to enhance interactions with the specific T cell.

As already discussed, an antigen/Ia association is not sufficient for the activation of all T cells. Other membrane molecules may play a role in these cases by helping to stabilize the interaction between APC and T cell in some way. For example, any membrane molecule which aids binding of the antigen (after processing if necessary) to the APC (for instance, various receptors) might enhance such interaction. Antibodies to the human T4 or mouse L3T4 membrane molecules have been shown to block activation of a variety of class II MHC-restricted T cells. It has been suggested that this surface molecule interacts with a non-polymorphic region of class II molecules during T cell activation, and this acts as a stabilizing mechanism. However, this is not certain since some results have suggested that anti-L3T4 antibodies can also inhibit activation of T cells by mitogenic stimuli which act in the absence of APCs and not via the T cell receptor. Experiments by Roska and Lipsky have shown that antigen-bearing guinea-pig macrophages fail to activate freshly primed T cells if they are fixed before testing. This defect could be overcome by providing metabolically active cells which would be Ia-negative (for example, fibroblasts), and which did not work by providing IL-1. This effect was shown to require cell-cell contact and was thought to function by the active cells in some way interacting with both T cell and antigen-bearing APC, thus stabilizing the T cell receptor-Ia/antigen interactions. As suggested earlier, these Ia-negative cells could also aid presentation by releasing processed forms of the antigen which subsequently interact with Ia molecules on the APC.

Other membrane molecules may also be found to influence the stability of T cell/APC interactions. For example, it has been suggested that the LFA-1 (lymphocyte functional antigen) molecule can be important for antigen presentation by some APCs. One could also conceive of other molecules having an adverse effect on antigen presentation if these have a tendency to repel the approach of other cells. In conclusion, it seems that although antigen/Ia-T cell receptor interactions are the minimal requirement for T cell activation, many cells, particularly in their original resting form, may have other requirements, depending on the affinity of the T cell receptor for antigen/Ia. In addition, different responses of the T cell may have different requirements, even though all are mediated through the same receptor.

ANTIGEN PRESENTATION *IN VIVO*

Despite the rapid advancement of our understanding of the mechanisms and cell types involved in antigen presentation to T cells *in vitro*, we are still rather ignorant about antigen presentation *in vivo*. The relative importance of different APC types is a matter of controversy. It is probably reasonable to assume that the importance of an APC type depends upon the conditions under which the body encounters the antigen. For example, in immune responses initiated in the skin, it is likely that Langerhans cells play an important role in presenting the antigen locally to T cells. Keratinocytes and fibroblasts, which can be induced to express Ia antigens, may also play a role. Langerhans cells bearing antigen may also migrate into peripheral lymphatic tissues where they may become dendritic cells and present antigen to T cells in these sites (see Chapter 14). It has been suggested that dendritic cells (also called interdigitating cells when observed *in situ* in extrafollicular sites in lymphoid tissues) are the most important cells for presenting antigen to virgin T cells. Follicular dendritic cells are a different cell type which do not bear MHC class II molecules, and are thus unable to present antigen to T cells. However, they play an important role in localizing antigen in immune complexes by binding via CR1 and 3 complement receptors, and presenting the antigen to B cells. These cells appear to be particularly important for the generation of memory B cells.

The role of B cells as APCs *in vivo* is still not certain. Their ability to concentrate and present antigen at low levels once they have been activated suggests that they may be very important at least in amplifying and maintaining immune responses. Recent studies on mice depleted of B cells from birth by treatment with anti-IgM antisera have shown that the loss of B cells results in a greatly diminished capacity of cells in the spleen to present antigens to T cells *in vitro*. One could speculate that non-specific polyclonal activation of B cells *in vivo* (for instance, during bacterial infections) might lead to the activation of self-reactive B cells which could present self antigens (perhaps those present in concentrations too low for effective presentation by other APCs, for instance, thyroglobulin) to self-reactive T cells, thus initiating an autoimmune disease. Other cell types may also play a significant role in presenting antigens if they become Ia-positive during the course of an immune response. This is most likely to occur locally, serving to enhance and maintain the local immune response to antigen. However, it is also possible that primary aberrant Ia expression by different cell types could be important, particularly in the presentation of self antigens.

SUMMARY

Unlike B cells, T helper cells cannot recognize soluble antigen directly. They require antigen to associate at the surface of antigen-presenting cells with class II molecules of the MHC. For this to be achieved, it seems that the antigen must attain a relatively stable binding at the cell membrane. For many protein and bacterial antigens this is achieved by processing events performed by the APC which, in most cases, involves proteolytic degradation of the antigen. Very small antigens or antigens which can bind to membrane receptors on the APC (for example, hormones) may not need such processing mechanisms because they can form a stable association with Ia at the cell surface more easily. How the T cell receptor interacts with antigen and Ia at the surface of an APC is still not clear, but several models have been suggested. The major argument currently focuses on the nature of antigen and Ia association. Some processed antigens may directly bind to polymorphic regions of the Ia molecule, to form a complex ligand which interacts with the T cell receptor in the form of a ternary complex. Alternatively, antigen and Ia may have no intrinsic affinities for one another, but they are forced into interactions by the T cell receptor with which they both interact. Evidence from different systems is available to support both of these models, and it is still possible that both mechanisms can occur: this would serve to enhance the diversity of the T cell repertoire.

Whilst macrophages were once considered to be the main cell involved in antigen presentation, it is now clear that many different Ia-positive cells can play this role (for example, dendritic cells, B cells, endothelial cells). The mode of interaction between antigen, Ia and the T cell receptor may be the same for different APCs, but they can still differ in their ability to activate T cells. Some T cells, probably those with a high affinity receptor, can be stimulated directly by interacting with antigen and Ia. Others, particularly resting T cells, appear to have further requirements such as IL-1 or stabilization of membrane interactions before they can be stimulated. Different APCs may vary in their ability to provide these additional needs of

the T cell. They may also differ in their ability to process a complex antigen, and this may result in different epitopes being predominant at the surface of different APCs. B cells may be particularly important in this regard, since they can bind and concentrate antigens present in very low amounts through their specific Ig receptor. They may then selectively process the antigen in such a way that certain T cell epitopes may be selected depending on their relationship to the specific epitope recognized by the Ig receptor of B cells.

In vivo, very little is actually known about the contributions made by different potential APCs. It is perhaps likely that the potential APCs available in a particular region in contact with antigen may all play at least a secondary role in antigen presentation to T cells. Whether or not they are capable of presenting antigen to virgin or memory T cells may be critical for the initiation of a response, and this still remains to be determined.

FURTHER READING

Abbas A.K., Haber S. & Rock K.L. (1985) *Antigen presentation by hapten-specific B lymphocytes. II. Specificity and properties of antigen-presenting B lymphocytes, and function of immunoglobulin receptors.* J. Immunol. **135**, 1661.

Allen P.M., McKean D.J., Beck B.N., Sheffield J. & Glincher L.H. (1985) *Direct evidence that a class II molecule and a simple globular protein generate multiple determinants.* J. Exp. Med. **162**, 1264.

Ashwell J.D., Fox B.S. & Schwartz R.H. (1986) *Functional analysis of the interaction of the antigen-specific T cell receptor with its ligands.* J. Immunol. **136**, 757.

Ashwell J.D. & Schwartz R.H. (1986) *T-cell recognition of antigen and the Ia molecule as a ternary complex.* Nature **320**, 176.

Babbitt B.P., Allen P.M., Matsueda G., Haber E. & Unanue E.R. (1985) *Binding of immunogenic peptides to Ia histocompatibility molecules.* Nature **317**, 359.

Baumhüter S., Bron C. & Corradin G. (1985) *Different antigen-presenting cells differ in their capacity to induce lymphokine production and proliferation of an apocytochrome c-specific T cell clone.* J. Immunol. **135**, 989.

Berzofsky J.A. (1983) *T-B reciprocity: an Ia-restricted epitope-specific circuit regulating T cell-B cell interaction and antibody specificity.* Surv. Immunol. Res. **2**, 223.

Buus S. & Werdelin O. (1980) *A group-specific inhibitor of lysosomal cysteine proteinases selectively inhibits both proteolytic degradation and presentation of the antigen dinitrophenyl-poly-L-lysine by guinea-pig accessory cells to T cells.* J. Immunol. **136**, 452.

Chesnut R.W., Colon S.M. & Grey H.M. (1982) *Requirements for the processing of antigens by antigen-presenting B cells. I. Functional comparisons of B cell tumours and macrophages.* J. Immunol. **129**, 2382.

Chesnut R.W. & Grey H.M. (1981) *Studies on the capacity of B cells to serve as antigen-presenting cells.* J. Immunol. **126**, 1075.

Coeshott C. & Grey H.M. (1985) *Transfer of antigen-presenting capacity to Ia-negative cells upon fusion with Ia-bearing liposomes.* J. Immunol. **134**, 1343.

Dekruyff R.H., Cantor H. & Dorf M.E. (1986) *Activation requirements of cloned inducer T cells. II. The failure of some clones to respond to antigen presented by activated B cells.* J. Immunol. **136**, 446.

Durum S.D., Gershon R.K. & Higuchi C. (1984) *Regulation of IL-1 release: role of the I-A glycoprotein.* J. Cell Biochem. **8a** (suppl.), 204.

Goodman J.W. & Sercarz E.E. (1983) *The complexity of structures involved in T cell activation.* Ann. Rev. Immunol. **1**, 465.

Grey H.M. & Chesnut R. (1985) *Antigen processing and presentation to T cells.* Immunology Today **6**, 101.

Grey H.M., Colon S.M. & Chesnut R.W. (1982) *Requirements for the processing of antigens by antigen-presenting B cells. II. Biochemical comparison of the fate of antigen in B cell tumours and macrophages.* J. Immunol. **129**, 2389.

Guidos C., Wong M. & Lee K.-C. (1984) *A comparison of the stimulatory activities of lymphoid dendritic cells and macrophages in T proliferative responses to various antigens.* J. Immunol. **33**, 1179.

Hansburg D., Heber-Katz E., Fairwell T. & Appella E. (1983) *Major histocompatibility complex-controlled, antigen-presenting cell-expressed specificity of T cell antigen recognition. Identification of a site of interaction and its relationship to Ir genes.* J. Exp. Med. **158**, 25.

Hayglass K.T., Naides S.J., Scott C.F., Benacerraf B. & Sy M.-S. (1986) *T cell development in B cell deficient mice. IV. The role of B cells as antigen-presenting cells in vivo.* J. Immunol. **136**, 823.

Inaba K., Steinman R.M., Van Voorhis W.C. & Muramatsu S. (1983) *Dendritic cells are critical accessory cells for thymus-dependent antibody responses in mouse and man.* Proc. Natl. Acad. Sci. USA **80**, 6041.

Kaye J., Gillis S., Mizel S.B., Shevach E.M., Malek T.R., Dinarello C.A., Lachman L.B. & Janeway C.A. Jr. (1984) *Growth of a cloned helper T cell line induced by a monoclonal antibody specific for the antigen receptor: interleukin 1 is required for the expression of receptors for interleukin 2.* J. Immunol. **133**, 1139.

Lanzavecchia A. (1985) *Antigen-specific interaction between T and B cells.* Nature **314**, 537.

Lechler R.I., Norcross M.A. & Germain R.N. (1985) *Qualitative and quantitative studies of antigen-presenting cell function by using I-A-expressing L cells.* J. Immunol. **35**, 2914.

Lechler R.I., Ronchese F., Braunstein N.S. & Germain R.N. (1986) *I-A-restricted T cell antigen recognition. Analysis of the roles of A_α and A_β using DNA-mediated gene transfer.* J. Exp. Med. **163**, 678.

Malynn B.A., Romeo D.T. & Wortis H.H. (1985) *Antigen-specific B cells efficiently present low doses of antigen for induction of T cell proliferation.* J. Immunol. **135**, 980.

Malynn B.A. & Wortis H.H. (1984) *Role of antigen-specific B cells in the induction of SRBC-specific T cell proliferation.* J. Immunol. **132**, 2253.

Matis L., Longo D.L., Hedrick S.M., Hannum C., Margoliash E. & Schwartz R.H. (1983) *Clonal analysis of the major histocompatibility complex restriction and the fine specificity of antigen recognition in the T cell proliferative response to cytochrome c.* J. Immunol. **130**, 1527.

Mizel S.B. (1982) *Interleukin I and T cell activation.* Immunol. Rev. **63**, 51.

Parham P. (1984) *A repulsive view of MHC-restriction.* Immunology Today **5**, 89.

Pernis B. & Axel R. (1985) *A one and a half receptor model for MHC-restricted antigen recognition by T lymphocytes.* Cell **41**, 13.

Puri J., Abromson-Leeman S. & Cantor H. (1985) *Antigen processing by macrophages: definition of the ligand recognized by T-inducer cells.* Eur. J. Immunol. **15**, 362.

Ramila G. & Erb P. (1983) *Accessory cell-dependent selection of specific T cell functions.* Nature **304**, 442.

Rock K.L., Benacerraf B. & Abbas A.K. (1984) *Antigen presentation by hapten-specific B lymphocytes. I. Role of surface immunoglobulin receptors.* J. Exp. Med. **160**, 1102.

Rosenthal A.S. & Shevach E.M. (1973) *Function of macrophages in antigen recognition by guinea pig T lymphocytes. I. Requirement for histocompatible macrophages and lymphocytes.* J. Exp. Med. **138**, 1194.

Roska A.K. & Lipsky P.E. (1985) *Dissection of the functions of antigen-presenting cells in the induction of T cell activation.* J. Immunol. **135**, 2953.

Schwartz R.H. (1985) *T-lymphocyte recognition of antigen in association with gene products of the major histocompatibility complex.* Ann. Rev. Immunol. **3**, 237.

Shimonkevitz R., Colon S., Kappler J.W., Marrack P. & Grey H.M. (1984) *Antigen recognition by H-2 restricted T cells. II. A tryptic ovalbumin peptide that substitutes for processed antigen.* J. Immunol. **133**, 2067.

Shimonkevitz R., Kappler J.W., Marrack P. & Grey H.M. (1983) *Antigen recognition by H-2 restricted T cells. I. Cell-free antigen processing.* J. Exp. Med. **158**, 303.

Siliciano R.F., Keegan A.D., Dintzis R.Z., Dintzis H.M. & Shin H.S. (1985) *The interaction of nominal antigen with T cell antigen receptors I. Specific binding of multivalent nominal antigen to cytolytic T cell clones.* J. Immunol. **135**, 906.

Steinman R.M. & Nussenzweig M.C. (1980) *Dendritic cells: Features and functions.* Immunol. Rev. **53**, 125.

Sunshine G.H., Gold D.P., Wortis M.H., Marrack P. & Kappler J.W. (1983) *Mouse spleen dendritic cells present soluble antigens to antigen-specific T cell hybridomas.* J. Exp. Med. **158**, 1745.

Szakal A.K., Gieringer R.L., Kosco M.H. & Tew J.G. (1985) *Isolated follicular dendritic cells: cytochemical antigen localization, Nomarski, SEM, and TEM morphology.* J. Immunol. **134**, 1349.

Unanue E.R. (1984) *Antigen-presenting function of the macrophage.* Ann. Rev. Immunol. **2**, 395.

Unanue E.R., Beller D.I., Lu C.Y. & Allen P.M. (1984) *Antigen presentation: comments on its regulation and mechanism.* J. Immunol. **132**, 1.

Watts T.H., Gaub H.E. & McConnel H.M. (1986) *T-cell mediated association of peptide antigen and major histocompatibility complex protein detected by energy transfer in an evanescent wave-field.* Nature **320**, 179.

Weinberg D.S. & Unanue E.R. (1981) *Antigen-presenting function of alveolar macrophages: uptake and presentation of Listeria monocytogenes.* J. Immunol. **126**, 794.

Ziegler K. & Unanue E.R. (1981) *Identification of a macrophage antigen-processing event required for I region-restricted antigen presentation to T lymphocytes.* J. Immunol. **127**, 1869.

7 Cytotoxic Lymphocytes

In 1960, Govaerts reported the first demonstration of cytotoxic activity by lymphoid cells. In his experiments on the mechanism of rejection of kidney allografts in dogs, he noted that thoracic duct lymphocytes from animals which had previously rejected an allograft were able to specifically kill donor kidney epithelial cells *in vitro*. These observations were soon confirmed by many other investigators, and extended to include killing of syngeneic tumour and virally infected cells. The effector cells involved in this killing of specific target cells were later found to be a subset of T cells, now known as cytotoxic T lymphocytes (Tc).

After the initial observations demonstrating the immunological specificity of cytotoxicity, a certain amount of confusion arose out of reports that lymphoid cells from non-immune individuals could non-specifically kill a variety of target cells, particularly following activation with mitogens. Furthermore, normal lymphocytes were shown to kill cells precoated with anti-target cell antibodies. It has subsequently become clear that these cytolytic activities are largely due to cells present in a subpopulation of mononuclear cells, known as large granular lymphocytes (LGL) because of their prominent azurophilic cytoplasmic granules. Non-specific killing of various tumour target cells is attributed to natural killer (NK) cells, and killing of antibody-coated target cells is due to killer (K) cell activity. Some cells within the LGL population can display both activities.

With the recent advent of techniques for cloning T cell populations, rapid advances of our understanding of the mechanisms of target cell killing by different cytotoxic cells have been made. It is now clear that the killing process can be separated into three distinctly recognizable phases:

1. Effector/target cell interaction involving cell/cell contact (Target Cell Recognition).
2. Effector cell preparation for delivery of its 'lethal hit' (Programming For Lysis).
3. Killer cell-independent destruction of the target cell (Target Cell Death).

The events involved in phases 2 and 3 appear to be very similar whether killing is mediated by Tc, NK or K cells. However, these three killer cell activities are distinguishable by their mode of target cell recognition. In this chapter the three phases of the killing process will be covered separately after a brief discussion of the different cytotoxic cell types. Target cells can also be killed non-specifically by a variety of mediators released by lymphocytes and macrophages during an immune response (see Chapters 11 and 15). Since this killing does not involve target cell recognition by the effector cell, it will not be considered further in this chapter.

CYTOTOXIC CELL TYPES

Cytolytic T Lymphocytes

Cytotoxic T lymphocytes (Tc) are a subpopulation of small lymphocytes which are important in the killing of virally infected cells, tumour cells and cells in both allogeneic and xenogeneic transplants. The majority of Tc belong to a subset of T cells, $CD8^+$ in humans and $Ly2^+$ in mice, which recognize antigens in association with class I molecules of the major histocompatibility complex (or foreign class I molecules directly on allogeneic/xenogeneic cells). However, a minority (probably no more than 10%) of Tc are $CD4^+$ ($L3T4^+$ in mice) and recognize antigen in association with class II MHC molecules (see Fig.7.1 overpage). Both types of Tc are derived from a pool of non-lytic precursor cells which are extremely radiosensitive. The frequency of precursor cells for a given antigen specificity has been estimated by limiting dilution analyses and found to fall in the range 0.02-0.2%. In most cases, these precursor cells need the cooperation of TH cells before they can mature into functional Tc in the presence of their specific antigen. The importance of TH cells appears to be primarily for the provision of IL-2, without which most Tc fail to mature and proliferate (see Chapter 10).

Experiments involving micromanipulation of individual cells have shown that a single cytotoxic T lymphocyte can sequentially kill several target cells. This implies that the Tc itself is resistant to the effects of its cytotoxic mediators. This is a very important observation, and it must be taken into account in any proposed killing mechanism, as will be seen later.

Natural Killer and Killer Cells

Natural killer (NK) cells are defined as cells which can spontaneously kill certain susceptible target cells in a manner which is apparently not restricted by MHC gene products (see Fig.7.1). These cells may play an important role in natural resistance against cancer and infectious diseases. NK cell activity is closely associated with the LGL sub-population of lymphocytes which represent about five percent of human peripheral blood lymphoid cells and which have been found in all vertebrates examined to date. These cells are non-phagocytic, non-adherent and lack certain markers characterizing T cells, macrophages and granulocytes. The majority of LGL possess high affinity receptors for the Fc region of IgG (Fc_γ) and often bear the glycolipid asialoGM1, a marker also found on granulocytes and macrophages. The possession of Fc_γ receptors enables the cells to mediate antibody-dependent cellular cytotoxicity (ADCC) reactions (K cell activity; see Fig.7.1). Some human cytotoxic T cells possess Fc_γ receptors, and thus can also mediate ADCC. Although many LGL can mediate both NK and K cell activity, some cells are only capable of killing target cells by one of these mechanisms. As will be seen below, the difference between NK and K cell activity is only at the level of target cell recognition. Once effector/target interactions have been established, killing appears to be the same for both types of effector activity. Thus, LGLs share a common killing mechanism which is activated through different target cell recognition events. The same mechanism also appears to account for killing by Tc.

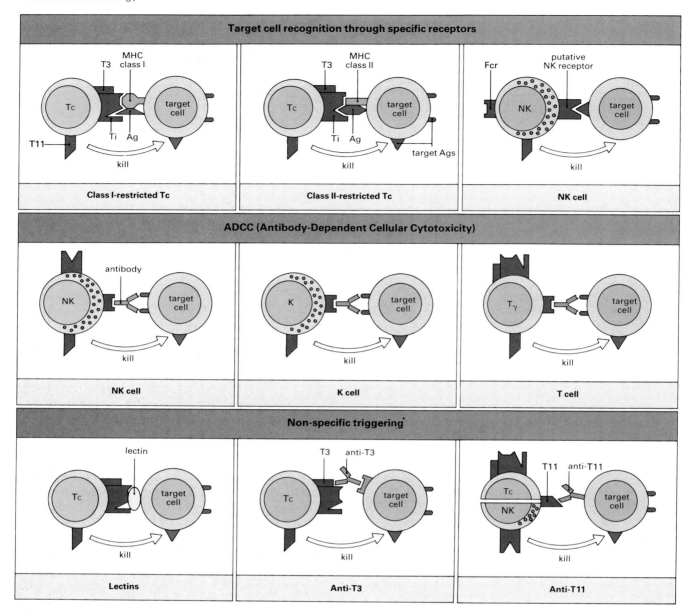

Fig.7.1 Modes of target recognition by cytolytic lymphocytes. The upper panels show target cell recognition through specific receptors (the αβ complex of the T cell receptor of Tc and a postulated distinct receptor of NK cells). In the middle panels, target cell recognition is mediated through Fc receptor binding to specific antibody (ADCC). This can be performed by cells with NK and K cell activities, as well as by a subpopulation of T cells (in humans) which bear Fcγ receptors (Tγ). The lower panels show non-specific interaction of Tc and NK cells with target cells through lectins or anti-T cell antibodies (T3 and T11).

TARGET CELL RECOGNITION

Cytotoxic T Cells

Tc utilize the α and β chains of their T cell receptor to recognize specific antigen in association with the appropriate class I and II molecules on the target cell. The lack of direct involvement of other molecules (for example, the T cell receptor γ chain) in the specific recognition of antigen has been proven recently by transfection experiments. In these studies, Dembic and colleagues transfected the α and β chain genes of a fluorescein (FL)-specific, H-2D^d-restricted cytolytic clone into a cytolytic T cell hybridoma specific for the hapten SP (3-[p-sulphophenyldiazo]-4-hydroxy-phenylacetic acid) in association with H-2K^k.

Transfectants were obtained which could lyse FL-coupled H-2D^d targets, as well as SP-coupled H-2K^k cells. As with antigen recognition by TH cells (see Chapter 6), the minimal requirements for Tc activation appear to be recognition of antigen associated with the appropriate MHC molecule, with many T cells also requiring other membrane molecules such as CD8/Ly2, CD4/L3T4 and LFA-1 to stabilize their interaction with the target cell.

As mentioned in Chapter 3, the CD8/Ly2 molecule appears to be important for stabilizing receptor-mediated interactions of class I-restricted T cells, whereas CD4/L3T4 is important for class II-restricted cells. Antibodies to these molecules are thought to have an inhibitory effect on T cell activation by preventing the stabilizing interactions they provide. However, activation of T cells by anti-CD3 antibodies or mitogens (which do not work through the T

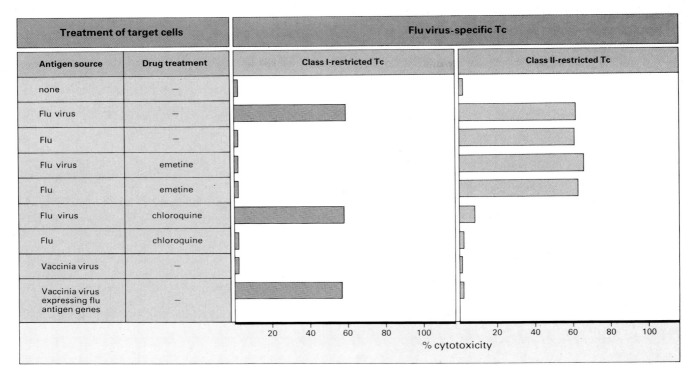

Treatment of target cells		Flu virus-specific Tc	
Antigen source	Drug treatment	Class I-restricted Tc	Class II-restricted Tc
none	−		
Flu virus	−		
Flu	−		
Flu virus	emetine		
Flu	emetine		
Flu virus	chloroquine		
Flu	chloroquine		
Vaccinia virus	−		
Vaccinia virus expressing flu antigen genes	−		

% cytotoxicity

Fig.7.2 Recognition of influenza virus-infected cells by class I- and II-restricted Tc. Target cells expressing both class I and II molecules were infected with virus (Flu virus), or incubated with inactivated antigen preparations (Flu) in the presence or absence of emetine (irreversible inhibitor of protein synthesis) or chloroquine (to inhibit antigen processing) as indicated. Target killing by class I-restricted Tc cells required *de novo* protein synthesis but was unaffected by chloroquine. Class II-restricted killing, on the other hand, was inhibited by chloroquine but did not require protein synthesis. Thus, class I-restricted Tc appear to recognize Flu antigens newly synthesized by the infected target cell, whereas class II-restricted Tc seem to only recognize a processed form of the added viral antigens. This conclusion is supported through the use of target cells infected with Vaccinia virus carrying Flu antigen genes; only class I-restricted Tc cells recognized these targets. Based on data of Morrison *et al.* (1986).

cell receptor) can also be blocked by anti-CD4 and anti-CD8 antibodies. It has been suggested that the CD4 and CD8 molecules can transmit a negative signal to the T cell whose effect is inversely proportional to the strength of the positive signal mediated through the T cell receptor.

The models outlined in Chapter 6 concerning the recognition of antigen and class II molecules by TH cells have also been put forward to explain the correcognition of antigen and MHC molecules (both class I and II) by Tc. Studies with alloreactive Tc clones have indicated that class I-specific cells recognize conformational determinants and not primary amino acid sequences. Exon-shuffling experiments with class I genes have shown that both the α_1 and α_2 domains of the class I molecule contribute to the formation of most of these epitopes. It seems likely that these conformational epitopes on allogeneic class I molecules are mimicking epitopes formed by a combination of antigen and self class I molecule, since many antigen-specific class I-restricted T cells have been shown to have distinct allospecificities. Furthermore, Hünig and Bevan identified several T cell clones which recognized one antigen in association with self class I molecules of H-2^k mice and a second, distinct antigen associated with allogeneic (H-2^d) class I molecules. These studies do not rule out the possibility that Tc recognize a new epitope on the class I molecule which is formed following conformational changes induced by interaction with antigen. This seems unlikely, however, since the exquisite specificity of Tc endows them with fine discriminatory powers. For example, Tc have been described which can distinguish between isomeric forms of the same hapten; it is difficult to imagine that different isomers would induce different conformational changes in a class I molecule.

How, then, do class I and II molecules associate with antigen for recognition by Tc cells? Since most studies of class I-restricted Tc have used cells specific for viruses, hapten-modified self antigens or allogeneic MHC molecules, it was thought that exogenous antigen becomes inserted in the cell membrane and then associates with the MHC molecule where it can be recognized by the T cell receptor. However, recent experiments indicate that this is not true in may cases. Townsend and colleagues have studied murine Tc clones specific for the nucleoprotein (NP) of influenza virus in association with class I MHC molecules. These cells were able to recognize and lyse L cells cotransfected with the NP gene and the appropriate class I gene. Through the use of deletion mutants and synthetic peptides, short peptide regions of NP were identified as being recognized by the Tc. This suggested that recognition of antigen by these class I-restricted Tc required some form of antigen processing events, perhaps akin to those required by TH cells. Morrison and colleagues have compared the recognition of influenza virus polypeptides by class I- and class II-restricted Tc clones (Fig.7.2). Their results indicate that class II-restricted Tc only recognize exogenously added viral polypeptides which may require some form of processing, since their recognition is blocked by treating the target cells with chloroquine (see Chapter 6). Thus, they appeared to have the same requirements as TH cells. In contrast, class I-restricted Tc recognizing the same viral polypeptides required *de novo* synthesis of viral proteins within the target cell, and they were completely unable to recognize exogenously added antigen (see Fig.7.2). Whether these newly synthesized polypeptides also required processing was not clear, but their recognition was insensitive to chloroquine treatment of the target cells.

It thus seems that recognition of antigen by class II-restricted Tc may follow similar rules to recognition of antigen by TH cells, whereas recognition of antigen in association with class I molecules may differ in some cases. It is likely that, as with TH, the formation of a stable association of antigen and class I molecule at the surface of the target cell is the most important factor in recognition by these Tc. How this occurs is also likely to vary from one antigen to the next depending on how the target cell 'handles' the antigen and which forms of antigen can associate with class I molecules. It may be that some viral antigens can become inserted into the cell membrane and associate directly with a class I molecule, whereas others only associate following intracellular processing or if they have been newly synthesized within the cell. In the latter case, one suggestion has been that newly synthesized viral polypeptides may associate intracellularly, and be coexpressed at the cell surface, with newly synthesized class I molecules.

Cytolysis by Tc requires intimate contact between a viable effector cell and its target. Clearly, this is normally mediated through T cell receptor interaction with specific ligands on the target cell. However, this can be bypassed experimentally such that non-specific killing can be triggered. For example, a specific Tc can be 'glued' to a non-specific target by various lectins and the targets will be killed, provided the effector cell is activated. This activation may be achieved with the same lectin, since many are mitogenic, or through the use of antibodies to CD3 or CD11 which activate T cells by bypassing the requirements for T cell receptor triggering (see Fig.7.1).

The effective adhesion of Tc cells to their targets is an active process, since it is inhibited by low temperature and metabolic inhibitors such as azide. It also has a requirement for divalent cations, with Mg^{++} being more effective than Ca^{++}. Although effector/target interactions occur in the absence of Ca^{++}, no lysis occurs because later events are Ca^{++}-dependent. Adhesion is also inhibited by cytochalasin B, suggesting that microfilaments are involved. It has been proposed that the microfilamentous structures are involved in recognition events, perhaps through movement of receptors into the region of membrane contact, whereas Mg^{++} is important for further non-specific stabilization of the effector/target interaction.

NK Cells

In contrast to Tc, very little is known about the nature of target cell recognition by NK cells. Some cloned cell populations with NK activity have been shown to have mRNA for, and rearrangements of, T cell receptor β-chain genes. However, this may be the result of *in vitro* differentiation (or maturation?), since freshly isolated NK cells do not appear to have rearranged their T cell receptor genes. Thus, it seems that target cell recognition by NK cells is normally mediated by a distinct receptor, although such a structure has not yet been identified. Also unlike Tc, NK/target cell conjugation is not inhibited by low temperature or metabolic inhibitors. However, the LFA-1 molecule does appear to be important for stabilizing these interactions. Although NK cells will lyse a wide spectrum of tumour target cells, there is

a selective killing pattern, with some targets being sensitive and others resistant to NK activity. It is not clear whether the apparent non-specificity of target cell recognition by NK cells reflects sharing of a determinant by susceptible cells, or whether multiple subsets of NK cells exist which have different target specificities. However, experiments utilizing the adsorption of NK cells onto monolayers of different target cells, cold-target inhibition studies and the use of cloned cell populations, have indicated that at least several subsets of NK cells exist.

The nature of the target structure also remains obscure. Treatment of target cells with various enzymes and specific metabolic inhibitors such as tunicamycin (which blocks carbohydrate synthesis) has indicated that NK cells may recognize a glycoprotein structure. The use of solubilized membrane proteins from susceptible target cells to inhibit NK-mediated lysis of target cells has also supported this conclusion. Since NK-resistant target cells can be transformed to susceptibility with certain oncogenes, it has been suggested that the target antigens involved in NK cell recognition may be viral or oncogene products. Transferrin receptors were also thought to be the target antigens of NK cells but, although they seem to play a role in effector/target conjugate formation, evidence for their absolute necessity is still controversial. Another unsubstantiated suggestion has been that Qa antigens represent NK cell target structures.

A unifying concept has been proposed by Kaplan to account for the nature and specificity of NK cells. According to his hypothesis, NK cells are prethymic T cells which express germline T cell V gene-encoded receptors, specific for either self or non-self histocompatibility antigens. Such histocompatibility antigens would include MHC molecules, minor histocompatibility antigens and differentiation antigens. Whether or not this hypothesis proves to be correct will depend on the outcome of experiments designed to characterize the NK cell receptor and the target structures it recognizes.

K Cells

Cells with K cell activity recognize target cells through binding of their high affinity Fc_γ receptor to anti-target cell antibodies. Thus, the anti-target cell antibody acts as an adapter allowing cytolytic cells bearing Fc_γ receptors to recognize and lyse target cells. Although many (but not all) NK cells bear Fc_γ receptors and can therefore also kill target cells by ADCC, blocking of the Fc_γ receptor only inhibits ADCC activity with little or no effect on NK activity. Thus, the same cell can enter into conjugate formation with a target through two distinct recognition structures. However, whichever recognition route is used, the same cytolytic mechanism is triggered.

PROGRAMMING FOR LYSIS

Effector Cell Triggering

For the second, Ca^{++}-dependent, phase of cytolysis (programming for lysis) to be activated, the effector cell must be triggered. For Tc, and probably also for NK and K cell activity, effector cell activation is usually mediated through the specific recognition receptors discussed above. However, T cells and NK cells may also be activated by other means to enter their cytolytic programme. For example, Tc can be activated to non-specifically lyse target cells by antibodies to the T3/Ti receptor complex or by certain

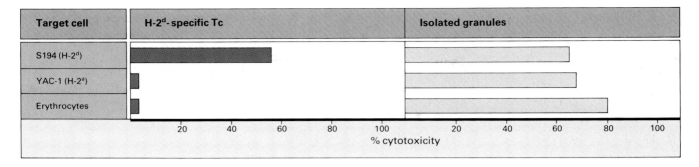

Target cell	H-2^d- specific Tc				Isolated granules				
S194 (H-2^d)									
YAC-1 (H-2^a)									
Erythrocytes									

% cytotoxicity

Fig.7.3 Granules isolated from cytotoxic cells can non-specifically kill target cells. Killing of three target cell types (S194 and YAC-1 tumour cells and erythrocytes) by a H-2^d-specific alloreactive Tc and cytoplasmic granules prepared from these effector cells is shown. Whilst the intact effector cells only kill the specific target, isolated granules can kill all three targets. Similar results have been obtained with NK cells, where isolated granules can kill NK-resistant targets (not shown).

mitogenic lectins such as concanavalin A (Con A). Such activation need not involve binding to the T cell receptor complex. For example, a pair of monoclonal antibodies recognizing distinct epitopes on the human T11 (CD2) molecule (the sheep erythrocyte receptor) can activate T cytotoxic and natural killer (NK) cells to kill non-specific or NK-resistant targets respectively. A monoclonal antibody recognizing the murine Thy1 molecule may also function in a similar way.

This evidence suggests that, although the T cell receptor is normally needed for specific recognition of targets and activation of the effector cell, it is probably not directly involved in the lytic process. Recent experiments by Lanzavecchia have confirmed this by showing that, once triggered (for example, through binding to the specific target), a Tc cell can kill any other susceptible cell that actively binds to it.

Cytolytic Granules in Tc and LGL
The membrane-bound cytoplasmic granules which are characteristic features of LGLs contain material which is darkly stained by the osmium used in electron microscopic (EM) studies. Such granules were also observed in the earliest EM studies of Tc/target cell conjugates, but their relevance was not appreciated, perhaps because they are not readily apparent by light microscopy. However, recent studies have shown that these granules are critical to the lytic process.

Grossi and colleagues demonstrated a marked correlation between the presence of cytoplasmic granules and the lytic capacity of a variety of cloned cell populations. Subsequently, granules have been isolated from Tc and NK cells by the groups of Podack and Henkart. These isolated granules were shown to non-specifically lyse a variety of targets in a Ca^{++}-dependent manner (Fig.7.3). Targets included erythrocytes and synthetic liposomes. In contrast, granule preparations from non-cytolytic T cells failed to lyse target cells. The granules contain a variety of lysosomal enzymes (including β-glucuronidase, aryl sulphatase and acid phosphatase), but these do not appear to be the source of the cytolytic activity. Antibodies raised against purified granules react with several major granule proteins and are capable of blocking granule-mediated target cell lysis. More importantly, F(ab′)$_2$ fragments of these same antibodies could block cell-mediated lysis of targets. Since these antibodies would not gain access to the granules in the cytoplasm of the effector cells, this observation supports the hypothesis that granule exocytosis is involved in the lytic

event (see below). Quantitative analysis of target cell lysis by granules has indicated that cell-mediated lysis could be completely accounted for by the activity of effector cell granules.

Cytoplasmic Rearrangements leading to Granule Exocytosis
Immediately following target cell binding, the cytolytic effector cell begins to reorganize its cytoplasmic constituents such that the Golgi apparatus and cytoplasmic organelles lie between the nucleus and the area of contact with the target cell. In addition, the microtubule organizing centre and the associated cytoskeletal proteins, tubulin and actin (but not myosin), become polarized within the cell in order to face the target. Such rearrangements do not occur subsequent to binding to non-specific or resistant target cells. A broadening of the region of membrane contact with specific targets is also seen and involves interdigitations of the two membranes. The reason for this is not known, but it provides a greatly increased area of contact with the target and thus probably improves the efficiency of cytolysis.

In an outstanding series of experiments, Yanelli and colleagues used high resolution cinematographic techniques to study the early events in the interaction of Tc with specific target cells. Tc cells were seen to move randomly by extending pseudopods from the broad leading edge of the cell which was largely organelle-free. Behind the nucleus, cells tapered to form a uropod containing many granules. Upon contact with another cell, pseudopodia were formed to extend the region of interaction, but further changes were only seen if the cell contacted a specific target. These began after one or two minutes and involved a 'rounding up' of the cell as well as reorientation of the cytoplasmic granules into the region of contact (Fig.7.4 overpage). Granule reorientation was completed within 6-10 minutes, consistent with the time required for delivery of the lethal hit. Fusions of granules with the cell membrane were also observed.

Other morphological studies have also followed the fate of granules after effector/target cell conjugate formation. For example, acid phosphatase and aryl sulphatase, originally found in granules, were seen deposited at the effector/target junction after cytoplasmic rearrangements had occurred. Apparently empty granules were also observed. Such observations all suggested that secretion of granule contents is involved in the cytolytic mechanism. The Ca^{++} requirement of cytolysis, particularly the programming for lysis phase, also points to the importance of a secretory mechanism since an increase in free cytoplasmic Ca^{++} is required

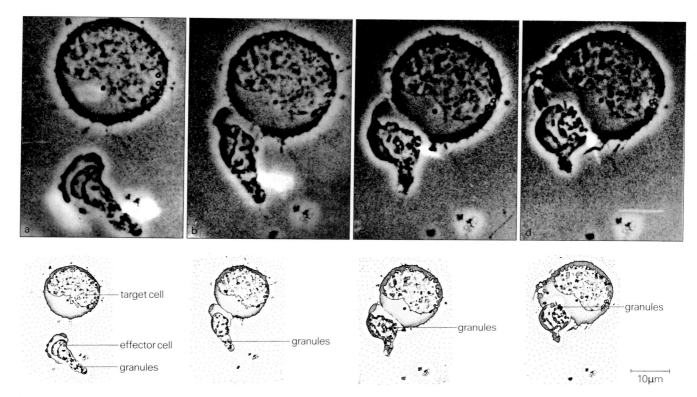

Fig.7.4 Photomicrographs of effector-target cell interaction. Early events in the interaction of Tc with specific target cells were studied with high resolution cinematographic techniques. The figure shows four frames taken at different times of a Tc cell interacting with its specific target. The location of granules within the effector cell is indicated in each case. Before contact with the target (a), the effector has an organelle-free, broad leading edge with granules located in a uropod at the rear. The effector Tc contacts the target (b) and within two minutes (c) has begun to round up and initiate granule reorientation. After ten minutes (d), the granules occupy a position in the zone of contact with the target where they are in the process of emptying their contents into the intercellular space between the two cells. By courtesy of Dr. V. H. Engelhard.

for most secretory processes. A Ca^{++} influx into the cell could be triggered through the T3/Ti complex, as with TH cells. Transmembrane chloride fluxes are also required for Tc effector function (not target cell binding), and such fluxes are known to participate in stimulus-secretion coupling. Pretreatment of effector cells with strontium, which promotes leucocyte degranulation, will reduce the cytolytic activity of the cell, further supporting a role for granule exocytosis. Thus, the balance of evidence presently available indicates that the programming for lysis phase of cytolysis by Tc cells and LGLs involves the activation of a polarized secretory process aimed at releasing cytolysins to the effector/target cell junction, to deliver the lethal hit (Fig.7.5). The nature of these cytolysins and the mechanism of target cell death will be discussed in the next section.

Fig.7.5 Granule exocytosis of perforins leads to transmembrane channel formation in target cells. Killing of target cells by cytolytic lymphocytes involves the secretion of granule contents into the intercellular environment between the closely apposed effector and target cells. Perforins, monomeric pore-forming proteins (PFP), are one of the major constituents of granules; in the presence of Ca^{++} they bind to the target cell membrane and polymerize to form polyperforins which become inserted into the membrane to create transmembrane channels. This appears to be essential, although not sufficient, for target cell killing by cytotoxic effector cells. However, the nature of other mediators and whether or not they also come from the granules, is not yet known.

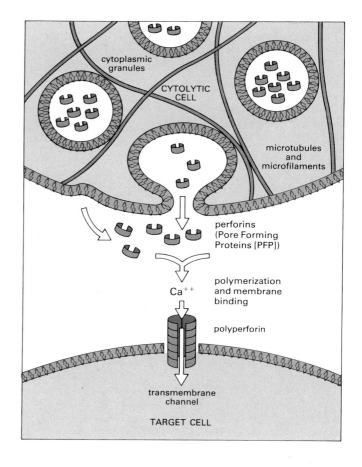

TARGET CELL DEATH

Nature of the Lethal Hit

Incubation of target cells with cytolytic lymphocytes (or cytoplasmic granules isolated from them) in the presence of Ca^{++} results in membrane lesions on the target cell, which are seen as ring structures of two different sizes and appear to be formed by polymerization of monomeric precursors (perforins) found in granules. Podack and colleagues have called the large (160Å) lesions 'polyperforin 1' (polyP1), and the smaller (50-70Å) lesions 'polyperforin 2' (polyP2). These are tubular complexes which perforate the target membrane and form non-selective transmembrane channels for ions (see Fig.7.5), in a similar way to lesion formation by polymerization of complement component C9.

PolyP1 is a tubular complex of approximately 160Å internal diameter and of similar length, with an estimated molecular weight of $1.5-2 \times 10^6$D composed of 18-20 pertorin monomers. Approximately 120Å of polyP1 appears to project out from the target cell membrane, with 40Å penetration into the membrane. The smaller polyP2 has an internal diameter of 50-70Å and a shorter length of 100-120Å. The Ca^{++} requirement for target cell lysis by isolated granules probably reflects the absolute need for calcium in polymerization and membrane binding of perforins. The assembly of the polyperforin channels is also pH- and temperature-dependent, and can occur on lipid vesicles, implying that there is no requirement for target cell macromolecules for insertion of these membrane channels. Some cytolytic lymphocytes, for example the rat LGL tumour cells studied by Henkarts group, appear to only produce membrane lesions of the polyP1 type. This implies that the polyP2 lesions are not essential for target cell lysis. Perforins have now been purified and shown to be a single protein (pore-forming protein [PFP]) of 62-66kD which alone is capable of forming membrane lesions morphologically and functionally similar to those produced by cytolytic cells and their granules.

As mentioned above, lesion formation by cytotoxic cells seems to have similarities with that produced by complement activation. Recent experiments have indicated that perforins share a common antigenic determinant with C9 and complexes of C7 and C8, and that this site may be involved in polymerization of the monomeric proteins. The activation of the complement system is complex and involves six different serine proteases. Evidence now beginning to accumulate indicates that perforin polymerization, and thus cell-mediated lesion formation, may involve a similar set of enzymes. For example, Pasternak and colleagues have described a membrane-associated serine protease which is secreted during cytolytic attack. It is a disulphide-linked dimer having trypsin-like properties,

although its restricted proteolytic activity is more characteristic of regulatory proteases such as those involved in the complement cascade. Molecular analyses of Tc-specific inducible mRNA transcripts have also revealed at least two which code for molecules having considerable homology with complement serine proteases.

As will be discussed in the following section, pore formation alone probably does not account for the death of the cell. However, the nature of other cytolytic mediators is still very controversial. It has long been debated whether soluble cytolytic molecules such as lymphotoxin (LT; see Chapter 11) might play a role in cell-mediated cytolysis. However, the observations that bystander target cells (i.e. not directly bound to the effector) are not lysed and that LT-mediated lysis takes a minimum of five hours, argues against a role for this molecule. Similar arguments apply to a soluble lytic factor which is secreted by NK cells (NK cytotoxic factor [NKCF]), although this factor sometimes appears to retain the target specificity of the cell it was released from. Current evidence suggests that NKCF may in fact be tumour necrosis factor (TNF; see Chapter 11). The slow kinetics of these lytic molecules when tested in free solution could be an artefact of the culture system. It is possible that high and effective concentrations of such cytolytic molecules could be achieved in the microenvironment of the space between the effector and target cell membranes. However, attempts to substantiate a role for these molecules by using specific antibodies have produced only conflicting results. Various lysosomal enzymes, including two serine esterases present in granules, have been postulated to be important in target cell killing. Although direct addition of purified enzymes to target cells is ineffective, it has been suggested that they could pass into the target via polyperforin channels to have their effect. This possibility still awaits experimental verification. It is more

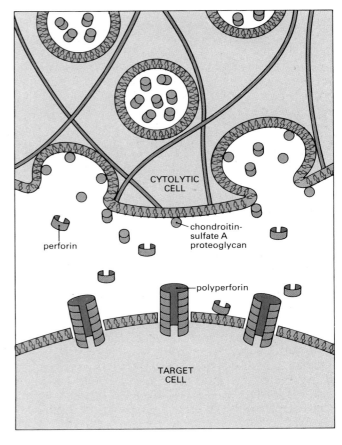

Fig.7.6 Postulated role for chondroitin sulphate A proteoglycans in protecting effector cells from cytolytic mediators. It is suggested that perforins bind to the negatively charged proteoglycans found in the cytoplasmic granules of effector cells. Upon granule exocytosis, perforins dissociate in the higher pH of the intercellular milieu and polymerize to form polyperforins. The proteoglycans remain bound to the fused granule membrane (or only diffuse very slowly because of their large size) and prevent perforin polymerisation (and thus killing) of the effector cell.

likely that these enzymes are involved in the formation of polyperforins, as discussed above.

Whatever the nature of the lytic mechanism, effector cytolytic cells are resistant to it; indeed they can lyse several successive target cells. However, cytolytic cells can be lysed when they are themselves specifically recognized by an effector Tc cell. Thus, killing occurs in one direction only, and it seems that activation renders the effector cell temporarily resistant to cytolysis. The mechanism of this resistance is unknown at the present time, but possibilities have been suggested. Kupfer and colleagues have shown that the cytoskeletal protein talin (215kD) becomes concentrated at the membrane of the effector cell in the region of conjugation during the cytoplasmic rearrangements which occur following specific target cell recognition. This appeared to be true for both Tc and NK cells. They suggested that this deposition of talin may protect the effector cell from cytotoxic mediators secreted into the intercellular space. An alternative model, proposed by Tschopp and Conzelmann, suggests a role for the chondroitin sulphate A proteoglycans found in the cytoplasmic granules of cytolytic cells. They extended earlier suggestions of MacDermott and colleagues to propose that perforins bind to the proteoglycans within the granule and this, together with the low pH, may help protect the cell from autolysis. Upon exocytosis, the perforins dissociate from the proteoglycans (because of the higher pH of the extracellular milieu) and polymerize in the presence of Ca^{++} to participate in the lysis of the target cell. The large proteoglycans diffuse much more slowly and some may remain attached to the fused granule membrane to bind any perforins diffusing back towards the effector cell, thus protecting it (see Fig.7.6, previous page). In support of this model, binding of perforins to chondroitin sulphate A proteoglycans at pH5 (the probable pH of cytoplasmic granules) is much stronger than at neutral pH.

Death of the Target Cell

There are two distinct modes of death in nucleated cells: necrosis and apoptosis (Fig.7.7). Necrosis, which is the result of complement-mediated immunological attack, occurs through an increase in the permeability of the cell membrane. An equilibration of ions across the membrane occurs, and cytoplasmic macromolecules exert an unbalanced osmotic pressure so that water is taken up and nuclear chromatin is seen to flocculate. Initially the changes are reversible, but they are quickly followed by irreversible disruption of the integrity of the cell. A cell undergoing apoptosis is seen to round up, and the endoplasmic reticulum dilates and forms vesicles which often fuse to the cell membrane. This gives a characteristic 'bubbling'

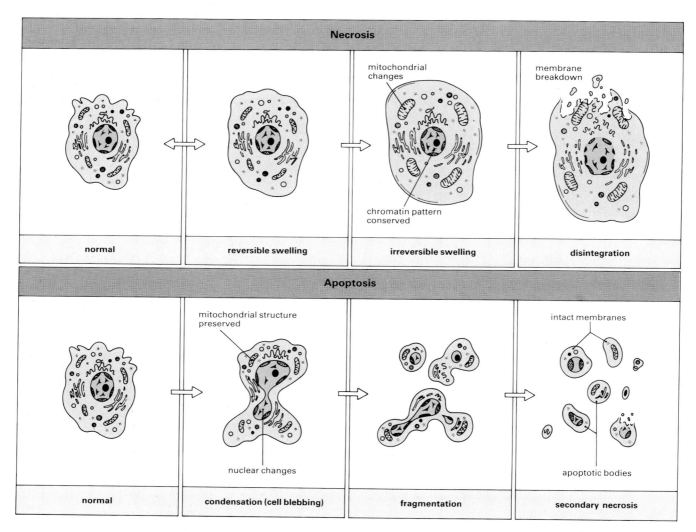

Fig.7.7 Two mechanisms of cell death: necrosis and apoptosis. Contrasting features of the morphology of necrosis and apoptosis are shown. Cellular cytotoxicity appears to occur by the mechanism of apoptosis, unlike killing by complement attack which is a necrotic mechanism.

appearance under EM. In contrast to necrosis, the chromatin forms dense aggregates and the nuclear membrane invaginates. Convolution of the plasma membrane leads to the cell separating into small membrane-bound segments called 'apoptotic bodies'. This may be seen experimentally as blebbing of the cell surface. Accompanying the nuclear changes, the chromatin is rapidly degraded into discrete fragments which have multiples of about 200 base pairs of DNA. This pattern of cleavage may be because of the vulnerability of the DNA between nucleosomes to endonuclease attack. In necrosis, DNA degradation is a late phenomenon.

Early studies of cell-mediated attack indicated that ions and small molecules are the first to be lost from target cells. This very early release of small ions suggested that cell death occurred by necrosis. However, this damage may only represent non-lethal perturbation of the membrane. Shortly after effector cell attack (within ten minutes), extensive DNA breakdown occurs in the target cell to produce fragments of multiples of 200 base pairs. This breakdown was seen to be dependent on Ca^{++} and inhibitable by Zn^{++}. The pattern of DNA fragments depends on the target cell type. It is suggested that the activation of Ca^{++}-dependent endonucleases may be involved in this DNA breakdown. Whether these are target cell endonucleases, activated during the cytolytic attack, or of effector cell origin (perhaps from granules) is still open to speculation.

Time-lapse cinematographic studies have shown that target cells attacked by Tc and ADCC effector cells undergo cytoplasmic bulging movements called zeiosis (membrane blebbing). This is only observed after effector/target conjugation, but occurs before the loss of target cell cytoplasmic contents. Such events were not observed during lysis with

specific antibody and complement. Thus, cell-mediated killing of target cells seems to occur by apoptosis and not by necrosis (lysis). Strictly speaking, therefore, the term 'lysis' should not be used to describe the death of target cells caused by cytotoxic cell attack.

SUMMARY

Target cell killing can be effected by two major populations of lymphocytes: cytotoxic T cells (Tc) and large granular lymphocytes (LGL) which do not bear classical T and B cell markers. Killing by the LGL population can be separated into two types: natural killer (NK) and killer (K) activities which differ in their mode of target cell recognition, although many individual cells can exhibit both activities. The different cytotoxic cell types differ in their recognition of target cells but, once they have been activated, they appear to utilize the same process for killing their targets (Fig.7.8).

The majority of Tc cells utilize α and β chains of their T cell receptor to recognize antigens associated with class I MHC molecules on the target cell membrane, although a minority see antigen associated with class II molecules. NK cells recognize a wide variety of target cells, probably through the use of a distinct receptor, although this has yet to be identified. Target cell recognition for K cell activity (antibody-dependent cellular cytotoxicity [ADCC]) is mediated by Fc receptor binding to IgG anti-target cell antibodies.

Following conjugation with a specific target cell, cytolytic cells undergo a process of cytoplasmic rearrangement in order to direct the secretion of cytolysins, present in

Fig.7.8 Summary of proposed mechanism of target cell killing by cytolytic lymphocytes.

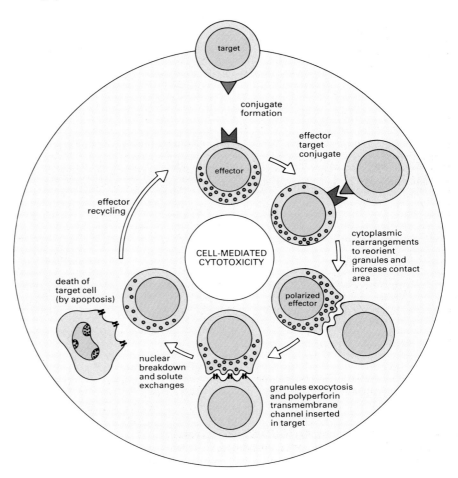

granules, towards the target cell. Perforin monomers released from the granules polymerize on the target cell membrane (in the presence of calcium) to form tubular complexes (polyperforins), which insert into the membrane to form transmembrane channels. Unlike cell killing by complement, these membrane lesions alone are not enough to kill the cell. However, the nature and relative importance of other cytolytic molecules is still unclear. Target cell death appears to occur by the mechanism of apoptosis (rather than true lysis), where nuclear degradation occurs very early and produces distinct patterns of DNA fragmentation. The effector cells themselves are in some way 'immune' to their own cytolytic mediators and can, therefore, kill more than one target cell.

FURTHER READING

Brunet J.F., Dosseto M., Denizot F., Mattei M.-G., Clark W.R., Haqqi T.M., Ferrier P., Nabholz M., Schmitt-Verhulst A.-M., Luciani M.-F. & Goldstein P. (1986) *The inducible cytotoxic T-lymphocyte-associated gene transcript CTLA-1 sequence and gene localization to mouse chromosome 14.* Nature **322,** 268.

Dembić Z., Haas W., Weiss S., McCubrey J., Kiefer H., von Boehmer H. & Steinmetz M. (1986) *Transfer of specificity by murine a and b T cell receptor genes.* Nature **320,** 232.

De Waal L.P., Nathenson S.G. & Melief C.J.M. (1983) *Direct demonstration that cytotoxic T lymphocytes recognize conformational determinants and not primary amino acid sequences.* J. Exp. Med. **158,** 1720.

Duvall E. & Wyllie A.H. (1986) *Death and the cell.* Immunology Today **7,** 115.

Glasebrook A.L., Kelso A. & MacDonald H.R. (1983) *Cytolytic T lymphocyte clones that proliferate autonomously to specific alloantigenic stimulation. II. Relationship of the Lyt-2 molecular complex to cytolytic activity, proliferation, and lymphokine secretion.* J. Immunol. **130,** 1545.

Govaerts A. (1960) *Cellular antibodies in kidney homotransplantation.* J. Immunol. **85,** 516.

Grossi C.E., Zicca A., Cadoni A., Mingari M.C., Moretta A. & Moretta L. (1983) *Ultrastructural characteristics of human T cell clones with various cytolytic activities.* Eur. J. Immunol. **13,** 670.

Henkart P.A., Millard P.J., Reynolds C.W. & Henkart M.P. (1984) *Cytolytic activity of purified cytoplasmic granules from cytotoxic rat LGL tumours.* J. Exp. Med. **160,** 75.

Henkart P.A. (1985) *Mechanism of lymphocyte-mediated cytotoxicity.* Ann. Rev. Immunol. **3,** 31.

Herberman R.B., Reynolds C.W. & Ortaldo J. (1986) *Mechanisms of cytotoxicity by natural killer (NK) cells.* Ann. Rev. Immunol. **4,** 651.

Hünig T.R. & Bevan M.J. (1982) *Antigen recognition by cloned cytotoxic T lymphocytes follows rules predicted by the altered self hypothesis.* J. Exp. Med. **155,** 111.

Kaplan J. (1986) *NK cell lineage and target specificity: a unifying concept.* Immunology Today **7,** 10.

Kupfer A., Singer S.J. & Dennert G. (1986) *On the mechanism of unidirectional killing in mixtures of two cytotoxic T lymphocytes. Unidirectional polarization of cytoplasmic organelles and membrane-associated cytoskeleton in the effector cell.* J. Exp. Med. **163,** 489.

Lanier L.L. & Phillips J.H. (1986) *Evidence for three types of human cytotoxic lymphocyte.* Immunology Today **7,** 132.

Lanzavecchia A. (1986) *Is the T cell receptor involved in T-cell killing?* Nature **319,** 778.

Lukacher A.E., Morrison L.A., Braciale V., Malissen B. & Braciale T.J. (1985) *Expression of specific cytolytic activity by H-2I region-restricted, influenza virus-specific T lymphocyte clones.* J. Exp. Med. **162,** 171.

MacDermott R.P., Schmidt R.E., Caulfield J.P., Hein A., Bartley G.T., Ritz J., Schlossman S.F., Austen K.F. & Stevens R.L. (1985) *Proteoglycans in cell-mediated cytotoxicity. Identification, localization, and exocytosis of a chondroitin sulphate proteoglycan from human cloned natural killer cells during target cell lysis.* J. Exp. Med. **162,** 1771.

Milanese C., Siliciano R.F., Schmidt R.E., Ritz J., Richardson N.E. & Reinherz E.L. (1986) *A lymphokine that activates the cytolytic program of both cytotoxic T lymphocyte and natural killer clones.* J. Exp. Med. **163,** 1583.

Millard P.J., Henkart M.P., Reynolds C.W. & Henkart P.A. (1984) *Purification and properties of cytoplasmic granules from cytotoxic rat LGL tumors.* J. Immunol. **132,** 3197.

Morrison L.A., Lukacher A.E., Braciale V.L., Fan D.P. & Braciale T.J. (1986) *Differences in antigen presentation to MHC class I- and class II-restricted influenza virus-specific cytolytic T lymphocyte clones.* J. Exp. Med. **163,** 903.

Nabholz M. & MacDonald H.R. (1983) *Cytolytic T lymphocytes.* Ann. Rev. Immunol. **1,** 273.

Ortaldo J. & Herberman R.B. (1984) *Heterogeneity of natural killer cells.* Ann. Rev. Immunol. **2,** 359.

Owen J.A., Scinto L.A.F., Klein L. & Kline C.J. (1986) *Cytotoxic T lymphocytes discriminate between isomeric forms of the same hapten.* Immunology **57,** 499.

Pasternak M.S., Verret C.R., Liu M.A. & Gisen H.N. (1986) *Serine esterase in cytolytic T lymphocytes.* Nature **322,** 740.

Podack E.R. & Konigsberg P.J. (1984) *Cytolytic T cell granules. Isolation, structural, biochemical and functional characterization.* J. Exp. Med. **160,** 695.

Podack E.R. (1985) *The molecular mechanism of lymphocyte-mediated tumour cell lysis.* Immunology Today **6,** 21.

Reid K.B.M. (1986) *Complement-like cytotoxicity.* Nature **322,** 684.

Townsend A.R.M., Goth R.M. & Davey J. (1985) *Cytotoxic T cells recognize fragments of the influenza nucleoprotein.* Cell **42,** 457.

Tschopp J., Masson D. & Stanley K.K. (1986) *Structural/functional similarity between proteins involved in complement- and cytotoxic T lymphocyte-mediated cytolysis.* Nature **322,** 831.

Tschopp J. & Conzelmann A. (1986) *Proteoglycans in secretory granules of NK cells.* Immunology Today **7,** 135.

Yanelli J.R., Sullivan J.A., Mandell G.L. & Engelhard V.H. (1986) *Reorientation and fusion of cytotoxic T lymphocyte granules after interaction with target cells as determined by high resolution cinematography.* J. Immunol. **136,** 377.

Young J.D.-E., Podack E.R. & Cohn Z.A. (1986) *Properties of a purified pore-forming protein (perforin 1) isolated from H-2-restricted cytotoxic T cell granules.* J. Exp. Med. **164,** 144.

Young J.D.-E., Hengartner H., Podack E.R. & Cohn Z.A. (1986) *Purification and characterization of a cytolytic pore-forming protein from granules of cloned lymphocytes with natural killer activity.* Cell **44,** 849.

8 Antigenicity of Proteins

The most fundamental feature of the immune system is its ability to specifically respond to a multitude of foreign antigens. In most cases, both T cells and B cells are involved in mounting this response. The nature of the T and B cell receptors involved in the specific recognition of antigens has been described in Chapters 2 and 3. In this chapter, the structural basis of protein antigenicity at both the T cell and B cell level will be discussed, since proteins are amongst the most diverse and profuse antigens encountered by the immune system; some of these have been studied in great detail. Carbohydrate, lipid and nucleic acid antigens (for example, many T independent antigens, tumour-associated antigens, DNA) can be recognized by the B cell component of the immune system. However, as the currently available information on determinants recognized by T cells is almost exclusively restricted to protein antigens, discussion of antigenicity will be restricted to these molecules. The basic principles of antibody recognition of proteins can, however, also be applied to non-protein antigens.

Before proceeding to a detailed description of protein antigenicity, it is important that some of the terms which will be encountered are clarified. Antigenicity is currently defined as the ability of a particular molecular structure to be recognized by B cell (antibody) and T cell receptor molecules. It should not be confused with immunogenicity, which is the ability of a molecule to induce an immune response. Immunogenicity is dependent upon the host's ability to respond, which in turn depends upon a variety of regulatory influences: the balance of activity of T helper (TH) and T suppressor (TS) cells, idiotype networks, MHC antigens, antigen presentation, as well as the available B and T cell repertoires. Such regulatory mechanisms are also responsible for the phenomenon of immunodominance, where reactions to certain of the potentially antigenic regions of a protein predominate following immunization with the native molecule (internal antigenic competition). For example, animals immunized with foreign immunoglobulins produce antisera which primarily react with the Fc region. Yet, these animals are quite capable of responding to other regions as shown by immunizing them with $F(ab')_2$ fragments.

Antigenic determinants (epitopes) on protein molecules are those regions which interact with specific antibody molecules or T cell receptors. Early studies using polyclonal antisera to a variety of proteins led to the definition of two classes of epitopes, based on the ability of antibodies to native proteins to bind to denatured antigen or protein fragments: conformational determinants required the native protein folding in order to bind antibodies, whereas sequential determinants appeared to depend only on the correct linear amino acid sequence, as antibodies to them also bound to isolated linear peptides. However, many conformational determinants can be prevented from interacting with antibody if large amounts of corresponding linear peptide are present, since the conformation

recognized by antibody is one of the many configurations that a peptide can assume in solution. (All determinants are actually conformational, in that they require the appropriate spatial arrangement of amino acid side chains to interact with antibody). Since determinants recognized by antibody are all composed of surface features of the protein (see below), they have been termed 'topographic'. Assembled topographic determinants (sometimes also termed discontiguous epitopes) are comprised of residues lying far apart in the protein sequence, but brought together by folding in the native structure. Other topographic determinants (contiguous epitopes) are formed by short amino acid sequences, and this type can often be mimicked by large amounts of the appropriate linear peptides (Fig.8.1).

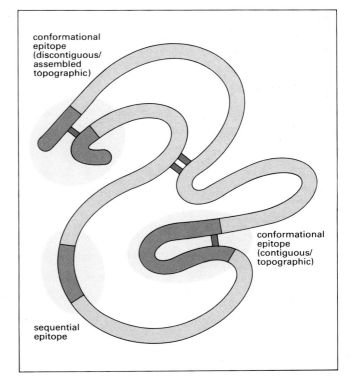

Fig.8.1 Epitopes of protein antigens. The terminology used to describe epitopes is shown in relation to the tertiary structure of a hypothetical protein antigen. Some antibodies can bind to linear peptides derived from a single region of the antigen (sequential epitopes). In some cases, antibodies bind to a linear peptide, but only if it retains sufficient tertiary structure to be recognized (contiguous/topographic conformational epitope). Some epitopes (discontiguous/assembled topographic) are formed from separate regions of the protein which lie close together when the protein is folded in its native conformation. Disulphide bonds (red) are often important for maintaining the conformational integrity of antigenic sites.

In recent years, rapid advances have been made in our understanding of protein antigenicity, particularly through the use of monoclonal antibodies and structurally well defined protein antigens having species variants with known amino acid sequence differences. The nature of epitopes recognized by T cells is now also being intensively investigated, through the recent availability of monoclonal T cell populations and genetically cloned MHC class I and II genes. The current understanding of the structural basis of protein antigenicity at both B and T cell levels is discussed below.

ANTIGENIC SITES RECOGNIZED BY ANTIBODIES

The first information available on the nature of the interaction between antigen and antibody came from the pioneering work of Landsteiner and Van der Scheer. These and subsequent studies focused on small molecules and haptens, such as dinitrophenol (DNP) and phosphoryl choline (PC), attached to macromolecular carrier proteins. Antibody binding to these rather rigid structures was seen to be independent of the carrier and to involve relatively small clefts or pockets in the Fab portion of the molecule.

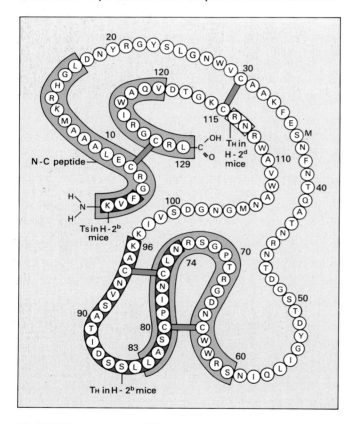

Fig.8.2 The structure of hen egg white lysozyme (HEL).
HEL consists of a single polypeptide chain of 129 amino acids (indicated in single letter code – see Fig.5.10) crosslinked by four disulphide bonds (red). Some of the regions containing epitopes recognized by murine antibodies and T cells are highlighted. The N-C peptide and 'loop' region (dark pink), which can be isolated following enzymatic cleavage of the molecule, bear epitopes recognized by antibodies. Major areas recognized by T_H (grey), and T_S (brown) cells in H-2^b mice and the major T_H determinant in H-2^d mice (white) are also shown.

Based on such observations, protein antigens were considered to consist of a number of discrete, non-overlapping regions (epitopes), each resembling a hapten in its interaction with the immune system. This concept appears to have been an oversimplification, as will be discussed below.

Most of the information which has led to our current understanding of antigen recognition by antibodies has come from the study of model protein antigens such as myoglobin, lysozyme, cytochrome c and myohaemerythrin. These model antigens are all very well characterized proteins, each having a known amino acid sequence and tertiary structure. In addition, species variants, peptide fragments and synthetic peptides with known amino acid differences have given insight into the importance of particular amino acids in an antigenic site.

Chicken lysozyme c from egg white (HEL), a small globular protein of 129 residues, has been used extensively in studies of protein antigenicity. HEL has four intrachain disulphide bonds, giving it a stable conformation in solution which is thought to be very similar to the crystalline structure used for X-ray analysis of its three-dimensional features (Fig.8.2). The antigenicity of HEL is largely dependent upon an intact conformation, since antibodies to the native protein show very little reactivity with the denatured molecule. Certain disulphide-bonded peptides derived from HEL, such as the 'loop' (residues 60-83) and the N-C peptide (residues 1-17; 120-129 disulphide-bonded between cysteines at positions 6 and 127), will react with anti-HEL antibodies but with much lower affinities. Non-disulphide-bonded peptides generally do not react with these antibodies. From these studies it has been concluded that most of the antigenic determinants on HEL are of the assembled topographic type. Detailed analysis of the binding of various polyclonal and monoclonal antibodies to different regions of the HEL molecule has indicated the importance of different amino acids in interactions with antibodies. For example, the fine specificities of antibodies to the 'loop' region of HEL has been examined by using different avian lysozymes, peptides derived from HEL, and synthetic peptide analogues with various amino acid differences from the 'loop' peptide. The results have clearly demonstrated that not all amino acid residues contribute to the antigenicity of this peptide. Arginine at position 68 seems to be a prime requirement for the binding of many antibodies. Monoclonal antibodies have been able to define at least three distinct, but overlapping, epitopes in this region (Fig.8.3). Interestingly, not all of these antibodies depended on the conformational restraints imposed by the disulphide bond in the 'loop' peptide. This does not necessarily imply that intact conformation is unimportant, as this particular region of HEL forms a hairpin bend with a β-turn involving Arg 68. Thus, it is possible that the non-disulphide-bonded 'loop' peptide maintains local conformational integrity, or antibody binds to molecules which have randomly adopted the correct conformation; this drives the equilibrium in the direction of the correctly folded structure.

A number of major conclusions can be drawn from these and other studies of model protein antigens. Most of the accessible surface of any globular protein appears to be potentially immunogenic (depending on the species immunized), and to consist of a continuum of multiple overlapping epitopes. A particularly good example is provided by one study investigating the specificity of binding of over 60 monoclonal antibodies to bovine serum

Fig.8.3 Overlapping epitopes in the 'loop' region of HEL. These space-filling models demonstrate topographic features involved in the antigenicity of the 'loop' region of HEL. The amino acids in the 'loop' are shown shaded (a) and sequence numbered (b). Three distinct, but overlapping, epitopes in the 'loop' region, defined by monoclonal antibodies, are shown in c, d and e. It can be seen that, whilst an antibody can be specific for a single amino acid residue, the side chains of many other amino acids are also involved in the binding of the antibody to its epitope. Courtesy of Darsley & Rees (1985).

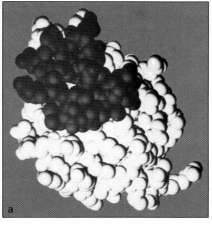
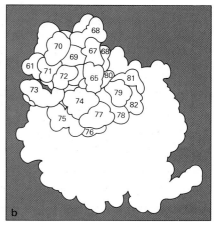
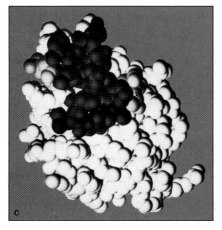
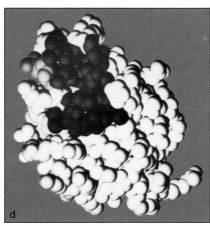
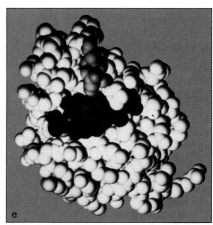

albumin: using ten different mammalian albumins with amino acid sequence differences, this study was able to define a minimum of 33 epitopes on bovine serum albumin. Only thirteen of these monoclonals recognized distinct non-overlapping sites; the remainder defined a series of overlapping antigenic determinants. It is not surprising to find that antibodies recognize determinants on the surface of proteins, since their function requires that they can bind to surface antigens of organisms which have compromised the host (on this point see Chapter 9). Although the repertoire of antibodies capable of binding a particular protein is often diverse, that expressed in serum is skewed by immunoregulatory influences to give certain dominant specificities. For example, in mice of the H-2^a haplotype immunized with HEL, at least 75% of the secondary response is directed to epitopes within the N-C peptide. Because of these regulatory influences on antibody responses, it is important to define the total antigenic structure of a protein by using a variety of responding individuals and species (see Fig.8.4). Of particular importance to the immunogenicity of a protein are the structural differences between it and any homologous protein in the

Cytochrome c species	Amino acid residue number		
	44	62	89
Rabbit	VAL	ASP	ASP
Mouse	ALA	ASP	GLY
Guanaco	VAL	GLU	GLY

Amino acid residue number	Rabbit antibodies to		Mouse antibodies to	
	mouse cytochrome c	guanaco cytochrome c	rabbit cytochrome c	guanaco cytochrome c
44	++	–	++	++
62	+	++	+	++
89	++	++	++	–

Fig.8.4 Recognition of cytochrome c epitopes by rabbit and mouse polyclonal antibodies. Cytochromes c from three epitope species (rabbit, mouse and guanaco) differ from one another at only two amino acid residues each (left panel of diagram). Rabbit antibodies to mouse and guanaco and mouse antibodies to rabbit and guanaco cytochromes c were tested for their ability to bind to regions containing the varying amino acids. The results (right panel of diagram) indicated that both species produce distinct antibodies which recognize epitopes on the immunizing cytochrome c, each containing a varying amino acid (++). Interestingly, residue 62 (aspartic acid in both rabbit and mouse cytochrome c) could also be recognized by antibodies (autoantibodies) present in both the rabbit anti-mouse cytochrome c and mouse anti-rabbit cytochrome c antisera (+ shaded red).

immunized host. In most cases, species variants of a protein differ in certain amino acids, but have a highly conserved peptide backbone structure in order to maintain function. The amino acid sequence differences thus confer minor structural differences, normally on the surface of the protein. It is these regions of amino acid differences which provide immunodominant epitopes in the immunized host, since there will be more stringent control over responses to shared epitopes (see Chapter 12). However, responses to shared epitopes are often detected, particularly when there are only a few amino acid differences between the host and the immunizing proteins. A good example is cytochrome c, a small, highly conserved single chain haemoprotein of 103-111 amino acids. Rabbit, mouse and guanaco (a type of llama) cytochromes c differ from each other at only two residues, as shown in Figure 8.4. Rabbit antisera to mouse and guanaco cytochromes c, and mouse antisera to rabbit and guanaco cytochromes c in each case had antibodies reacting to the appropriate regions containing the varying amino acids. In addition, antibodies specific for the region of residue 62 were found in both rabbit anti-mouse and mouse anti-rabbit cytochrome c antisera, even though both have aspartic acid at this residue. Rabbit antibodies raised to pigeon cytochrome c were found to be directed against four sites in the molecule, and these involved all seven of the amino acids differing between the host and the immunizing protein. These and other similar observations indicate that most amino acid substitutions in proteins have the potential to be detected immunologically. It has been suggested that amino acid sequence variations could influence the antigenicity of distant epitopes by long-range conformational changes, such as occur in allosteric interactions (for example, aspartate transcarbamylase or haemoglobin). However, this is probably uncommon as most evolutionary sequence changes appear to produce only local conformational changes leaving distant epitopes unaltered.

The Molecular Basis of Antigen-Antibody Interactions
Operationally, protein antigenic sites recognized by antibodies consist of three-dimensional arrays of amino acid side chains presenting particular electron cloud shapes capable of forming ionic interactions with the antibody combining site, and which require native conformation for their integrity. Recent work on the molecular basis of antigen-antibody interactions has shown that antigenicity correlates with a relatively high local mobility in those regions of the protein molecule. Although many antibodies directed against antigenic peptides fail to bind the native protein, those that do so appear to bind to regions of local flexibility. The observations underlying these conclusions will now be discussed.

X-ray crystallographic studies of protein molecules can identify individual atoms and provide information on the relative mobility (degree of freedom from conformational constraints) of these atoms in the form of atomic temperature factors. High temperature factors reflect regions of high mobility, as there are lower energy barriers between different conformations at biological temperatures. Conversely, regions of low mobility have low temperature factors, as more energy is required to move from one conformation to another. For simplicity, regions of high and low mobility are termed 'hot' and 'cold' respectively. Recent studies indicate that many protein antigenic determinants are located in the 'hot' regions of the molecule.

One particularly thorough study by Lerner and colleagues utilized myohaemerythrin (MHr) as a model antigen.

MHr is an invertebrate oxygen-carrying molecule of 118 amino acids, with two iron atoms at the active site, whose three-dimensional structure has been well characterized. Furthermore, the temperature factors related to this protein indicate that it has surface areas of both low and high mobility, including contiguous regions. Peptides of 10-14 amino acids representing different regions of the MHr molecule were synthesized, coupled to carrier proteins and used to immunize rabbits. The resulting antisera were then tested for their ability to react with the immunizing peptide and the native MHr molecule. As shown in Figure 8.5, only antisera raised to 'hot' peptides were able to interact significantly with the intact protein, although all except one (42-51, which was apparently non-immunogenic) reacted well with the immunizing peptide. A similar study by Westhoff and colleagues of tobacco mosaic virus coat protein (TMV) showed that the seven contiguous epitopes identified on the molecule were all localized to 'hot' regions.

Retrospective studies of previously well characterized antigenic sites in proteins such as myoglobin, lysozyme, insulin and lactate dehydrogenase, have subsequently shown that these sites are often found in 'hot' regions of the molecule. Furthermore, the ability of anti-peptide antibodies to bind native protein appears to correlate better with the mobility of the target sites than with the surface exposure of these sites. In fact, it has been suggested that the relationship between surface exposure and antigenicity at least partly reflects the increased mobility of loops and turns in exposed areas. In addition, many antigenic determinants involve N- and C-terminal residues (for example, cytochrome c and bovine pancreatic ribonuclease), and these regions frequently have a high intrinsic mobility.

Because it is difficult, or even impossible, to crystallize most proteins for X-ray studies, accurate information on site mobility is at present restricted to a few model proteins. However, reasonable predictions of sites of high mobility can be made through analysis of secondary structures and hydrophilicity profiles of molecules whose tertiary structure is known. For other proteins, clues might be gleaned through studies at the DNA level, as amino acid residues encoded at exon-intron boundaries are often associated with relatively high mobility.

The realization that mobility of amino acid side chains is associated with antigenicity has led to the suggestion that the old idea of antibody binding to antigen through an 'induced fit', represented originally as a conformational change in the antibody, might in fact be partly true, but with conformational changes also occurring in the antigen. It is clear that major rearrangements of protein tertiary structure do not occur following binding of antibody. However, some recent experiments support the view that small local conformational changes in the antigen and/or antibody may take place in some instances and lead to an improved complementarity between antibody and antigen. For example, the binding of antibodies raised to a modified form of myoglobin (apomyoglobin) provokes conformational changes resulting in the release of haem when bound to myoglobin itself. X-ray crystallographic studies of the binding of N-formylated peptides to a model binding site created in a light chain dimer indicated that these peptides assume the best conformation to fit with the antibody. In addition, the antibody binding site undergoes

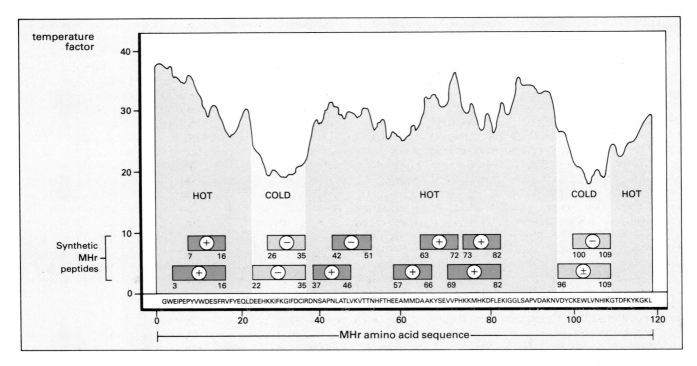

Fig.8.5 Correlation of antigenicity of peptides of myohaemerythrin (MHr) with regions of high atomic mobility. Temperature factors (as a measure of relative atomic mobility) are plotted against the sequence of the myohaemerythrin polypeptide chain. Peptides of ten to fourteen amino acids representing different areas of the molecule (sequence-numbered bars) were synthesized, coupled to carrier proteins and used to immunize rabbits. The antisera thus obtained were then tested for their ability to bind the immunizing peptide and the native myohaemerythrin molecule. Whilst all but one (42–51, which was apparently non-immunogenic) reacted well with the appropriate peptide, only the antisera raised to peptides from 'hot' regions of the molecule (red bars) were significantly positive (+) with MHr. Peptides representing 'cold' regions (grey bars) were either negative (−) or only marginally positive (+/−). The one-letter code used to represent the amino acid sequence of myohaemerythrin is shown in Chapter 5, Fig.5.10. Data modified from Tainer *et al.* (1984).

conformational changes to improve complementarity with the peptide. The changes involved include rotations and translations of amino acid side chains, as well as an expansion of the binding site by positional adjustments of the first, second and third hypervariable regions. Other studies of Fab binding to lysozyme have found no obvious conformational changes in the antigen. For example, one crystallographic study, utilizing a monoclonal Fab with high affinity for HEL, showed that the binding site interacted with a large area of the surface of the molecule with Gln 121 essential for binding. This region of HEL is not one of the highly mobile regions, therefore it may not be surprising that there was no evidence for 'induced fit'. This may well turn out to be an exception, as many other Fab molecules could not be studied because they did not form proper crystals; perhaps they were unable to do so precisely because of their binding to mobile regions of the antigen. Binding of antibody to a mobile site will involve a reduction of its conformational freedom at the expense of its association energy. Thus, antibody binding to rigid sites will be stronger, but mobility has the advantage of allowing small shifts in conformation to improve the complementarity of binding.

It seems likely that there exists a spectrum of antigenic sites on most protein antigens, with rigid and highly mobile regions thought to be the more extreme cases. However, which type of antigenic site finally dominates will be dependent on the regulatory elements directing the immune response.

The recognition of antigen by antibodies can now be viewed as a multistep process, rather than as a simple lock-and-key complementarity. At least three stages have been suggested to be involved: firstly, electrostatic forces and perhaps the breaking of salt bridges in the protein serve to orient the antibody to the epitope. Secondly, specific amino acids interact through their side chains, and this may be followed by an induced fit involving small local changes in both epitope and paratope.

EPITOPES RECOGNIZED BY T CELLS

Most T cells respond to antigen when it is associated with MHC proteins. T_H cells only respond when antigen is presented to them in association with the appropriate class II molecule, whereas cytotoxic T cells generally utilize MHC class I molecules. In view of this, it is not surprising that antigenic determinants recognized by T cells are often quite different from those reacting with antibody. As an exception, some suppressor T cells can apparently bind specifically to free antigen, but as yet the mechanism whereby Ts cells respond to antigen is uncertain.

Early experiments using polyclonal T cell populations indicated that native, denatured and often fragmented forms of the antigen could be recognized by many T cells. It later became apparent that this reflected the requirement of many T cells that the antigen is processed into a form that can interact appropriately with MHC proteins, and subsequently interact with the T cell receptor (see Chapter 6). In this section, discussion will be confined to which regions of proteins are involved in activating Tн cells (referred to as 'T cell epitopes' for convenience), either because they directly interact with the T cell receptor or because they are important for other reasons (i.e. interacting with class II molecules). The recognition of antigens by cytotoxic T cells has been dealt with in the previous chapter; information concerning antigen processing and presentation, including the association of antigen with class II molecules, has been covered in Chapter 6.

The recent advent of techniques for obtaining monoclonal T cell populations, coupled with the use of model protein antigens, has rapidly advanced our understanding of antigen recognition by Tн cells. However, because recognition necessarily involves a three-way interaction between antigen, class II molecule and the T cell receptor (as far as it is known there is no secreted form of the T cell receptor), no simple ligand-binding assay yet exists. Instead, biological responses of the T cells, such as proliferation or IL-2 secretion, have to be used as a measure of antigen recognition. Thus, it will be some time before molecular information, akin to that available for antigen-antibody interactions, will be obtained for T cell-class II-antigen interactions.

The same model proteins used to study epitopes recognized by antibody are often used to investigate T cell epitopes, and for the same reasons. It is clear that different regions of a protein are recognized by the T cells of different species and even individuals within a species. For example, mice of different MHC haplotypes recognize a distinct epitope or epitopes on HEL. Tн cells of H-2^b strains predominantly respond to a determinant(s) in the region of amino acids 74-96, whereas Tн cells from H-2^d mice mainly recognize an epitope involving amino acids 113 and 114 (see Fig.8.2).

The epitopes recognized by T cells are, in many cases, different from the antibody-reactive determinants on the same molecule, and are quite often fewer. The epitopic specificities of predominant Tн cells can significantly influence the specificity of the B cells stimulated to produce antibody during the immune response. The B cell specificity might equally well influence the Tн cell specificity if it is involved in presenting antigen during the response. This would occur if the processing is influenced by antigen being complexed with a surface Ig molecule (see Chapter 6). When the immunizing antigen is very closely related to an equivalent host protein, as with cytochrome c, predominant T and B cells may see the same region of the protein. However, even in these cases the conformational requirements will probably differ because the T cells need to see the epitope in association with class II antigens.

Studies on lysozyme, β-galactosidase, myelin basic protein and others indicate that epitopes recognized by Tн and Ts cells are also different in many cases. Ts cells reacting to HEL, in non-responder B10 (H-2^b) mice, recognize a single determinant contained within the N-C peptide region of the molecule (see Fig.8.2), requiring the N-terminal tripeptide Lys-Val-Phe. These suppressor cells dominate the response of B10 mice to HEL so that Tн cell activation is blocked. Removal of this tripeptide with aminopeptidase, or replacing the Phe with Tyr (as found in the related ring-necked pheasant lysozyme), changes the molecule such that it no longer induces suppression but is able to activate Tн cells reactive to other regions of the

molecule; it is also still able to bind most monoclonal antibodies to HEL. This same region of the molecule was also found to be a Ts determinant involved in maintaining experimentally induced tolerance in responder B10.A (H-2^a) mice.

Because many T cell epitopes remain intact in small peptide segments of the antigen, it is possible to synthesize peptides of different sizes and to change various amino acids in order to investigate the requirements for activity. This is well illustrated in studies of Berzofsky on sperm whale myoglobin. Mice of the B10.D2 (H-2^b) strain have T cells which recognize an immunodominant epitope centred around Glu 109 in the amino acid sequence, and others reactive to a minor determinant around Lys 140.

Myoglobin peptide	Reactivity with T cell clones
132 134 136 138 140 142 144 146	
N K A L E L F R K D I A A K Y	++
K A L E L F R K D I A A K Y	++
A L E L F R K D I A A K Y	+
E L F R K D I A A K Y	+
L F R K D I A A K Y	−
N K A L E L F R K D I A A K	++
N K A L E L F R K D I A A	−

Fig.8.6 Reactivity of T cells of B10.D2 (H−2^b) mice with synthetic peptides of sperm whale myoglobin. T cell clones, reactive with a determinant centred around a lysine at position 140, were tested (in a proliferation assay) for their ability to respond to different synthetic peptides of myoglobin (shown in sequence-numbered one-letter code). Results are represented as very positive (++), positive but requiring high doses of peptide (+) and negative (−). The figure shows that, whilst Lys 140 is known to be recognized by these T cells, other amino acids (Lys 133, Glu 136 and Lys 145) are also important for the antigenicity of this epitope. The importance of these amino acid residues may be for stabilizing the peptide in the correct conformation for interacting with the T cell receptor and/or the class II MHC molecule.

The use of different synthetic peptides of the Lys 140 region of myoglobin has indicated that Lys 133, Glu 136, Lys 140 and Lys 145 are all important in the antigenicity of this particular epitope (Fig.8.6).

Similar studies by Schwartz and colleagues on cytochrome c have also provided useful information on the nature of structures recognized by T cells. In B10.A (H-2^a) mice, the T cell response to pigeon cytochrome c is directed largely towards an epitope at the C terminus of the molecule. In this case, lysine at position 99 appears to be critical for interaction with the T cell receptor. In addition, amino acids at position 103 and 104 appear to be important for T cell stimulation, but in this case they were found to be necessary for the peptide to interact with the class II MHC molecule (a possible 'agretope'; Chapter 6). By using synthetic peptides of different lengths to stimulate a cytochrome c-reactive T cell clone, the minimum size of the epitope appeared to be the seven amino acids 97-103. However, the addition of further residues to the N terminus led to a marked increase in the stimulatory potency of the peptides (Fig.8.7). Residue 95 appeared to have the greatest effect, but there was considerable flexibility in the choice of amino acid. Replacement of isoleucine with large, uncharged amino acids such as valine and phenylalanine had little effect, but charged molecules such as glutamic acid or lysine markedly reduced the efficacy of the peptide. Since the T cell clone could clearly be stimulated by peptide 97-103, although at high concentrations, residues at positions 95 and 96 were clearly not essential for binding to either the T cell receptor

or the class II molecule. Why, therefore, are these amino acids important? Computer-assisted calculations for predicting preferred conformations indicate that peptide 94-103 assumes an α-helical configuration, whereas 99-103 (still containing the T cell and class II contact amino acids) does not. This suggests that residues 94-98 are stabilizing an α-helical configuration required for correctly orientating the contact residues. Subsequent measurements of the various peptides to ascertain their percentage α-helical configuration (using circular dichroism) have shown that antigenicity does, indeed, correlate with the increased α-helical content of longer peptides. This would also account for the increased antigenicity of 89-103 over 94-103.

Fig.8.7 Amino acid requirements for an epitope recognized by a pigeon cytochrome c specific T cell clone. Synthetic peptides of different lengths (shown in one-letter code) representing part of the C-terminal region of pigeon cytochrome c were used to stimulate a specific T cell clone from a B10.A (H-2ᵃ) mouse. The response of the cloned T cells (measured in a proliferation assay) to the different peptides is shown as dose-response curves (upper panel) and summarized (lower panel) as the potency relative to the longest peptide (89-103). This value (relative potency) is calculated as the ratio of the peptide concentrations required to give a response of 100,000 c.p.m. The lysine (K) residue (shaded red) is known to be critical for this epitope to interact with the T cell receptor of this clone. Peptide 98-103 did not stimulate the clone at any concentration N.R. (not recognized). The shortest peptide to stimulate the clone was 7 amino acids in length (97-103). However, the addition of two amino acids to the N-terminal region (peptide 95-103) led to a marked increase in potency of the peptide. Changing the N-terminal isoleucine (I) residue of peptide 95-103 to a range of different amino acids (shown only in lower panel) had a variable effect on the potency of the peptide. Large uncharged residues, such as valine (V) and phenylalanine (F), had little effect, whereas charged amino acids such as glutamic acid (E) and lysine (K) markedly reduced the potency of the peptide. Since residue 95 is clearly not essential for activity of the peptide (peptide 97-103 is still active, albeit at high concentration), it is thought to be important for stabilizing the peptide in the best conformation for contacting the T cell receptor and/or MHC class II molecules. Based on the data of Schwartz et al., 1985.

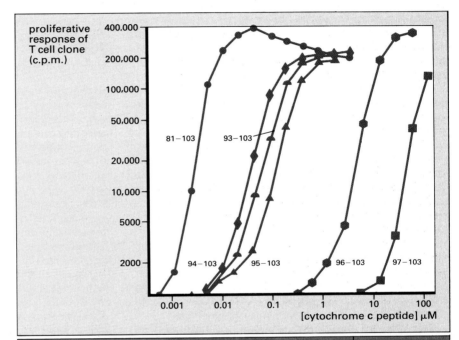

Amino acid sequence of peptide		Relative potency
81 83 85 87 89 91 93 95 97 99 101 103 V F A G L K K A N E R A D L I A Y L K Q A T K		1
98-103 L K Q A T K		N.R.
97-103 Y L K Q A T K		9500
96-103 A Y L K Q A T K		1400
95-103 I A Y L K Q A T K		26
94-103 L I A Y L K Q A T K		7
93-103 D L I A Y L K Q A T K		20
95V-103 V A Y L K Q A T K		23
95F-103 F A Y L K Q A T K		65
95M-103 M A Y L K Q A T K		338
95Q-103 Q A Y L K Q A T K		172
95E-103 E A Y L K Q A T K		1508
95K-103 K A Y L K Q A T K		7150

Data on the myoglobin T cell epitope centred on Lys 140 (see Fig.8.6) can also be explained in a similar way, as can the other major myoglobin epitope recognized by H-2^b mice (centred on Glu 109). In these cases, the appropriate peptides may fold into an amphipathic α-helix; this has hydrophilic amino acid side chains on one side of the structure and hydrophobic side chains on the other. It has been suggested that this type of structure (or amphipathic β-turns) is common to many T cell epitopes. Indeed, analysis of known T cell epitopes on HEL, cytochrome c, ovalbumin and insulin has shown that a number of them have the right periodicity of hydrophilic and hydrophobic amino acids to adopt amphipathic conformations when isolated from the native molecule (which perhaps resembles more closely the 'processed' form of the antigen). However, this is not uniformly true, as some known T cell epitopes (such as on the influenza virus haemagglutinin) do not fit this model. It is also clear that not all potentially amphipathic regions of a molecule provide T cell epitopes.

Although the T cell epitopes of many proteins appear to be dependent only on the linear peptide sequence, tertiary structure may also be important in some cases. For instance, recent studies wth pig insulin-reactive T cell hybridomas have indicated that a particular conformation in the native molecule is important. In addition, some cytotoxic T cells have been shown to recognize conformational determinants on class I molecules. In view of these observations, and of the requirements for antigen/class II interaction in stimulating T$_H$ cells (discussed below), it is most likely that T cells, like antibody, actually recognize a conformational structure. However, in the case of T$_H$ cells this is a composite of antigen and class II molecules. Whether or not an antigen is seen in native or fragmented (processed) form(s) would, thus, depend on which forms are most capable of associating with class II MHC molecules to provide a suitable composite determinant.

It is apparent that there are more constraints on the regions of a protein capable of stimulating T cells, and this may be one reason why there are often fewer T cell epitopes than B cell epitopes. Perhaps one or two MHC haplotype/T cell epitope combinations are so strongly favoured that other possible combinations do not form to a significant degree. Amino acid residues in the region of the epitope can be important for at least three reasons. Firstly, they may be critical for contacting the T cell receptor along with appropriate regions of the MHC protein: this would be considered as the true epitopic region. Secondly, certain regions may be required for interaction with the class II molecule ('agretopes'). Finally, other amino acids

may be important for stabilizing the epitope in the best configuration (for instance, an α-helix), in order to make contact with both the class II molecule and the T cell receptor. Other regions of the native protein could also influence which of the potential T cell epitopes are recognized. For example, it has been suggested that certain regions of the protein constitute 'processing determinants' in that they somehow influence the way the protein is processed and presented to T cells. Obvious candidates for such determinants would be enzyme cleavage sites. Finally, it must be emphasized that, as with the antibody response, host regulatory mechanisms influence T cell responses in such a way that certain epitopes dominate. The final outcome of the response will depend on whether this determinant stimulates T$_S$ or T$_H$ cells (see Chapter 10).

SUMMARY

Both B and T cells can recognize antigenic determinants of proteins. The number of potential antigenic determinants which could be recognized by antibody is generally large, covering the entire surface of the molecule. Most of these determinants require intact conformation, as they consist of a three-dimensional array of amino acid side chains assembled at the surface by folding of the protein chain. Antibodies to native proteins will only bind to peptides of the molecule if these peptides are capable of retaining or adopting the correct conformation. T cells also recognize conformational determinants, but in this case they are usually formed by interactions between the protein (often in a 'processed' form) and the appropriate MHC molecule. T cells, like antibody, are highly specific in their ability to distinguish single amino acid differences. Certain regions of the molecule, closely associated with the true epitope, are also important in stimulating T cells because they interact with class II molecules, or enable the processed antigen to adopt the correct configuration for interacting with the T cell receptor and the MHC molecule.

Although the potential repertoire of antigenic determinants is large, particularly with respect to antibody, the response of an individual is normally skewed such that certain epitopes are dominant. Which regions dominate depends on structural differences between the immunizing antigen and the hosts' proteins, as well as the complex regulatory mechanisms employed by the immune system to direct and control the response. Dominant epitopes recognized by T and B cells can also influence the selection of responding B and T cells respectively.

FURTHER READING

Ada G. & Skehel J.J. (1985) *Are peptides good antigens?* Nature **316**, 764.

Allen P.M., McKean D.J., Beck B.N., Sheffield J. & Glimcher L.H. (1985) *Direct evidence that a class II molecule and a single globular protein generate multiple determinants.* J. Exp. Med. **162**, 1264.

Atassi M.Z. (1984) *Antigenic structures of proteins. Their determination has revealed important aspects of immune recognition and generated strategies for synthetic mimicking of protein binding sites.* Eur. J. Biochem. **145**, 1.

Benjamin D.C., Berzofsky J.A., East I.J., Gurd F.R.N., Hannum C., Leach S.J., Margoliash E., Michael J.G., Miller A., Prager E.M., Reichlin M., Sercarz E.E., Smith-Gill J.J., Todd P.E. & Wilson A.C. (1984) *The antigenic structure of proteins: a reappraisal.* Ann. Rev. Immunol. **2**, 67.

Berkower I., Kawamura H., Matis L.A & Berzofsky J.A., (1985) *T cell clones to two major T cell epitopes of myoglobin: effect of I-A/I-E restriction on epitope dominance.* J. Immunol. **135**, 2628.

Carbone F.R. & Paterson Y. (1985) *Monoclonal antibodies to horse cytochrome c expressing four distinct idiotypes distribute among two sites on the native protein.* J. Immunol. **135**, 2609.

Darsley M.J. & Rees A.R. (1985) *Three distinct epitopes within the loop region of hen egg white lysozyme defined with monoclonal antibodies.* EMBO J. **2**, 383.

Fotedar A., Boyer M., Smart W., Widtman J., Fraga E. & Singh B. (1985) *Fine specificity of antigen recognition by T cell hybridoma clones specific for poly-18: a synthetic polypeptide antigen of defined sequence and conformation.* J. Immunol. **135**, 3028.

Geysen H.M. (1985) *Antigen-antibody interactions at the molecular level: adventures in peptide synthesis.* Immunology Today **6**, 364.

Glimcher L.H., Schroer J.A., Chan C. & Shevach E.M. (1983) *Fine specificity of cloned insulin-specific T cell hybridomas: evidence supporting a role for tertiary conformation.* J. Immunol. **131**, 2868.

Hannum C.H. & Margoliash E. (1985) *Assembled topographic antigenic determinants of pigeon cytochrome c.* J. Immunol. **135**, 3303.

Hannum C.H., Matis L.A., Schwartz R.H. & Margoliash E. (1985) *The B10.A mouse B cell response to pigeon cytochrome c is directed against the same area of the protein that is recognized by B10.A T cells in association with the $E^k_\beta:E^k_\alpha$ Ia molecule.* J. Immunol. **135**, 3314.

Oki A. & Sercarz E.E. (1985) *T cell tolerance studied at the level of antigenic determinants. I. Latent reactivity to lysozyme peptides that lack suppressogenic epitopes can be revealed in lysozyme-tolerant mice.* J. Exp. Med. **161**, 897.

Schulze-Gahmer U., Prinz H., Glatter U. & Beyreuther K. (1985) *Towards assignment of secondary structures by anti-peptide antibodies. Specificity of the immune response to a β-turn.* EMBO J. **4**, 1731.

Schwartz R.H., Fox B.S., Fraga E., Chen C. & Singh B. (1985) *The T lymphocyte response to cytochrome c.V. Determination of the minimal peptide size required for stimulation of T cell clones and assessment of the contribution of each residue beyond this size to antigenic potency.* J. Immunol. **135**, 2598.

Sercarz E.E., Yowell R.L., Turkin D. , Miller A., Araneo B.A. & Adorini L. (1978) *Different functional specificity repertoires for suppressor and helper T cells.* Immunol. Rev. **39**, 108.

Shastri N., Miller A. & Sercarz E.E. (1984) *The expressed T cell repertoire is hierarchical: the precise focus of lysozyme-specific T cell clones is dependent upon the structure of the immunogen.* J. Mol. Cell Immunol. **1**, 369.

Tainer J.A., Getzoff E.D., Paterson Y., Olson A.J. & Lerner R.A. (1985) *The atomic mobility component of protein antigenicity.* Ann. Rev. Immunol. **3**, 501.

Tainer J.A., Getzoff E.D., Alexander H., Houghten R.A., Olson A.J. & Lerner R.A. (1984) *The reactivity of anti-peptide antibodies is a function of the atomic mobility of sites in a protein.* Nature **312**, 127.

9 Immune Recognition of Pathogens

When the immune response against a single antigen is compared to that against a microorganism, it soon becomes evident that the reaction to microorganisms is generally very complex. Even the simplest viruses express several different antigens, and eukaryotic parasites can have hundreds of different antigens on their surface. Each of these molecules contains several epitopes, sometimes repeated (as in the case of bacterial carbohydrates) and sometimes distinct. It has been shown (Chapter 8) that T and B cells usually recognize different parts of a particular antigen, and the same is true for recognition of antigens on microorganisms. There is an additional complication associated with the antigens of pathogens in that a molecule expressing several epitopes in solution may only express one or two when the same molecule is set in a particular orientation on the pathogen's surface.

It is clear that the immune response to each individual pathogen is a major area of study in its own right. Nevertheless, this chapter aims to bring together some of the unifying principles governing the development of antibody and cell-mediated immune responses to pathogens, by reference to particular examples. A distinction should be drawn at this stage between the overall composition of the immune response and those components which are important in the resolution of infection, as well as the components which are responsible for the prevention of reinfection. In many cases, particular elements of the immune response are critically important; for example, cell-mediated immunity in leprosy. Even when considering a particular effector system, the response directed against some antigens is often much more effective than that directed to others. Sometimes the response may be only marginally beneficial, or even positively detrimental. Detrimental immune responses may be broadly divided into two categories: a) where they prevent other elements of the immune system from engaging the pathogen effectively, and b) where they induce greater damage to the host than that caused by the organism itself, that is, autoimmunity and hypersensitivity. In other words, immune responses to particular microbial antigens have different degrees of relevance to antimicrobial immunity, depending on the nature of the organism, its pathogenicity, and the nature of the immune response it initiates.

A further complication is added by the organisms themselves: apart from their basic antigenic complexity, their antigenic composition is not always stable. Organisms which have a stable structure survive by evading the immune response as a whole, by localizing inside cells (for example, the prions of Scrapie), by lurking on the periphery of the body (for instance, superficial fungi), or by relying on a sufficiently large population of non-immune individuals to allow continuous cycles of acute infection in different subjects (for example, measles). The alternative route to pathogen survival is evasion of immune effector systems by changing surface antigens. Sometimes this occurs at the level of the pathogen population (as in the case of influenza); in other cases, individual pathogens have the capacity to switch their surface antigens during their own life cycle (for instance, African trypanosomes). Selective pressure from the host immune system favours modulation of the parasites' surface antigens to allow survival in the host. Consequently, the continuous battle between microorganisms and the corporate immune system of the host population provides the driving force for evolution of the parasites and the selective pressure for improvement of the immune system. Theoretically, the rapid evolution rate of microorganisms should allow them to quickly evolve in order to evade the body's defences, but the enormous flexibility of the immune system, intrinsic in the T and B cell antigen receptors, prevents them from gaining the upper hand.

CRITICAL SITES

Immune responses directed towards some antigens on a pathogen are more effective than the responses to others, in bringing about destruction of that pathogen. Such antigens are termed 'critical sites'. This concept is well illustrated when considering viruses. Viruses have both internal and external protein antigens. The internal antigens are most often associated with the viral nucleic acid, or they form part of the internal structure of the virus; they may also be viral proteins required for the initiation of an infective cycle within the cell (for example, nucleic acid polymerases). The external antigens include the outer coat, or envelope proteins, of the virus: particularly important here are the proteins required for attachment to the host cell (Fig. 9.1 overpage).

Since attachment to the host cell is the very first step in the viral replicative cycle, antibodies directed towards these proteins are most effective in preventing transmission of the virus to new cells. Different viruses attach to their target cells via different cell surface molecules. For example, HIV (the causative agent of AIDS) attaches to helper T cells via the T4 molecule, while Epstein-Barr virus attaches to human B cells via their C3b receptor. The influenza A virus attaches to a number of cell types via the haemagglutinin molecule in its envelope. Antibodies directed towards the haemagglutinin are most effective at preventing infection of a cell and reinfection of an individual by the same strain of influenza. By comparison, antibodies to the neuraminidase, which is also present in the envelope, are less effective at neutralizing viral infectivity, and antibodies to the internal M protein are virtually ineffective. For the same reason, the haemagglutinin molecule is most subject to variation in different strains of influenza, the neuraminidase less so, and the M protein not at all.

It is also possible to pinpoint critical antigens on some bacteria. The simplest examples are the toxins produced by the causative agents of diphtheria and tetanus, and by

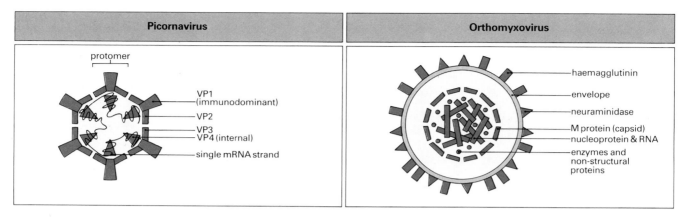

Fig.9.1 Antigenic structure of viruses. The antigens of a non-enveloped and an enveloped virus are illustrated diagramatically. Picornaviruses have a capsid consisting of only four proteins (VP1-VP4) arranged as 60 protomers, and contain a single RNA strand. Neutralizing antibodies bind to the external proteins, particularly VP1, while VP4, which is associated with the RNA, is not normally accessible to antibody. Orthomyxoviruses (here represented by influenza A) have a core containing nucleocapsid associated with RNA and several non-structural proteins. This is enclosed in a capsid consisting of the M protein, which is in turn surrounded by an envelope derived from the host cell plasma membrane. The envelope contains two viral proteins, the haemagglutinin and neuraminidase. Neutralizing antibodies recognize epitopes on the haemagglutinin, although antibody to the neuraminidase can also contribute to immunity.

enteric clostridia. The damage produced directly by the infectious agent in these diseases is slight in comparison with that produced by the secreted toxins. Consequently, immunization against these agents involves vaccination with toxoids. Nevertheless, the immune system must still eradicate the primary site of the bacterial infection if the disease is to be resolved. The target antigens for bactericidal antibodies are extremely diverse. These antigens include lipopolysaccharides (LPS), capsular polysaccharides and other outer membrane proteins. Many of the enterobacteria have a common antigen in their outer membrane which can be the target of antibody-mediated attack. When considering the important target antigens on these bacteria, the prime effector system in bacterial lysis or cytostasis must be taken into account. Complement-mediated damage to the outer membrane of Gram-negative bacteria is particularly important in the resolution of infections with these organisms. For this reason, antibodies directed towards proteins in the outer membrane are often most effective. By comparison, antibodies to flagellae or pilae are often ineffective, since these structures are too far from the outer membrane to precipitate classical pathway complement-mediated attack on the outer membrane. In this case, the effectiveness of the antibodies is limited by the range (related to half-life) of activated C4b and C3b. Bacterial defence systems, such as capsules and surface polysaccharide chains, also play a large part in determining the susceptibility of bacteria to antibody/complement-mediated damage.

Immune recognition of parasites is extremely complex, due to their diverse surface antigens and life cycles. Nevertheless, the antibody response to some antigens appears to be more effective than to others. Taking *Plasmodium falciparum* as an example, it is found that hyperimmune antiserum to this malarial parasite precipitates at least 21 separate proteins when the precipitated antigens are analysed by polyacrylamide gel electrophoresis in the presence of SDS (SDS PAGE). Of these, eight are schizont-specific antigens (the infected red cell stage), and are not found on the parasites at other stages of their life cycle. The reaction spectra of these immune sera differ for parasites cultured *in vitro* and for those that are freshly isolated. It is difficult to assess which of these antibodies are critical in host defence, as IgG fractions of immune sera which inhibit parasite growth *in vitro* are ineffective in preventing infection in squirrel monkeys. However, sera which are most effective at conveying immunity to the monkeys precipitated antigens of molecular weights 96, 90 and 72 kD.

P. falciparum infection has certain similarities to viral infection, since the parasite must enter the host red cells to complete its life cycle. The attachment phase is mediated by a protein consisting of two peptides (155 and 133kD), which binds to glycophorin on the surface of the red cell. There are 5000 such proteins on the surface of a merozoite (red cell infective stage), and both free glycophorin and antibody to the glycophorin-binding protein inhibit merozoite invasion of red cells. When considering *P. knowlesi* it is found that antibody to a 66 kD protein is capable of stopping red cell invasion. In this case, however, it has been shown that mouse monoclonal antibody to the protein can block infection, while rabbit polyclonal antibody to the same protein cannot. This indicates that even when an animal produces antibodies to a critical antigen, some may be more effective than others by virtue of being directed towards critical epitopes on that antigen. Other stages of malaria parasite life cycles are also susceptible to immune protection by antibodies. Some of these inhibit growth of the parasite within the red cell, others block different stages of the parasite life cycle (see below), and others can outmanoeuvre the parasite's own defence mechanisms. An example of this is again seen with *P. falciparum*: it is thought that in this disease infected red cells may be destroyed in the spleen and liver. The parasite has developed a way of avoiding this by placing proteins on the surface of the infected red cell, which cause it to attach to the venous endothelium and thus prevent passage of the infected cell through the spleen. Red cells with this capacity have small knobs on their surface. Sera which block this antigen reverse the adherence to the endothelium and permit the parasitized cell to be cleared by cell-mediated immune effector systems in the spleen.

LOCATION OF EPITOPES

Recent advances in our knowledge of the structure of some animal viruses have made it possible to locate the precise antibody binding sites on these viruses. One of the first to be thoroughly examined was human rhinovirus 14. This cold virus is a member of the picornaviruses which include the causative viruses of polio and foot-and-mouth disease (FMDV). They have a relatively simple structure consisting of a protein capsid containing a strand of RNA associated with an internal protein. Rhinovirus 14 (HRV) has 60 protomers, each consisting of only four proteins, VP1, VP2, VP3 and VP4; VP2 and VP4 are generated by the cleavage of a larger polypeptide, VP0, at the time of virion assembly. This occurs when the RNA is inserted into the developing capsid, and VP4 is associated with this RNA on the inside of the capsid. As it is normally inaccessible to antibody, VP4 may be considered a non-critical antigen (see Fig.9.1).

The main strategy for locating epitopes on viruses is to culture the virus in the presence of a monoclonal antibody, and to isolate mutant strains which develop in spite of the antibody. The rationale behind this procedure is as follows: wild type virus is unable to develop in the presence of neutralizing monoclonal antibody to one of its critical antigens, but if a mutation should occur in this antigen at the epitope, then the neutralizing antibody will no longer be able to bind and the mutant virus will proliferate. When the amino acid sequences of the wild type and mutant viruses are compared, they will differ at only one position (usually) and, by implication, this is one of the residues which constitute the epitope in the wild strain. This strategy has been used to identify the epitopes of HRV and those of the influenza haemagglutinin.

When this technique is applied to the proteins of HRV, four epitopes are identified (Fig.9.2). Two of these are on VP1, one on VP2 and one on VP3. As might be anticipated from its internal position in the virion, these neutralizing antibodies do not bind VP4. Furthermore, when the location of the epitopes is seen in relation to the overall virion structure, it is immediately apparent that each of the epitopes is on the outside of the capsid. None face the RNA core (Fig.9.3). Of the two sites on VP1, one of them is constituted of a single peptide loop, whereas the other

Epitope-associated mutations	Amino acid number	Wild type	Observed mutations
NIm–IA			
VP1	91	D	A,E,G,H,N,V,Y
VP1	95	E	G,K
NIm–IB			
VP1	83	Q	H
VP1	85	K	N
VP1	138	D	E, G
VP1	139	S	P
NIm–II			
VP2	158	S	F
VP2	159	A	V
VP2	161	E	D, V*, K
VP2	162	V	M, A*
VP2	136	E	G
NIm–III			
VP3	72	N	I
VP3	75	R	G, K, M
VP3	78	E	K, V
VP1	287	K	I
VP3	203	G	D

Fig.9.2 Identification of antiviral antibody-binding sites on a human rhinovirus. Binding sites for antibodies on a human rhinovirus were determined by antibody-induced selection of mutants. This technique identifies four epitopes on the virus, two on VP1 (NIm-IA and NIm-IB) and one each on VP2 and VP3 (NIm-II and NIm-III). The amino acid sequence of viral mutants which fail to bind monoclonal antibodies directed to these epitopes is compared with that of the wild type virus which does bind the antibodies; e.g. one set of variants has a change at position 91 of VP1, while another set of variants has mutations at position 95. The amino acid in the wild type (column 3) is indicated, next to those which occur in the same position in the mutants (column 4). Amino acids are shown in single letter code (see Fig.5.10). This technique identifies an epitope recognized by antibody to site NIm-IA at position 95 of VP1. There is another site in VP1 formed by residues around position 84 and 139 (NIm-IB), and also sites in VP2 and VP3, but none in VP4. In one case (*) a viral mutant contained two changes within a single epitope. From Rossman et al., 1985.

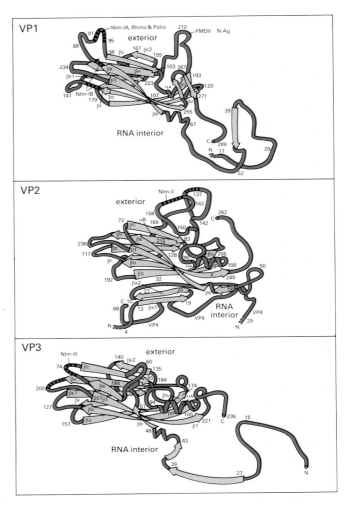

Fig.9.3 Identification of epitopes on HRV14. The locations of the epitopes on the three capsid proteins of human rhinovirus 14 are shown (NIm-IA, NIm-IB etc.). Note that each of the epitopes is on an exposed loop on the outside of the virus. Polioviruses have an epitope in an analogous position to NIm-IA, while the neutralizing antibody to foot-and-mouth disease virus (FMDV) binds elsewhere.

depends on two adjoining segments of β-pleated sheet. One can compare which parts of VP1 form epitopes on different picornaviruses, since the overall structure of this protein is very similar for different viruses. Neutralizing antibodies to poliovirus are similar to the anti-HRV antibodies, as they bind to a site around position 93. It is notable that this region forms a prominent external loop of residues in both HRV and polio. By contrast, FMDV lacks the external loop around position 93: antibodies to the immunodominant determinant of FMDV-VP1 bind to a different external loop corresponding to position 210 on HRV, and they do not neutralize FMDV. In effect, the epitope recognized by antibodies to virus proteins depends in part on the virus proteins and in part on the strain of the animal infected. In this respect the viral antigens are similar to other protein antigens.

Another feature of these viruses is worth mentioning. It has been stated that there are 60 protomers in the capsid, meaning that there are 60 sets of epitopes and 60 target cell attachment sites. Nevertheless, it is found that as few as four immunoglobulin molecules can neutralize a virion. It is quite likely that the antibody-binding sites described above do not correspond to the virus's binding site for the cell. This means that antibodies do not need to bind exactly to some functional site to neutralize the virus, nor do they need to completely coat the virus. In other words, a few antibodies are sufficient to sterically interfere with the viral life cycle, or to recruit other immune effector systems in order to destroy the virus. The same is true of antibacterial immunity; thus, it is not necessary to neutralize more than a proportion of the bacterial surface antigens to have effective immune reactions.

T AND B CELL RECOGNITION OF EPITOPES

It was shown in the previous chapter that T and B cells recognize different parts of protein antigens, reflecting the carrier/hapten recognition of artificial antigens. This can also occur with antigens from microorganisms. One example of this which has been well studied is the haemagglutinin (HA) of influenza A. The HA molecule formed by the virus is cleaved after production into two disulphide-linked subunits, HA-1 and HA-2. The HA-1 subunit binds sialic acid residues and is responsible for the binding of virus to the host cell. It contains several neutralizing epitopes identified by antibody-induced mutagenesis (see above). This technique has demonstrated four major antibody-binding regions in the head of the molecule (Fig.9.4). These regions are the most structurally diverse parts of the molecule in naturally occurring isolates of influenza which arise by a process of genetic drift, generated by the selective pressure of antibody in the host population. Of course, T and B cells cannot recognize the same molecular entity of any particular antigen, since T cell recognition is MHC-restricted whereas antibody binding is not. Nevertheless, it is valid to ask whether particular segments of the haemagglutinin contribute residues to epitopes recognized by T or B cells. To examine T cell recognition of influenza antigens, T cell clones reactive to the whole virus have been raised in mice. In one such study, 37% of TH clones recognized the matrix (M) protein, 45% the neuraminidase (NA), 9% the nucleoprotein (NP), and 9% the haemagglutinin. If this is a true reflection of the entire T cell response, it means that a

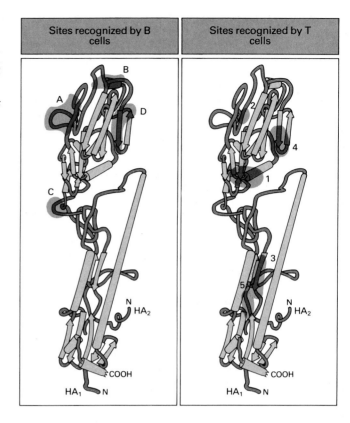

Sites recognized by B cells	Sites recognized by T cells

Fig.9.4 T and B cell recognition of influenza A haemagglutinin. The structure of the influenza haemagglutinin is shown. Antibody-binding sites on the haemagglutinin have been identified by site-induced mutagenesis. There are four such major regions in the head of the molecule (A-D). Other techniques have identified sites which are involved in T cell activation (1-5) and some have identified 'T cell epitopes' in the stalk part of the antigen, while it has also been shown that T cells can recognize the same region as B cells (i.e. site D and site 4).

substantial proportion of T cells recognize relatively invariant antigens of the virus. In fact, it has been shown that T cells specific for the M protein can help B cells specific for the haemagglutinin, so that the relative lack of HA-specific T cells may not limit the level of help delivered to HA-specific B cells. This is difficult to understand in terms of traditional models of T cell help, where B cells interact with T cells via an antigen bridge. However, if an HA-specific B cell takes up virus via its surface antibody and then processes it, it will be able to present all of the viral antigens to T cells (see Chapter 6). Consequently, it will be able to receive help from MHC-restricted TH cells specific for any of the viral antigens (not just from TH cells specific for HA).

Cytotoxic T cell clones have also been raised recognizing NP and HA. Unlike the HA-specific antibodies, HA-specific Tc cells cannot usually distinguish viral subtypes. Since antibodies to the HA do not prevent Tc cells from recognizing virally infected target cells, this also suggests that antibodies and T cells recognize different parts of the molecule. A number of T cell lines appear to react with determinants on the stalk part of the HA, nearest to the virus envelope. This region is less variable than the globular head and does not contain antibody-binding sites (see Fig.9.4). Using synthetic peptides corresponding to the putative antigenic sites, it has been found that HA-specific T cells respond to peptides equivalent to their supposed determinants, but studies using peptides which correspond to the B cell epitopes have failed to produce antibody binding. This may reflect the fact that for epitopes to be recognized by antibody greater conformational stability is often required. Other studies have shown that the T and B cell epitopes need not be different. When TH clones which were specific for the HA of strain A/X31 were isolated and then tested for reactivity against antibody-induced mutant strains, several of the mutants were unable to stimulate TH cells. This shows that alterations in the amino acids at the antibody-binding site also prevented T cells from recognizing HA. In this instance, the Asp residue at position 63 appeared to be mandatory for T cell stimulation; this residue is also an essential part of an immunodominant B cell epitope. The T cells were specifically selected on the basis of their ability to discriminate between strains, but this shows that the normal T cell response includes cells which react to the same determinants as B cells, as well as those that react elsewhere.

A similar situation occurs in the response to glycoprotein D (gD) which is present on herpes simplex virus (HSV) types I and II. This antigen induces neutralizing antibodies for both viruses and can activate T cells. Some individuals have the virus-specific T cells but lack the anti-gD antibody. An immunodominant antibody-reactive epitope of gD is formed by the N-terminal 23 amino acid residues of the protein, and this region also stimulates T cells from infected individuals. The T cell response is maximal when there are at least 16 amino acids in the stimulating peptide fragment, which must also contain the N-terminal part of this region if it is to retain full activity (Fig.9.5).

Strictly speaking, it is very difficult to determine with certainty whether particular amino acids are recognized by the T cell antigen receptor, or whether they are mandatory for some other part of the T cell recognition process. In the example below (Fig.9.5), it might at first appear that the T cell receptor binds amino acids in the first 16 residues, and that a peptide of this length is required to maintain conformation of the T cell-binding epitope. However, it is equally possible that these requirements are determined by the process of antigen presentation, that is, the antigen must be sufficiently large to be taken up by the APC, and of such a structure that it can be associated with MHC class II molecules. In other words, the apparently essential residues are not recognized by the T cell antigen receptor, but form a part of the antigen's agretope. Only if the critical residues are present will the peptide associate with MHC molecules in such a configuration as to be recognized by the T cells (see Chapters 6 and 8).

When considering simple protein antigens such as lysozyme, it is known that different T cell subpopulations recognize different parts of the molecule. This also occurs with microbial antigens, as has been demonstrated in vitro with a streptococcal protein antigen. Two antigen fragments have been obtained from the microorganism, one 4 kD and the other 185 kD. Although the level of T cell help or suppression obtained with these fragments depends on the dose used to stimulate the cells, it is notable that, using moderate antigen doses (10-100µg/ml), the 4 kD fragment induces help while the 185 kD fragment induces suppression. At high antigen doses, the 185 kD fragment induces help and its ability to induce Ts diminishes. This study suggests that the smaller fragment contains determinants which induce TH cells, but it lacks the necessary determinants to induce suppressors (either as agretopes or epitopes). The 185 kD fragment contains both helper and suppressor epitopes, and which type of cell will be induced depends on several factors. By analogy with the T cell responses to well studied antigens, it might be anticipated that the ability of B and T cells to respond to different parts of an antigen would depend on the species, the way the antigen is processed by APCs, and on the individual's MHC haplotype. That is to say, immune recognition of microorganisms is governed by the same principles which determine responses to simple antigens, and is strictly dependent on immune response genes — both those linked to the MHC and those at other loci. These factors determine the mode of the immune reaction as well as its type. In experimental systems great emphasis is placed on the level of the immune reaction, but as regards the response to microorganisms the modality is even more important, since only some of the available immune effector systems are effective against particular pathogens.

Antigen fragment		Donor reaction				
		A(+)	B(+)	C(+)	D(−)	E(−)
1–23	KYALADASLKMADPNRFRGKDLP	+	+	(+)	+	+
1–16	KYALADASLKMADPNR	+	(+)	−	+	+
1–16'	KYALAD**P**SLKMADPNR	+	(+)	−	+	−
3–23	ALADASLKMADPNRFRGKDLP	+	+	−	−	(+)
8–23	SLKMADPNRFRGKDLP	+	+	−	−	−
11–23	MADPNRFRGKDLP	−	(+)	−	−	−

Fig.9.5 T cell recognition of herpesvirus. Fragments of the N-terminal end of glycoprotein D of HSV were used to stimulate T cells from different immune donors (A-E), some with herpes-specific antibodies (+). All donors responded to a fragment containing the first 23 amino acid residues (1-23), but the precise site within the peptide appears to vary for different T cells. Donor E responds to a 16 residue fragment with aspartic acid in position 7 (1-16), but not to one with proline (1-16'), suggesting the importance of this residue for these cells; for donor D this appears unimportant, as it requires some part of the N-terminal segment (amino acids 1 and 2), although A and B do not. This suggests that antigen processing and presentation vary between individuals. From De Freitas et al., 1985.

ANTIGENIC STRUCTURE OF BACTERIA

Up to this point the discussion has centred mainly on viruses having well-defined antigens and a relatively simple structure. By comparison, bacterial cell surfaces are generally more antigenically complex, and it is often more difficult to pinpoint critical antigens for two reasons: a) bacteria usually have a greater variety of surface molecules, each of which is potentially capable of activating immune effector mechanisms, and b) the effectiveness of the immune response to bacteria is largely dependent on a balance between the activity of the appropriate immune effector systems and the protective mechanisms developed by the pathogen to deflect them.

Bacterial cell envelopes fall into three major groups: Gram-positive, Gram-negative and mycobacterial. Spirochaetes and corynebacteria have characteristics intermediate between these simple categories. All three groups have an inner cytoplasmic membrane and a peptidoglycan cell wall. Gram-negative organisms also have an outer membrane containing proteins and lipopolysaccharide (LPS; endotoxin), while mycobacteria have an outer glycolipid layer consisting of mycolic acid residues linked to arabinogalactan which is anchored to the cell wall peptidoglycan via phosphate linkages. Many bacterial species also have an outer capsule which is antiphagocytic and makes a major contribution to the virulence of the microorganism. Most bacteria, therefore, provide both carbohydrate and protein antigens for the immune system to grapple with. As in the case of viruses and parasites, those antigens which are of greatest importance in pathogen virulence (hence in host defence) are also most likely to vary between strains.

The antigenic structure of Gram-positive bacteria is exemplified by *Streptococcus pyogenes* (Fig.9.6). This bacterium often has a capsule consisting of hyaluronic acid which acts as a shield. Hyaluronic acid is a normal constituent of host connective tissue, and consequently the outer capsule of the bacterium is non-antigenic. Attached to the cell wall peptidoglycan are three major protein antigens: M, R and T, as well as the C antigen (carbohydrate). The M protein is the main target for opsonizing antibody. This protein forms the fimbriae which are antiphagocytic. Antibacterial immunity depends almost entirely on anti-M antibodies and, as might be anticipated, there are at least 55 variants of the M protein on different strains of this species. The C antigen, formed of rhamnose and N-acetyl glucosamine units, is covalently attached to the cell wall peptidoglycan and also varies, different types depending on the precise structure of the carbohydrate units in each species.

The antigenic structure of Gram-negative bacteria is illustrated by *Neisseria gonhorroeae* (see Fig.9.6). In contrast to streptococci, the capsule of the gonococcus is a polysaccharide which is antigenic and type-specific. The outer membrane contains pili formed of type-specific protein antigens. These pili have an antiphagocytic function, and they are essential for adherence of the bacteria to host cells in the urogenital tract. Invasion of epithelial cells follows the attachment. Antibodies to the pili prevent adherence and facilitate bacterial opsonization. Antibodies are also formed to the outer membrane proteins and to lipopolysaccharide endotoxin. The nature of the infection means that specific immunoglobulin A antibodies to capsule and pili are a major host defence mechanism. However, the organism's defences include an IgA-specific protease.

From these two examples it is clear that effective antibodies must be of the right class in order to activate appropriate effectors, and the important antigens are those involved in evasion of immune effector mechanisms (pili, fimbriae and capsular antigens) which constitute the major antigens of the outer layer of the bacteria. In some cases, the epitope specificity of the antibodies is also important, as it determines whether complement becomes deposited on the bacteria in a position capable of causing damage to the outer membrane. Some antibodies ('blocking antibodies') are actually detrimental to the overall immune response by

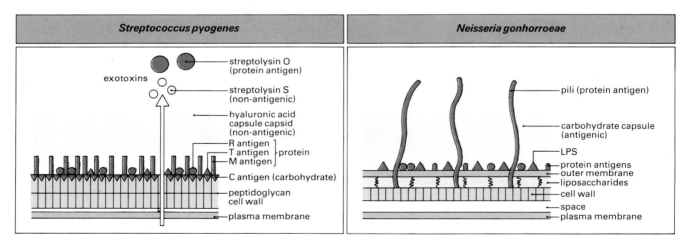

Fig.9.6 Antigenic structure of bacteria. The surface antigens of representative Gram-positive (*Streptococcus pyogenes*) and Gram-negative (*Neisseria gonhorroeae*) bacteria are shown. *S. pyogenes* has carbohydrate (C) antigens attached to its peptidoglycan cell wall and an outer set of protein antigens (M, R and T), of which the antibodies to M are most important for immunity. The antiphagocytic capsule of hyaluronic acid is non-antigenic, as is the exotoxin streptolysin S (too small to stimulate a response). Antibodies to streptolysin O also occur and can be diagnostic for infection, but they do not eliminate the bacterium. *N. gonhorroeae* has an outer membrane containing several antigenic proteins and LPS, but the important component of the antibody response is directed to the antiphagocytic carbohydrate capsule and the pili required for attachment to epithelial cells.

causing complement deposition to non-critical sites on the bacteria. Also, serum-resistant strains of enterobacteria actually evade complement-mediated damage by presenting an external surface which diverts the complement deposition from the outer membrane itself.

Mycobacteria have an unusual envelope with a surface of esterified mycolic acids. These microbes have numerous protein antigens which can induce an antibody response, but the antibody response to these bacteria is largely irrelevant to immunity. This is most obvious in lepromatous leprosy where the patients have weak cell-mediated immunity, high levels of specific antibody and tissues heavily infected with bacteria. It is difficult, if not impossible, to identify critical antigens in mycobacterial infections; PPD, an immunogenic extract of mycobacteria, contains several antigenic proteins. Surprisingly, the immune mechanisms which lead to the destruction of mycobacteria by recognition of mycobacterial antigen need not be antigen-specific. In this case, intracellular killing depends on activation of the macrophage microbicidal activity (see Chapter 15). IFN$_\gamma$ released by activated T cells stimulates macrophage oxidative metabolism, and has been shown to facilitate killing of intracellular parasites. The antigen-non-specificity of this immune effector system has been properly demonstrated using T cell lines specific for PPD, or a control antigen (thyroglobulin). It was found that PPD-specific T cells stimulated with mycobacterial antigens could induce macrophages to stop the growth of their intracellular mycobacteria, but thyroglobulin-specific T cells stimulated with thyroglobulin could also do so.

From these studies it may be concluded that, in many cases, it is not so important that the response is directed to a particular antigen but, rather, that an appropriate immune effector system is activated. This principle is critically important in the response to virtually all pathogens; indeed, the activation of an inappropriate effector mechanism can sometimes shield the pathogen from the full onslaught of the appropriate effectors.

EFFECTOR SYSTEMS

The effectiveness of the response to most bacterial and parasite pathogens depends on whether an appropriate defence system becomes activated. For example, the neutralizing antibodies to influenza surface proteins prevent reinfection of cells with that strain of virus, but they do not destroy virally infected cells. In fact, the rate of clearance of virus from the lungs of experimentally infected mice is proportional to the level of specific cytotoxic T cell activity, and does not relate to antibody levels. Furthermore, Tc cells do not generally distinguish between influenza virus strains, and as they persist for several years after infection this also shows their limited effect because reinfection in successive years is not prevented. This situation is true for many viral infections which have a viraemic phase: antibody prevents transmission between cells, while Tc cells destroy infected cells. This is quite logical in view of the way antibody and T cells recognize antigen, and it also explains why the critical antigens recognized by the antibodies (that is, HA and NA) change their structure frequently so as to evade the immune response and thus reinfect an otherwise immune host. On the other hand, some antigens recognized by Tc cells (matrix, nucleoprotein) change rarely or not at all.

In some cases, a particular type of antibody response is mandatory for clearance of the pathogen. This is true of many bacterial infections, where specific antibodies to surface antigens are necessary to neutralize the bacterial defences and opsonize the bacteria for phagocytes. This is also the case in the immune reaction to schistosomes, but here IgE antibodies are essential. Although schistosomula acquire host MHC class I and II antigens on their surface shortly after infection of a host, they are impervious to the action of Tc cells. Destruction of the parasite is effected by antibody-dependent, cell-mediated cytotoxicity (ADCC), in which the prime participants are eosinophils, macrophages and, to a lesser extent, platelets. Immune sera can mediate the ADCC, but if they are depleted of IgE they become inactive. Protective IgE antibodies have been identified which bind to a protein of molecular weight 22-26 kD. Following infection, the schistosomes are susceptible to these mechanisms for two to three days, after which time the parasites' defence mechanisms (primarily antigenic disguise) become active.

The principle in these examples is that recognition of a particular antigen is not in itself sufficient to produce an effective immune response. In some cases a cell-mediated response is appropriate, in others antibody is required. Antibody class switching gives the immune system the flexibility to activate different effector systems. The mechanisms of class switching are currently under investigation (see Chapters 2 and 4), but the way in which particular types of infection induce switching to an appropriate subclass is still tantalizingly obscure.

ANTIGENIC VARIATION

In the preceding sections it has been shown that particular critical antigens of microorganisms often vary in such a way that the pathogen can evade the immune response. In general, viruses and bacteria do not carry enough genetic information for more than one set of surface antigens; consequently, antigenic variation in viruses and bacteria refers to that between different strains of the same species. Many protozoa and eukaryotic parasites which have more complicated life cycles change their surface antigens during the life cycle. This may be a result of different morphological stages in their development, as occurs during the ontogeny of *Plasmodia*, or it may include antigen switching by activation of genes for new surface antigen variants, as seen in *Trypanosoma brucei* infection. Some schistosomes disguise themselves by adopting MHC molecules from their host and incorporating them into their outer tegument so as to make themselves antigenically invisible.

One of the most interesting examples of strain variation is seen in influenza A, where the haemagglutinin and neuraminidase continually undergo slight alterations in their structure as a result of mutation. The new variants that develop cannot be neutralized by antibodies to the previous strain, and so the new variants can infect otherwise immune individuals. In fact, the sera induced by a later variant are often able to react with a previous variant strain, but not vice versa; in other words, last year's antibody does not neutralize this year's virus. This kind of variation is called 'antigenic drift'. Sporadically a major change of the surface antigens occurs, termed 'antigenic shift'. This is caused by recombination of genetic material

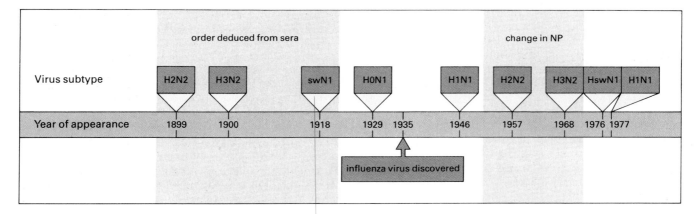

	order deduced from sera						change in NP		
Virus subtype	H2N2	H3N2	swN1	H0N1	H1N1	H2N2	H3N2	HswN1	H1N1
Year of appearance	1899	1900	1918	1929 1935	1946	1957	1968	1976	1977

influenza virus discovered

Fig.9.7 Antigenic shift in influenza A haemagglutinin and neuraminidase. Since its discovery in 1935, there have been sporadic major changes (shifts) in the surface antigens of the flu virus. The haemagglutinin has changed from type H0 to H1, H2, H3 etc. in successive shifts, during which time the neuraminidase has changed from type N1 to N2 and back again. By looking at the neutralizing antibodies present in the sera of people alive before the discovery of the virus, it has been possible to deduce the type of antigens present on the strains extant then (e.g. HSW). This suggests that antigenic types can recur as soon as the overall level of immunity in the population falls below a certain level, so that a new pandemic strain develops. Note also the changes in the nucleoprotein (e.g. N1-N2 in 1957).

between two completely different strains of the virus. The genetic material of the virus is in eight separate RNA strands, which readily permits gene reassortment if two different viruses should simultaneously infect the same cell. The shifts which have occurred in the HA and NA molecules during this century are illustrated in Figure 9.7. The nucleoprotein also underwent a minor variation in 1946. In the case of flu, the newly emergent variants tend to completely displace previous strains. This is dissimilar to the situation seen with rhinoviruses, coronaviruses and enterobacteria, where numerous variants coexist in the host population. However, for these viruses and bacteria a major part of the host's immunity is due to specific IgA, and this response tends to wane much more rapidly than the IgG-mediated immunity which is effective in preventing reinfection with flu. Consequently, a single strain of flu virus cannot regularly reinfect the same host. This, coupled with the virulence of flu epidemics, means that a large proportion of the host population is immune after an outbreak of the disease, and therefore this type of infection tends to be epidemic rather than endemic. The more complicated forms of antigenic variation seen in protozoa are considered below.

Antigenic Variation Within The Life Cycle
Parasites such as *Plasmodia*, *Trypanosoma* and some schistosomes have complicated life cycles, in which the parasites may infect different host species and pass through different morphological stages in each host. In this case, some of the antigens are retained between different stages while other antigens are specific for one or more stages. This can be seen in the pattern of antigens expressed on the surface of *P. knowlesi* (Fig.9.8). The complexity of the antigenic pattern of malarial parasites is also demonstrated in a study by McBride and colleagues concerning the antigens of *P. falciparum*: monoclonal antibodies were raised to two strains of the parasite (K1 and PB1), and their reactions on each strain were observed at different stages

Fig.9.8 Stage-specific antigens of P. knowlesi. SDS PAGE analysis of *P. knowlesi* parasites pulse-labelled at different stages of their life cycle, shows that some antigens (for example, 6) persist for more than one stage, whereas others (for instance, 7) are specific for a single stage of development. Courtesy of Dr. J Deans.

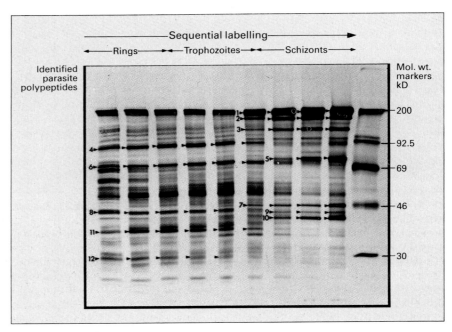

Location of antigens	Number of monoclonal antibodies to	
	Strain K1	Strain PB1
All asexual forms and gametocytes	4(0)	1(0)
Schizonts, merozoites and ring forms	7(0)	2(0)
All asexual stages	2(1)	0
Schizonts and merozoites	5(4)	9(8)
Trophozoites and schizonts	2(1)	0

Fig.9.9 Stage-specific antigens of *P. falciparum*.
Monoclonal antibodies were raised to two different strains of
P. falciparum (K1 and PB1), and binding to antigens at
different stages of the parasite was noted. Five groups of
antigens could be recognized by this means. Numbers
indicate the number of antibodies induced by (and binding to)
strain K1 and strain PB1. Numbers in parentheses indicate
the number of those antibodies which bound only to the
inducing strain. This shows both the diversity of the antigens
and that some are strain-specific while others are not. Data
from McBride *et al.*, 1982.

of the life cycle (Fig.9.9). This study demonstrates two
points. Firstly, that some antigens persist from one stage to
another and, secondly, that some of the antigens vary
between strains while others do not (inasmuch as these
antibodies can distinguish).

When considering the immune response to these parasites, antibodies to antigens of different stages may be
equally effective at destroying that stage of the parasite, but
they can have fundamentally different effects on the
outcome of the infection. For example, in the case of
malaria, antibody to the sporozoites already present in the
host could prevent the first stage of infection, which is the
invasion of host liver cells by sporozoites injected by the
Anopheles vector. Similarly, antibodies to the merozoite
prevent the cycles of reinfection of red cells, while
antibodies to gametocyte-specific antigens can break
the cycle of reinfection of the mosquito although they are
of little help in clearing infection in the original host
(Fig.9.10).

At least 14 different antigens are present on the asexual
blood stage of *P. falciparum*, differentiated according to
molecular weight. In some cases, single antibodies isolate
several antigens differing in molecular weight, but experiments on other malarial species indicate that some malarial
proteins undergo fragmentation into smaller peptides. An
example of this is the breakdown of a 230 kD protein of *P.
knowlesi* into 75, 55, 53 and 43 kD fragments, which
accompanies schizogeny. Also present in the blood stage
are antigens which are localized in the rhoptry proteins of
the paired organelles at the apex of the merozoite. These
organelles are internal, and are lost during merozoite
reinvasion of red cells. The antibody to them is able to
partially inhibit red cell invasion, but it is generally less
effective than antibodies to the glycophorin-binding
proteins on the outside of the parasite (mentioned above).
Antigens are also found associated with ring form-
parasitized red cells (early trophozoites). At the early stages
of infection, the antigen on the latter is derived from the

infecting merozoite which has fused with the red cell, but
later these antigens come from the developing internal
parasites. 90% of the sera from people living in endemic
areas react with ring forms, and these antibodies can
prevent parasite reinvasion *in vitro*. Another facet of the
developing schizont is the production of S antigens which
bathe the developing merozoites. This antigen appears at
the start of schizogeny, and it has been suggested that it
could act as a decoy protein for the immune system by
being, in effect, a large load of a non-critical antigen.

The preceding section illustrates the diversity of antigens
encountered on the asexual stages of the malaria parasite
and the infected red cell, but there has also been interest in
the sexual stages of the life cycle. Antibodies to antigens on

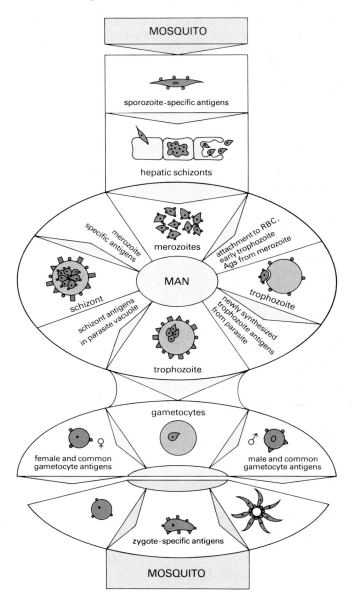

**Fig.9.10 Antigens at different stages of the malarial life
cycle.** Starting from the sporozoite injected into man by the
mosquito vector, antigen (red) expression is illustrated
schematically during different stages of the life cycle in man.
Antibodies to malaria can act at many stages. These include
the various asexual blood stage forms, the infected red blood
cells (RBC), and even the developing gametocytes and zygote
following ingestion by the mosquito. Antibodies to all the stages
shown have been detected.

the gametes can act in two ways at this stage: a) on gametes and zygotes shortly after ingestion by the mosquito, and b) by preventing development of zygotes into ookinetes within the gut of the vector. Antibodies have been identified which act at both these levels, recognizing antigens which develop on, and are common to, both male and female gametes. It is rather surprising that the host antibodies can still have some protective action for the human population as a whole, even after ingestion into the vector.

Although this section has dwelt on the stage-specific antigens present in malaria, many other parasite infections also express different antigens during each stage of development. This is particularly well illustrated in *Toxoplasma gondii* infection. This parasite may be acquired either by contact with oocysts in infected soil, or by eating bradyzoites in infected meat. Both routes of infection lead to parasitization with tachyzoites but, despite the different modes of infection and life cycle, tachyzoites acquired by either route are antigenically indistinguishable, although the antigenic profile of tachyzoites differs appreciably from the other stages. The complications introduced by these alternative routes of infection, hence of surface antigens, make it even more difficult to determine which are the critical antigens for immunity. Indeed, at this stage the organisms are so complex that the concept of critical antigens becomes too simplistic, since it is clear that responses to many different antigens can contribute towards disruption of parasite life cycles or parasite destruction.

Antigenic Variation in *T. Brucei*

Some pathogens show antigenic variation within a single phase of their life cycle. The most marked example of this is *Trypanosoma brucei*, the causative agent of 'sleeping sickness'. These organisms have a surface coat consisting of about seven million identical, closely packed glycoproteins of molecular weight 61 kD, called the 'variant surface glycoprotein' (VSG). As its name suggests, the VSG is expressed in antigenically different forms in different cells. Every organism carries approximately 1000 separate genes encoding variants of the VSG, although at any one time only one of them is expressed. Individuals can switch from the production of one variant to another, an event that occurs at low frequency. This kind of switching is often accompanied by gene rearrangement, which may bring the new variant gene into proximity with a promoter to allow its expression; the old variant is presumably switched out of the active site at the same time.

The ability to switch VSG gives the trypanosome a chameleon-like capacity of changing its surface appearance as far as the immune system is concerned. The immune system can successfully eradicate any particular variant by producing variant-specific antibody, but small numbers of new variants will have arisen which evade the immune response and rapidly replace the previously dominant variant. The parasite is always one step ahead of the immune system, therefore the disease is chronic. It is not that new strains arise under selective pressure, but that the same organism has an altered appearance. At one time it was thought that trypanosomes went through a particular ordered sequence of switching in each new infection, but this is not true. Some variants are selected more often than others during the switching process, hence infections tend to expose a particular sequence of variants, but the sequence is determined both by the parasite and the

immune status of the host. The importance of antigen switching to this parasite can be judged by the fact that 10% of the organism's genome is devoted to VSGs.

The antigenic structure of the VSG has been examined using monoclonal antibodies raised in mice to the isolated glycoprotein and some of its proteolytic fragments (Fig.9.11). These antibodies recognize five antigenic domains within the molecule. The domains were identified by seeing whether one monoclonal antibody blocked binding of another. Where blocking was only partial, it was inferred that the domains overlap, and a map of the antigenic structure was built up from this datum. Of the five domains, only one is expressed on the surface of intact organisms. This is formed from the N-terminal part of the molecule which is its most highly variable section. Indeed,

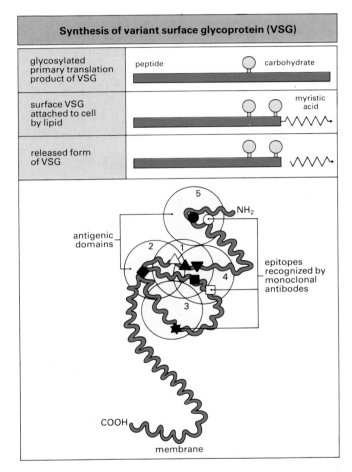

Fig.9.11 Variant surface glycoprotein (VSG) of *T. brucei*. The VSG of *T. brucei* covers the entire trypanosome surface. It is formed from a single peptide which becomes glycosylated and attached to the parasite surface via a myristic acid unit. The VSGs may be cleaved and released from the parasite surface to act as a decoy protein (upper). Miller and colleagues (1984) have shown that there are potentially five antigenic domains in the VSG which can be recognized by monoclonal antibodies. These antibodies fall into different groups which totally inhibit the binding of other members of the group, and partially inhibit binding of antibodies in adjacent groups. The latter are indicated on the structure by geometric shapes. Groups which fall within the same antigenic domain have the same shape. The domains have been correlated with the structure of the molecule, analysed by CNBr cleavage. Only one of the domains (5) is accessible on the intact parasite. From Miller *et al.*, 1984.

the C-terminal portion which contains the residues linking the VSG to the membrane is relatively constant. Hence the only portion of the molecule exposed to the immune system is the most variable part of it.

DECOY PROTEINS

An additional factor involved in parasite evasion of the immune response is the ability to release antigens which divert the immune reaction. *T. brucei*, for example, can shed its VSG into solution by proteolysis of the C terminus, which detaches the head portion from the myristic acid anchorage (see Fig. 9.11).

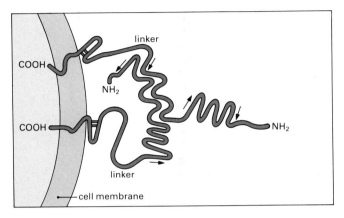

Fig.9.12 Proposed structure of the circumsporozoite (CS) antigen. The CS protein which occurs on malaria sporozoites is a candidate for an immune decoy protein. It contains sections of β-pleated sheet (arrows) with repeating epitopes, and it can be clipped from the parasite surface in the presence of immune sera to deflect specific antibody from the parasite. From Godson *et al.*, 1984.

The shed antigens can act as a decoy by preventing antibody binding to VSGs on the trypanosome itself. It has also been suggested that presentation of new spurious epitopes also diverts the immune system into producing antibodies which will be unable to react with epitopes on the viable undamaged parasite.

This type of decoy action is also used by malarial sporozoites which express a surface protein termed 'circumsporozoite' (CS) antigen. The CS protein of *Plasmodium knowlesi* contains 12 tandem repeats of a 12 amino acid residue sequence presenting a heavy antigenic load to the immune system (Fig.9.12). Also, when sporozoites are treated with immune serum containing anti-CS, they shed a morphologically distinguishable outer layer. This shedding reaction deflects the immunological attack from the sporozoite itself, and this delay enables it to reach an hepatocyte.

Reference has already been made to the S antigen of *Plasmodium falciparum*, shed by developing merozoites into the vacuole of the schizont. This too is a decoy protein and, like other decoy proteins, it contains repeated epitopes and undergoes antigenic variation. These kinds of decoy reactions are well suited to parasites or stages in parasite life cycles which are only briefly in contact with immune defences, whereas antigenic variation is a long-term solution to the problem of evasion of immunity.

CROSS-REACTIONS OF MICROBIAL AND HOST ANTIGENS

Cross-reaction between microbial and host antigens is an area of particular interest, since these may provide a trigger for the breakdown of self-tolerance following infection with a particular organism. It is sometimes difficult to determine whether an organism actually contains a particular cross-reactive antigen, or whether the reaction is to a host tissue antigen released by pathogen-induced damage. An example of this is the case of antibodies to cardiolipin, which occur in *Treponema pallidum* infection (causative agent of syphilis). These antibodies are also present in leprosy and the autoimmune disease systemic lupus erythematosus (SLE). Cardiolipin *does* occur in the envelope of treponemes, which explains the occurrence of the antibody in syphilis, but is not present in mycobacteria which cause leprosy. To explain the presence of this antibody in other infections, one can invoke the adjuvant properties of mycobacteria acting in association with host cell damage. In fact, when analysis of the specificity of the anti-cardiolipin antibodies which occur in syphilis and SLE is made, they differ in that the antibodies of syphilitics have a higher reactivity with phosphatidyl ethanolamine, while the antibodies in SLE react preferentially with phosphatidyl serine. This suggests that the breakdown of self-tolerance in the two groups occurs by different means. Free cardiolipin is not normally immunogenic, but it could become so when associated with treponemal antigens.

Antigen cross-reaction has also been used to explain the autoimmune reactions occurring in the heart muscles and valves, which develop in rheumatic fever following infection with streptococci. The same mechanism has also been proposed for the reaction to nerve and muscle tissue which occurs in Chagas disease (South American trypanosomiasis). Rheumatic fever is an infrequent sequel to streptococcal pharyngitis, occurring two to four weeks after bacterial infection. It has been explained in terms of cross-reaction between the bacterial carbohydrate and a structural protein on heart valves, as well as a cross-reaction between an M-associated antigen and cardiac muscle. This, however, is not an adequate account as it fails to explain pericarditis (no cross-reactive antigens are seen in the pericardium), nor does it explain why only a small proportion of infected individuals develop the disease which solely follows pharyngitis and not other streptococcal infections. It cannot be a simple matter of breakdown of self-tolerance. Indeed, it is notable that autoimmune reactions occur after many diseases, but it is only in rare instances that they develop into autoimmune disease. Immunoregulation of autoimmunity usually prevails.

Although the two examples above concern the breakdown of B cell tolerance, the damage which occurs in the late stages of Chagas disease is primarily cell-mediated, suggesting that T cell tolerance could also be broken by cross-reaction. It is possible that this mechanism could provide a trigger for other autoimmune diseases with otherwise unsuspected causes. If the triggering antigen occurred on several organisms, association between one disease and one single organism would not be marked, nor would the organism be thought of as the sole aetiological agent, but only as a contributory factor.

SUMMARY

Microorganisms and viruses have large numbers of different antigens, but from the aspect of immunity a number of these antigens are important while the remainder are not. These critical antigens are usually located on the outer surface of the pathogen. Viruses must attach to host cells to initiate infection, and antibodies to the attachment proteins are often the most effective at preventing infection. The same principle applies to intra-cellular parasites, such as malaria, which must attach to a host cell via specific cell-surface proteins. The response to bacteria is complicated by the production of bacterial exotoxins. While it is frequently essential that an adequate response is mounted to these toxins, elimination of the bacteria still depends on the production of antibodies to critical surface antigens. Since many pathogens deploy mechanisms to deflect the immune response (for example, antiphagocytic proteins, leucocidins and capsules), it is essential that these defences are neutralized so as to permit occurrence of adequate immune responses.

Both T and B cells recognize determinants on microbial antigens, and these may be different or common portions of the antigen. As with soluble proteins, the response depends on the antigen, the way it is processed and presented, as well as the animal's immune response genes.

One difference between microbial and artificial antigens is that the conformation of the microbial surface can limit which of the potential epitopes on the antigens are actually available. Another consideration in the response to microbes is the type of effector system that becomes activated, as only particular mechanisms are effective against some organisms. Thus, the outcome of an infection depends on the way the antigens are processed, whether cell-mediated or humoral responses occur, and on the class of antibodies produced.

The antigens of microorganisms are not static. Immunity within the host population places them under a continual pressure to change their critical surface antigens within the limitations of the functions of those antigens. In certain species this leads to the development of numerous variant strains, which presents a problem for scientists trying to devise vaccines. In some cases variants coexist within the host population, whereas in others new variants replace the old, thus producing epidemic outbreaks of disease. Complicated pathogens, including trypanosomes and malaria, deploy several different coats of antigens during their life cycle. Other strategies to evade immune responses include antigenic anonymity (for example, prions), lying low (for example, retroviruses and some herpes viruses), disguise (for example, schistosomes), and the active defensive counter-measures used by many pathogenic bacteria.

FURTHER READING

Carter R., Miller L., Rener J., Kaushal D., Kumar N., Graves P., Grotendorst C., Gwodz R., French C. & Wirth D. (1984) *Target antigens in malaria transmission blocking immunity.* Philos. Trans. R. Soc. Lond. (Biol) **307**, 201.

Cross G.A. (1984) *Structure of the variant glycoprotein and surface coat of T. brucei.* Philos. Trans. R. Soc. Lond. (Biol) **307**, 3.

Deans J.A. (1984) *Protective antigens of bloodstage Plasmodium knowlesi parasites.* Philos. Trans. R. Soc. Lond. (Biol) **307**, 159.

De Freitas E.C., Dietzschold B. & Koprowski H. (1985) *Human T-lymphocyte response in vitro to synthetic peptides of herpes simplex virus glycoprotein D.* Proc. Natl. Acad. Sci. USA **82**, 3425.

Godson G.N., Ellis J., Lupski, J.R., Ozaki L.S., Svec P. 1984 *Structure and organization of genes for sporozoite surface antigens.* Philos. Trans. R. Soc. Lond. (Biol) **307**, 129.

Hackett C.J., Hurwitz J.L., Dietzschold B. & Gerhard W. (1985) *A synthetic decapeptide of influenza virus haemagglutinin elicits helper T cells with the same five recognition specificities as occur in the response to the whole virus.* J. Immunol. **135**, 1391.

Heber-Katz A., Hollosi M., Dietzschold B., Hudecz F. & Fasman G. (1985) *The T cell response to the glycoprotein D of the herpes simplex virus: the significance of antigen conformation.* J. Immunol. **135**, 1385.

Howard R.J. (1985) *Antigenic variation of blood stage malaria parasites.* Philos. Trans. R. Soc. Lond. (Biol) **307**, 141.

Hurwitz J.L., Hackett C.J., McAndrew E. & Gerhard W. (1985) *Murine T$_H$ response to influenza virus: recognition of hemagglutinin, neuraminidase, matrix and nucleoproteins* J. Immunol. **134**, 1994.

Johnson A.M. *The antigenic structure of Toxoplasma gondii: a review.* Pathology **17**, 9.

Lehner T., Mehlert A., Avery J., Jones T. & Caldwell J. (1985) *The helper and suppressor functions of primate T cells elicited by a 185K streptococcal antigen, as compared with the helper function elicited by a 4K streptococcal antigen.* J. Immunol. **135**, 1437.

McBride J., Walliker D. & Morgan G. (1982) *Antigenic diversity in the human malaria parasite P. falciparum.* Science **217**, 254.

Miller E.N., Allan L.M. & Turner M.J. (1984) *Mapping of antigenic determinants within peptides of a variant surface glycoprotein of T. bruceii.* Mol. Biochem. Parasitol. **13**, 309.

Miller E.N., Allan L.M. & Turner M.J. (1984) *Topological analysis antigenic determinants of a variant surface glycoprotein of T. brucei.* Mol. Biochem. Parasitol. **13**, 67.

Mills K.H., Skehel J.J. & Thomas D.B. (1986) *Conformational dependent recognition of influenza virus haemagglutinin by murine T-helper clones.* Eur. J. Immunol. **16**, 276.

Minor P.D., Evans D.M., Ferguson M., Schild G.C., Westrop G. & Almond J.W. (1985) *Principal and subsidiary antigenic sites of VP1 involved in the neutralisation of polio virus type 3.* J. Gen. Virol. **66**, 1159.

Mitchell D.M. (1985) *The Immunology of Influenza.* Br. Med. Bull. **41**, 80.

Nestorowicz A. (1985) *Antibodies elicited by influenza virus haemagglutinin fail to bind to synthetic peptides representing putative antigenic sites.* Mol. Immunol. **22**, 145.

Pettersson R.F., Oker-Blom C., Kalkkinen N., Kallio A., Ulmanen I., Kääriäinen L., Partonen P. & Valeri A. (1985) *Molecular and antigenic characteristics and synthesis of rubella virus structural protein.* Rev. Infect. Dis. 7sl. s140.

Rook G.A., Champion B.R., Steele J., Varey A.M. & Stanford J.L. (1985) *I-A restricted activation by T cell lines of anti-tuberculosis activity in murine macrophages.* Clin. Exp. Immunol. **59**, 414.

Rossman M.G., Arnold E., Erichson J.W., Frankenberger E.A., Griffith J.P., Hecht H.-J., Johnson J.E., Komer G., Luo M., Mosser A.G., Rueckert R.R., Sherry B. & Vriend G. (1985) *Structure of a human common cold virus and functional relationship to other picornaviruses.* Nature **317**, 145.

Taussig M.J. (1984) *Processes in Pathology and Microbiology.* Chapters 3 and 4, Blackwell Scientific Publications.

Van der Ploeg L.H.T. & Cornelissen A.W. (1984) *The contribution of chromosomal translocations to antigenic variation in T. brucei.* Philos. Trans. R. Soc. Lond. (Biol) **307**, 13.

Wiley D.C., Wilson I.A. & Skehel J.J. (1981) *Structural identification of the antibody-binding sites of Hong Kong influenza haemagglutinin, and their involvement in antigenic variation.* Nature **289**, 373.

Yewdell J.W., Bennink J.R., Smith G.L., & Moss B. (1985) *Influenza A virus nucleoprotein is a major target antigen for cross-reactive anti-influenza A virus cytotoxic T lymphocytes.* Proc. Natl. Acad. Sci. USA **82**, 1785.

Young R.A., Mehra V., Sweetster D., Buchanan T., Clark-Curtis J., Davis R.W. & Bloom B.R. (1985) *Genes for the major protein antigens of the leprosy parasite M. leprae.* Nature **316**, 450.

INTERACTIONS OF IMMUNOLOGICALLY ACTIVE CELLS

10 Immunoregulation

The immune response, like all biological systems, is subject to regulation, and many factors can influence this response in a given individual. An effective immune response is the end-result of interactions between antigen and a network of immunologically competent cells. This response, once initiated, can be modulated in a variety of ways. The form and route of administration of the antigen, the genetic background of the individual, history of previous exposure to the antigen (or even antibody to this antigen) can all influence the response. Many of these factors have been mentioned in previous chapters, but they will be discussed more fully here. Emphasis will be given to the role of various cells and their products in integrating and modulating the immune response.

THE ROLE OF ANTIGEN

An immune response is initiated by antigen, and in most cases it requires the help of T cells. TH cells are activated when their T cell receptors interact with antigen presented in association with class II MHC molecules on the surface of an antigen-presenting cell. This interaction drives the T cell from a resting (G0) state into G1, and causes the production of IL-2 and IL-2 receptor expression. The transcription of IL-2 and IL-2 receptor genes is activated following specific antigenic triggering. This results in the expression of high affinity IL-2 receptors (Kd=10pM), binding of IL-2 and progression of the cell through to S phase and cell division. When these receptors bind IL-2 they are internalized and replaced by low affinity receptors (Kd=10nM). Therefore, as antigen is cleared *in vivo*, the driving force required to maintain the production of IL-2 and the generation of high affinity receptors disappears. A comparable scenario occurs for the B cell, since B cells are also triggered as a consequence of specific binding of antigen to the immunoglobulin receptor. These cells also move from G0 into the G1 phase of the cell cycle and become sensitive to a variety of growth factors produced by antigen-stimulated T cells (for example, B cell growth factors BSF1 [IL-4], IL-2, BCGFII and IFN; see Chapter 11). Clearance of antigen, the ultimate aim of the immune response, removes the stimulus for interleukin production and receptor expression, and thus the cells gradually return to a quiescent state.

GENETICS OF THE IMMUNE RESPONSE

It was apparent as early as the nineteenth century that there were genetic factors influencing the ability of an individual to make an immune response. The observed familial patterns of susceptibility to *Corynebacterium diphtheriae* infection gave rise to the suggestion that resistance or susceptibility might be an inherited characteristic. This was further investigated by studying the inheritance of resistance or susceptibility to a variety of pathogens and toxins, initially using outbred and later highly inbred strains of animals. It was conclusively demonstrated that genetic factors play a role in determining immune responsiveness, and that genes located within the MHC play a major role in influencing the immune response against an infectious agent.

MHC-Linked Immune Response Genes

It is now known that cooperative interactions between APCs, TH cells and B cells or T effector populations are required to produce an effective immune response against an antigen. It has been shown experimentally that productive cooperative interactions require identity between the MHC of the APC and the T cell. Furthermore, the ability of the T cell to recognize MHC is essentially an acquired characteristic which is dependent on the MHC of the thymus. This learnt ability of the T cell to recognize MHC manifests itself as associative recognition and MHC restriction: T cells can only recognize antigen in association with the MHC haplotype of the thymic epithelium to which they were exposed as they matured (Fig.10.1).

Early studies on the genetics of immune responsiveness employed very complex antigens, such as diphtheria toxin, and were limited by the lack of congenic mouse strains. Therefore, although important observations were made on

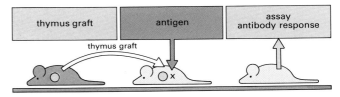

Thymus graft	Recipient haplotype (H-2)	Antibody response to	
		collagen	SRBC
–	(d × b)	–	–
b	(d × b)	+ +	+ +
d	(d × b)	–	+ +

Fig.10.1 The thymus affects the ability to generate an antibody response. BALB/c mice (H-2^d) are low responders to collagen, while C57BL/6 (H-2^b) are high responders. In the experiment, nude (athymic) F1 mice of haplotype H-2^{dxb} were given a thymic graft of either parental type and immunized with either collagen or sheep erythrocytes (SRBC). The antibody response was then measured. Animals grafted with no thymus could not respond to either antigen. Animals given a thymus from a donor of responder haplotype (H-2^b) could respond to collagen, while those that received a non-responder thymus (H-2^d) could not. (NB: x = irradiated). Data of Hedrick and Watson, 1979.

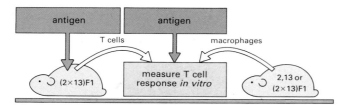

Antigen	Macrophages	Response
DNP - GL	(2×13)F1	+
	2	+
	13	−
GT	(2×13)F1	+
	2	−
	13	+
Mycobacterium tuberculosis	(2×13)F1	+
	2	+
	13	+

Fig. 10.2 Effect of immune response genes in antigen presentation. Strain 2 guinea-pigs respond to the antigen DNP-GL but not to GT, whereas in strain 13 animals the pattern of responsiveness is reversed. Both strains respond to *Mycobacterium tuberculosis*. T cells from a hybrid strain (2×13)F1 were cocultured with macrophages from the parental or F1 strains using different antigens. The T cell response was then measured by assessing cell proliferation. Although T cells from (2×13)F1 animals are potentially capable of responding to all these antigens, they do so only in the presence of macrophages from animals of the high responder haplotype. This implies that the immune response (Ir) genes are expressed on antigen-presenting cells. The observation that F1 macrophages present all these antigens indicates that these Ir genes are codominantly expressed. Data of Shevach and Rosenthal, 1973.

the heritability of responsiveness, the data often required elaborate statistical analysis to confirm the finding. Following the availability of synthetic polypeptides and purified small proteins (such as insulin), which were antigenically less complex, immunologists were able to make considerable advances in understanding the genetic basis of immune responsiveness (Fig. 10.2). It was found that responsiveness to many of these antigens was dominant, highly antigen-specific, and could be mapped to a single genetic locus. The genes controlling immune responsiveness were called Ir genes and were mapped, with the use of recombinant mouse strains, to the I region of the MHC. Numerous Ir genes were described which controlled responsiveness to a range of different antigens, but it should be emphasized that these were generally perceived by the mouse as being antigenically simple. The antigens employed to reveal Ir gene control were either cross-reactive with self such that the animal was tolerant to a majority of the epitopes, or they were synthetic polypeptides composed of a limited number of amino acids. However, Ir gene control to some complex antigens could be demonstrated when low amounts of antigen were administered. Presumably, at limiting antigen concentration only immunodominant epitopes are recognized by the immune system. In studying the Ir gene control of the immune response to sperm whale myoglobin, Bersofsky and his colleagues showed that the immune responses to two different epitopes were regulated by different

H-2-linked genes. Therefore, since different antigenic determinants on the same molecule can be influenced by different Ir genes, the aggregate response to any given complex antigen will tend to be positive.

Cell transfer and *in vitro* studies showed that T cells played an obligate role in Ir gene-controlled immune responses, and that the T cell Ir gene phenotype was an acquired characteristic determined by the thymic environment in which the T cell matured. The effect of Ir genes on macrophage function was shown in the early experiments of Shevach and Rosenthal in the guinea-pig, in which non-responder macrophages only failed to present antigens to which the donors were genetically unable to respond: a finding which has been amply confirmed. Ir genes were also shown to be expressed in B cells by both *in vivo* and *in vitro* studies. The experiments of Marrack and Kappler showed that high responder (R), but not low responder (NR), B cells could make antibody when presented with antigen on (RxNR)F1 macrophages in the presence of (RxNR)F1 T cells (Fig. 10.3). This apparent need for identity of responder status in the macrophage and the B cell suggests that cognate interactions play a fundamental role in antibody responses. The final solution to the Ir gene puzzle was provided by the observation that Ir genes were localized in the same genetic region as the genes coding for Ia, the restriction elements for DTH and TH. Alloanti-sera raised using recombinant mouse strains in which

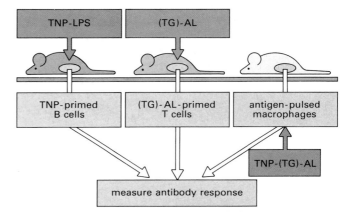

B cells	T cells	Macrophages	Response
H-2^k	H-2$^{(b×k)}$	H-2$^{(b×k)}$	−
H-2^b	H-2$^{(b×k)}$	H-2$^{(b×k)}$	+++

Fig. 10.3 B cells must be of the responder haplotype to produce an antibody response. B cells primed to TNP were isolated from mice immunized with TNP-LPS. T cells primed to (TG)-AL were obtained from animals immunized with (TG)-AL. Macrophages from normal animals were treated with the hapten/carrier antigen TNP-(TG)-AL, to act as antigen-presenting cells in coculture with the lymphocytes. The antibody response to the antigen TNP was measured. Both T cells and macrophages came from (TG)-AL high responder (R) H-2^k × H-2^b animals. When the B cells came from the (TG)-AL low responder (NR) strain (H-2^k) they could not produce an antibody response, whereas when using B cells from a high responder H-2^b strain a response was elicited. (Note that high and low responsiveness does not refer to the ability of the B cells to recognize TNP.) This implies that MHC-linked immune response genes are expressed on B cells. Based on data of Marrack and Kappler, 1978.

Strain	Response to		
	DNP-GL	GT	PPD
2	+++	−	+++
13	−	+++	+++
(2×13) F1	+++	+++	+++

T cells	(2×13) F1 macrophages pulsed with			Treated with
	DNP-GL	GT	PPD	
1	(2×13)F1	+++	+++	+++	control
2	(2×13)F1	−	+++	+	anti-strain 2 Ia
3	(2×13)F1	+++	−	+	anti-strain 13 Ia

Fig.10.4 Anti-class II antibody interferes with antigen presentation. Responses of strains 2 and 13 guinea-pigs to DNP-GL, GT and PPD antigens (upper panel). Proliferation obtained when strain (2×13) F1 responder T cells are cultured with (2×13) F1 responder macrophages in the presence of antisera to Ia molecules of either haplotype (lower panel). With no antibody to class II present, T cells proliferate to all antigens (1). Anti-strain 2 Ia abrogates the response to DNP-GL and reduces that to PPD, but leaves the response to GT unaffected (2). Anti-strain 13 Ia abrogates the response to GT and reduces that to PPD, but leaves the response to DNP-GL unaffected (3). In each case, only anti-Ia antiserum directed to the responder haplotype blocks antigen presentation. Data of Shevach et al., 1972.

Response to	B10.A donor (Ia^k)	(B10.A×B10.Q) F1 (Ia^k×Ia^q)
GL-Phe	−	+

T cells	Macrophages	Antigen	T cell response		
			−	anti-Ia^k	anti-
1	Ia^k	Ia^k × Ia^q	GL-Phe	−	−	−
2	Educated Ia^k	Ia^k × Ia^q	GL-Phe	+++	+++	−
3	Educated Ia^k	Ia^k	GL-Phe	−	−	−
4	Educated Ia^k	Ia^q	GL-Phe	+++	+++	−

Fig.10.5 Anti-class II antibody acts on APCs. B10.A (Ia^k) mice are low responders to GL-Phe, while (B10.A × B10.Q)F1 (Ia$^{k×q}$) animals respond. Irradiated F1 responder animals were repopulated with bone marrow cells of non-responder phenotype, and the response of the newly developed T cells to GL-Phe was measured in the presence of anti-class II antibodies directed to either haplotype. Normal Ia^k cells cannot respond to GL-Phe in these conditions (1), but Ia^k cells educated in an F1 responder animal can, if presented with antigen on either F1 macrophages (2) or on responder Ia^q macrophages (4). They will not respond when antigen is presented on non-responder Ia^k macrophages (3). In experiments 2 and 4, anti-class II antibody directed to the responder (but not to the non-responder) haplotype blocks the proliferation. Data of Longo and Schwartz, 1981.

differences lay within the H-2 locus (that is, antibodies against class II MHC antigens) were shown to block T cell proliferative responses to antigen-pulsed macrophages if the antisera recognized the MHC of the responder strain (Fig.10.4). Antisera against class I MHC antigens had no effect, nor did antisera against NR class II MHC. The identity of the Ir gene product with Ia molecules was further supported by gene complementation studies and confirmed by studies employing mice carrying the bm12 mutation (see Chapter 5). Thus, it now seems that the basis of MHC-linked control of responsiveness depends on whether or not a particular antigen can, following processing, interact appropriately with the Ia molecule for recognition by TH cells (see Chapter 6). The inability to effectively demonstrate MHC-linked Ir gene effects using complex antigens is because such antigens will usually generate at least one effective association with Ia (Figs.10.5 & 10.6).

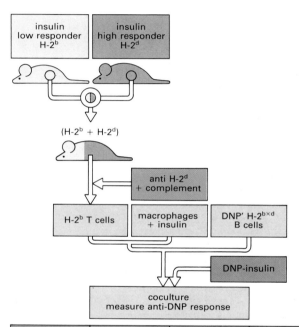

T cells	B cells	Macrophages	Anti-DNP response
H-2^b allophenic	H-2$^{b×d}$	H-2^b	(+)
H-2^b allophenic	H-2$^{b×d}$	H-2^d	+++

Fig.10.6 Immune responsiveness is an acquired characteristic. Allophenic (chimaeric) mice were made by fusing fertilized ova (8 cell stage) from H-2^b and H-2^d mice, reimplanting them and allowing them to develop. T cells taken from these mice were 82% of the H-2^b haplotype and 18% of the H-2^d haplotype. The H-2^b cells were isolated by killing H-2^d cells with antibody and complement. These cells were stimulated with antigen (insulin)-pulsed macrophages for four days, and then cocultured with B cells primed to DNP together with the hapten/carrier antigen DNP-insulin. The anti-DNP response was measured. H-2^b T cells are normally low responders to insulin. When they have developed in association with high responder H-2^d cells in the allophenic mouse they can respond to insulin, but only if it is presented by macrophages expressing the high responder (H-2^d) phenotype. This implies that low responder T cells can acquire responsiveness, if they develop in an environment with high responder APCs. Data of Erb et al., 1980.

Non-MHC-Linked Immune Response Genes

Non-MHC genes have also been shown to play an important role in the response to infectious organisms (Fig. 10.7). For example, non-MHC genes play a major role in the resistance to mycobacteria, and studies with congenic mice have mapped this resistance to a gene Bcg on chromosome 1. Similarly, studies on murine resistance to *Leishmania donovani* and *Salmonella typhimurium* have revealed that the non-MHC genes involved (Lsh and Ity respectively) also mapped to chromosome 1. It seems likely that the genes Bcg, Lsh and Ity are in fact identical, although this is not yet certain. The exact role of this gene in determining resistance is also not known, but it seems to be intimately involved in tissue macrophage function. It has been proposed that these genes influence the ability of macrophages to inhibit replication of the intracellular parasite. This gene therefore influences the course of an infection during the first few days, after which other genetic factors linked to the MHC may determine the subsequent outcome of the infection. This has been clearly established in studies on leishmaniasis. Thus, the disease profiles following either *L. donovani* or *L. tropica* infection appear to be determined by two genetic influences: the innate ability of the tissue macrophage to inhibit intracellular replication of the parasite, and the ability of the animal to develop effective T cell-mediated immunity (CMI). The former appears to be determined by the presence of the resistance-conferring allelic form of the Lsh gene, and the latter by the presence or absence of T suppressor cells which affect the development of CMI (Fig. 10.8). This latter variable is linked to the MHC. Studies on murine resistance to cytomegalovirus (HSV-5) infection showed that BALB/c congenic mice of the k haplotype were resistant, while BALB/c with b, d and q haplotypes were susceptible. Genetic analysis of the patterns of resistance and susceptibility of mice to herpesvirus infections showed that both H-2 and non-H-2 immune response genes are important. Indeed, with regard to DNA and RNA viral infections and parasitic diseases in mice, both H-2 and non-H-2 immune response genes regulate resistance to infection. Again, macrophages play a crucial role in these

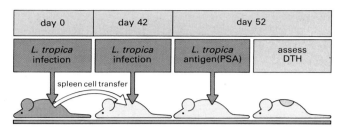

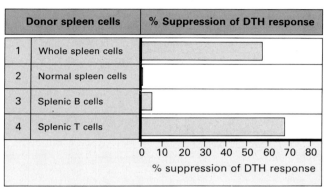

Fig. 10.8 Suppressor cells in leishmaniasis. BALB/c mice were infected with *Leishmania tropica*, and after 42 days the spleen cells from these animals were transferred to recipients which were then also infected. After 10 days, the ability of the recipients to mount a delayed type hypersensitivity (DTH) reaction was measured following sensitization with protein-soluble antigen (PSA) from *L. tropica*. DTH reflects the ability of these animals to resist the infection. Animals which had received whole spleen cells showed a 57% suppression of their DTH response (1), by comparison with control animals which received spleen cells from uninfected donors (2). When the splenocytes from the infected donors were fractionated before transfer, it was found that B cells could not produce the suppression (3) whereas T cells could (4). This indicates that T cells contribute to disease susceptibility. Based on data of Howard *et al.*, 1982.

responses, and some of these non-H-2 genes may be involved in macrophage function.

Another example of the role of non-H-2-linked immune response genes in determining the outcome of an immune response is found in an experiment utilizing 'Biozzi' mice. Biozzi originally noted that within an outbred population of mice there is a spread in the ability to respond to erythrocyte antigens. By selectively breeding high or low responder mice for twenty generations he was able to establish two lines of mice, one a high responder and the other a low responder to erythrocytes. These mice were also shown to respond differently to a variety of other antigens. Interestingly, the low responder mouse strain appeared to be able to clear intracellular parasites more effectively than the high responder strain. The genetic basis for the differences in immune responsiveness between these mice is complex, involving at least ten genetic loci. One or more of these genes affects the ability of the macrophage to process and present antigen; the high responder strain macrophages retain antigen on their surface for a markedly longer time than low responder macrophages which appear to have much more lysosomal activity.

It was noticed in 1962 that, unlike all other inbred mouse strains, the strain A2G was resistant to normally lethal infective doses of influenza virus. This resistant trait was shown to be inherited as a single dominant allele, now

Organism	Resistant		Susceptible	
	strain	haplotype	strain	haplotype
Mycobacterium lepraemurium	DBA/2J C3H/HeJ	d k	BALB/cJ C3H/A	d k
Salmonella typhimurium	DBA/2J	d	B10.D2, BALB/c	d d
M. tuberculosis	CBA, C3H	k	B10.BR	k
Listeria monocytogenes	B10.A B10.D2 B10.BR	a d k	A/J DBA/2, BALB/c CBA, C3H	a d k
Rickettsia tsutsugamushi	AKR SWR BALB/c	k q d	C3H, CBA DBA/1 DBA/2	k q d

Fig. 10.7 Role of non-MHC genes in resistance to infection. Different strains of mice vary in their resistance to the organisms listed. Since different strains with the same MHC haplotype can be susceptible or resistant, this shows that the MHC haplotype is not critical in determining resistance to infection. Modified from Krco and David, 1981.

designated MX⁺. In the mouse, resistance or susceptibility to influenza is known to be mediated by interferons α and β. Comparison of interferon-induced proteins of congenic MX⁺ and MX⁻ cells revealed only a single difference: the presence of a 75kD polypeptide, now termed 'the MX protein'. Analogous proteins have also been found in man and other animals, and it appears to be critical for the establishment of resistance to orthomyxoviruses and perhaps other viruses. Elegant experiments of Staeheli, Haller and colleagues have localized the MX gene to chromosome 16 in the mouse. This gene has been cloned, sequenced and shown to confer resistance when transfected into susceptible 3T3 cells.

Thymic Education of T Cells

A large number of studies have tried to determine the precise role of the thymus in T cell maturation, and the development of MHC restriction. It is well established that the thymus is essential for T cell development, since implanting syngeneic thymic grafts into nude mice restores their capacity to make T cell-mediated responses. The

contribution of the thymus to the development of MHC restriction is less certain. Some of the most sophisticated experiments to determine this, used chimaeric mice in which bone marrow stem cells were allowed to develop in a host with a genetically different thymus. The interpretation of these experiments can be very difficult, and in some cases they lead to conflicting conclusions. A main cause of these problems is that it is often difficult to distinguish the effects of the thymus on MHC restriction, from the effects exerted by the antigen-presenting cells present in the host.

To illustrate the kinds of experiments used, Figure 10.9 shows an experiment using radiation chimaeras. It shows that (AxB) cells developing in an irradiated animal containing a type A thymus can only kill virally infected target cells of type A. This implies that the haplotype of the thymus entirely determines the MHC restriction of cytotoxic cells developing within it, even though these cells would normally be able to react against both haplotypes if they developed in their own (AxB) haplotype thymus.

In contrast, Figure 10.10 shows a similar kind of experiment on nude mice. When haplotype A nude mice

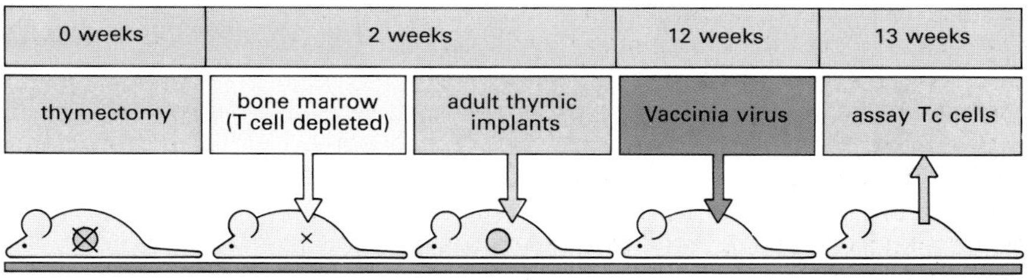

Fig.10.9 Importance of thymic haplotype in T cell development.

Eight-week-old mice of MHC haplotype A×B were thymectomized, irradiated and reconstituted with bone marrow which had been specifically depleted of T cells by treatment with anti-Thy 1, 2 and complement. Each mouse was then given a subcutaneous graft of adult thymus of either type A or type B haplotype (grafted tissue was first irradiated to destroy mature T cells). About 20% of animals survived this treatment and recovered immune function. Ten weeks after grafting, they were infected with Vaccinia virus and the spleen cells from these mice were tested one week later for their ability to specifically kill virally infected target cells of haplotype A or B. Animals reconstituted

Donor bone marrow	Recipient	Thymic donor	Killing of infected targets	
			type A	type B
A × B	A × B	A	+	−
A × B	A × B	B	−	+

with a type A thymus were able to kill targets of haplotype A, and those with a

type B thymus killed haplotype B targets. Data of Zinkernagel *et al.*, 1978.

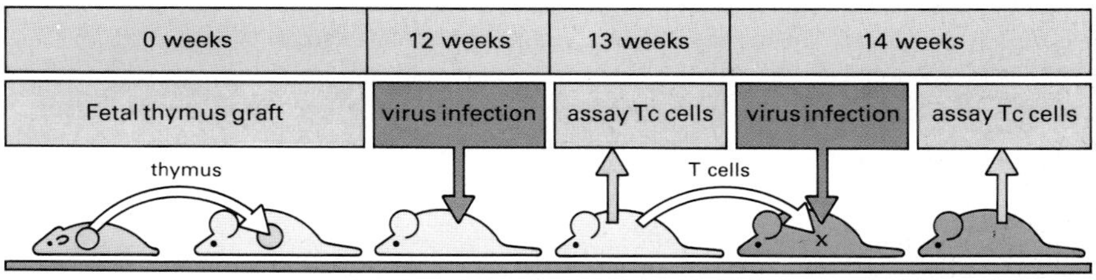

Fig.10.10 Peripheral tissues influence T cell MHC restriction.

Nude mice of A or A×B MHC haplotype were given fetal thymus grafts of the haplotypes shown. After 12 weeks they were infected with Vaccinia virus and one week later cytotoxic T cells were assayed against virally infected targets of different haplotypes. T cells from these animals were also transferred into irradiated infected mice, to see whether they changed their MHC restriction pattern when restimulated in an adoptive host. In these experiments the stem cells come from the nude mouse. In experiments 1-3, the T cells are restricted to the haplotype of the animal in which they mature and encounter virus, and are not restricted to the thymus haplotype. However, A×B stem cells preferentially react against type B targets if they mature in a type B thymus and encounter virus on A×B

Thymus donor	Nude recipient (stem cells)	Cytotoxicity in host to targets of		Cytotoxicity in recipient to targets of	
		type A	type B	type A	type B
A	A	+	−	+	−
B	A	+	−	+	−
(A×B)	A	+	−	+	−
B	(A×B)	−	+	−	+

peripheral antigen-presenting cells. The patterns of MHC restriction are

maintained after adoptive transfer. Data of Zinkernagel *et al.*, 1980.

10.5

are reconstituted with a fetal or neonatal thymus of haplotype (AxB), the cells which develop may be of a type A or type (AxB), but in each case they are able to only kill infected targets of haplotype A, following an *in vivo* challenge with virus. In this case the developing thymocytes do not acquire the ability to kill type B cells, even though the thymus in that animal expresses the B haplotype.

Through many series of experiments, irradiation chimaeras appear to act differently from thymically re-constituted nude mice. One set of data suggests that the haplotype of the thymus is important, while the other indicates that the host tissue type is critical. To try to resolve the contradiction, the T cells from irradiated chimaeras (as in Fig.10.9) were adoptively transferred to another infected (AxB) recipient, and their ability to kill infected target cells was then remeasured. In this case it was found that the T cells could now kill target cells of type B although they had been unable to do so before. One way to interpret these findings is to say that T cells develop MHC restriction both during thymic development and in their subsequent expansion. Cells which develop in a type A thymus will subsequently react well to targets of type A, but the development of cells recognizing type B plus antigen is not precluded by development in the type A thymus. Should these T cells repeatedly encounter virus on a type B antigen-presenting cell or target cells, then the type B-restricted populations can be expanded. This means of reconciling apparently conflicting data places equal emphasis on the thymic maturation period and subsequent stimulation in secondary lymphoid organs.

It is worth noting that when stable thymic chimaeras develop in nude mice, the lymphocytes are tolerant to the thymic haplotypes. This suggests that the development of self tolerance is an important function associated with thymic maturation.

THE ROLE OF T HELPER CELLS IN MODULATING THE IMMUNE RESPONSE

T Cells Provide Help by Recognition of Carrier Determinants

The requirement for T cells, as well as B cells, in the immune response to some antigens was first indicated by the finding that irradiated mice had to be repopulated with both thymus-derived cells and bone marrow cells before they could respond well to sheep erythrocytes (SRBC). Chromosomal and cell surface marker studies revealed that the antibody was made by the B cell, and that T cells were specifically primed by the antigen to provide help for these antigen-specific B cells. Further pioneering experiments by Mitchison, Rajewsky and their colleagues demonstrated that T and B cells recognized two different antigenic determinants on the same antigen: T cells were said to recognize carrier determinants, whereas B cells recognized haptenic determinants (Fig.10.11). This led to the proposition that specific (cognate) interactions between T and B cells occurred via an antigen-bridging mechanism. Further elucidation of the role of MHC antigens in T cell activation resulted in the definition of cognate interactions between T cells, B cells and macrophages. It now seems more reasonable to consider that cognate interactions between T and B cells occur in a similar manner to (and perhaps as a consequence of) specific presentation of antigen by the B cell (see Chapter 6).

T cells can obviously augment the immune response by providing help for B and other T cells. However, there is some suggestion, on the basis of phenotype, that the cell which helps a B cell may be different from that which helps a T cell. In addition, there is evidence to suggest that different B cell subpopulations, distinguishable by the presence or absence of the marker Lyb5, may require different kinds of T cell help. Singer and colleagues have found that Lyb5[+] B cells do not appear to have a strict requirement for genetic restriction in their interactions with T$_H$ cells.

Limit dilution analyses have given some measure of the numbers of T helper cells and the kinds of T cells activated following antigenic stimulation. Using carrier (KLH)-primed T cells in a limiting dilution analysis with hapten-primed B cells (primed to TNP-BSA) and SRBC-primed B cells, Marrack and Kappler found that the frequency of T cells providing cognate help was 7-15 per 10^6 cells, whereas T cells providing bystander help (through the release of a variety of B cell stimulating factors) were present at approximately twice that frequency. Waldmann and colleagues additionally discovered that T cells mediating cognate help only interacted with one B cell (that is, they were monogamous), but T cells providing bystander help interacted with more than one B cell. As we would now expect with some knowledge of the process of T$_H$ activation, cognate help was found to be MHC-restricted, whereas bystander help was not restricted. An antigen-stimulated B cell can respond to a variety of lymphokines produced by activated T cells (see Chapter 11), and in the local environment of a germinal centre the concentrations of these lymphokines may be high. Since responsiveness to these factors is only apparent following antigenic

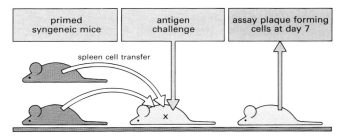

	Cells primed to	Antigen challenge	Anti-NIP response
1	NIP - OA / —	NIP - OA	+++
2	NIP - OA / —	NIP - BSA	—
3	NIP - OA / BSA	NIP - BSA	+++

Fig.10.11 Independent recognition of hapten and carrier. Irradiated mice were given spleen cells from antigen-primed donors and were then challenged. Animals receiving NIP-OA-primed cells make a strong response to the hapten NIP when challenged with this antigen (1). If the hapten is linked to another carrier (NIP-BSA), no response follows (2). However, if the recipient also receives spleen cells primed to the new carrier (BSA), the response is restored (3). This indicates that hapten and carrier are recognized independently by B and T cells. T and B cells can respond to separate parts of a single molecule, as demonstrated with lactate dehydrogenase in rabbits: T cells respond to one subunit of the enzyme and B cells to another. Data of Mitchison *et al.*, 1971.

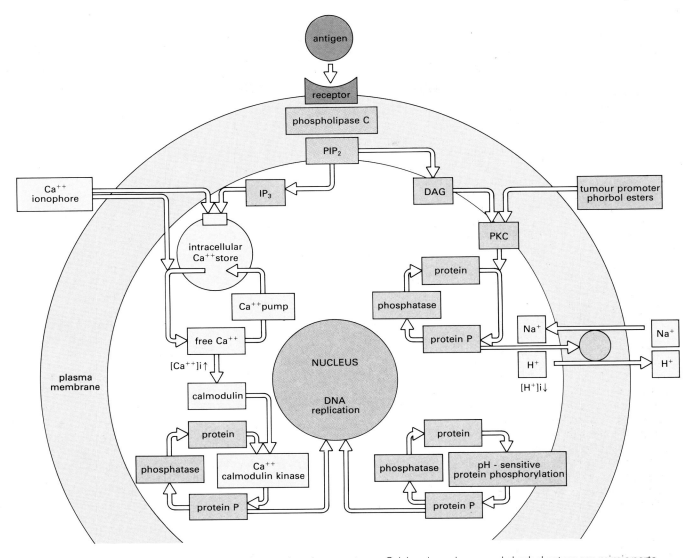

Fig.10.12 Lymphocyte triggering: transmembrane signal.
T and B cells appear to be activated in a similar way to other cells. Activation of the membrane receptor causes release of inositol triphosphate (IP₃) and di-acyl glycerol (DAG) from membrane phosphatidyl inositol biphosphate (PIP₂), by phospholipase C. DAG increases the activity of protein kinase C (PKC) by increasing its affinity for Ca⁺⁺, whereas IP3 releases Ca⁺⁺ from intracellular stores. Calcium ionophores and phorbol esters can mimic parts of the activation process. The increase in Ca⁺⁺ causes the activation of protein kinases which mediate the protein phosphorylation, which precedes DNA replication. Alteration in the activity of membrane ion pumps caused by phosphorylation affects the intracellular ion concentrations, and thus the activity of the protein kinases. Modified from Isakov *et al.*, 1986.

stimulation, some degree of specificity is retained. However, since cognate interactions between T and B cells have been shown to play a fundamental role in the immune response (the requirement for MHC restriction identity between T and B cells coupled with the finding of antibody production of restricted clonality by cultured splenic fragments), it is possible that bystander help is largely an *in vitro* occurrence.

Since there is now a wealth of evidence indicating that T cell-derived growth factors (several of which have now been gene cloned) are able to take an antigen-triggered B cell through all stages of differentiation to become a plasma cell, one may question the need for antigen-specific T helper factors. Indeed the way in which one of these factors (IL-4) appears to function resembles the triggering of a normal activation pathway utilized by a variety of cell types, when they transit from a non-growing to a growing phase (Fig.10.12). It could, therefore, be argued that in the local environment of a lymph node or spleen, where T and B cells may be intimately associated in a ternary complex with an

APC, antigen (by specifically triggering the appearance of receptors for lymphokines and monokines on the specific lymphocytes) confers specificity on the response to such non-specific factors.

Antigen-specific helper factors have been described, and a few laboratories have established T cell hybridomas making such factors specific for responses to amino acid copolymers and chicken gamma globulin (CGG). These helper factors selectively bind to antigen-coupled immunoadsorbents. They have been shown, in some cases, to express an idiotype shared with conventional antibodies raised to the same antigen. They have molecular weights in the range of 35-50kD, and two polypeptide chains, one of which appears to carry a determinant cross-reactive with frame work determinants of immunoglobulin Vн, and the other a determinant cross-reactive with Ia. They also appear to be MHC-restricted in that they can only help B cells sharing the same Ia. The way in which these helper factors function is unclear. It has been proposed that they may be shed or secreted forms of the T cell receptor, but this possibility has now been ruled out. Further biochemical and genetic analysis of these factors is still needed to shed light on their relevance to cellular interactions.

T Cells Can Help by Recognition of Immunoglobulin Determinants

Isotype-specific T cell help. Studies on the regulation of IgE synthesis suggested that T cells which provided help for B cells to make IgE were different from T cells which helped in an IgG response. It has been shown in rodent experiments that the IgE response is highly sensitive to the adjuvant employed with the antigen in initiating the response. Alum and pertussis are good adjuvants for IgE responses, whereas complete Freund's adjuvant leads to good IgG responses. Further analysis of the mechanism of this isotype bias elicited by adjuvant has revealed the essential role of specific T cell-derived factors (IgE-binding factors [Ebf]).

Nippostrongylus infection provides a powerful stimulus for IgE responses, and it has been shown that T cells (bearing $FC_\varepsilon R$ receptors) from infected rats produce a 15kD glycoprotein which binds IgE and specifically enhances the IgE response *in vitro* without affecting the IgG response. Comparable studies, carried out using complete Freund's adjuvant instead of parasite to stimulate T cells, revealed the production of an IgE-specific suppressor factor which also had a molecular weight of 15kD and bound to IgE. These two T cell products appear to play a critical role in determining whether IgE is produced by the B cell.

Recently, a rat T cell hybridoma has been obtained which produces Ebf. cDNA clones have been isolated from this hybridoma, and transfection experiments have shown that they code for a 15kD IgE-enhancing factor. Interestingly, it has also been shown that the enhancing and suppressive Ebf use the same polypeptide chain, their differential effects being achieved by glycosylation differences. When cells carrying the transfected gene were treated with tunicamycin (to inhibit assembly of N-linked oligosaccharides), production of enhancing factor switched to production of suppressive factor. Which factor is produced by the T cell is determined by other T cell-derived factors. Ishizaka and colleagues have shown that alum and pertussis (and presumably some parasites such as *Nippostrongylus*), stimulate rat $CD4^+$ cells to produce a glycosylation-enhancing factor (GEF), whereas complete Freund's adjuvant triggers $CD8^+$ cells to produce a glycosylation inhibition factor (GIF) (Fig.10.13). GIF appears to be a phosphorylated form of lipomodulin (a phospholipase inhibitory protein), currently called 'lipocortin', which is inactive against phospholipase A2. This regulatory circuit is not restricted to rodents, since comparable factors have been found in the human.

Another example of T cells influencing isotype expression is the observation that carrier-primed T cells from F1 male mice bearing the X-linked defect Xid fail to help B cells to make IgG3 antibody responses, whereas T cells from F1 female mice (and therefore normal) helped both male and female B cells to make IgG3.

Antigen-specific TH cell clones derived from Peyer's patches appear to fall into two categories: one which can help B cells to make IgM and IgG responses, and another which provides help for IgM, IgG1, IgG2 and IgA responses. Although both types of T cell clone were $Fc_\gamma R^+$, it has recently been shown that $sIgA^+$ B cells are preferentially stimulated by the T cell clones stimulating IgM and IgA production.

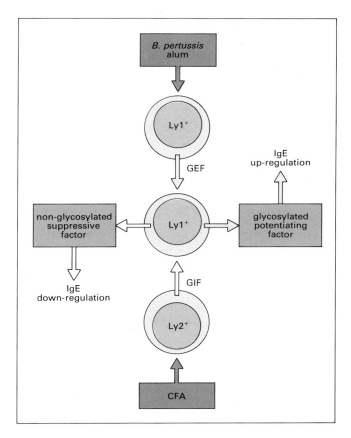

Fig.10.13 Isotype-specific factors. IgE production is potentiated by a glycosylated 15kD factor produced by $Ly1^+$ T cells. If the factor is not glycosylated, it suppresses IgE production. Glycosylation is modulated by glycosylation enhancing factor (GEF) produced by T cells stimulated with *B. pertussis* or alum; this enhances IgE production (grey arrows). Complete Freund's adjuvant acts on $Ly2^+$ cells to produce a glycosylation inhibition factor (GIF) which decreases IgE production (white arrows). Based on Gershwin and Gerswhin, 1986.

Allotype-specific T helper cells. The studies of Herzenberg and colleagues, carried out in 1976, have suggested that T cells are present which are allotype-specific. This was demonstrated using BALB/c x SJL F1 mice which are heterozygous for immunoglobulin allotype. The BALB/c mothers make IgG2a immunoglobulin of the Ig-1^a allotype, whereas the SJL fathers make immunoglobulin which is Ig-1^b. The SJA mouse is congenic with the SJL, but makes IgG2a immunoglobulin with the BALB/c allotype, Ig-1^a. Adoptive transfer studies using BALB/c x SJL F1 hapten (DNP)-primed B cells and carrier (KLH)-primed T cells, obtained from either BALB/c x SJL F1 or BALB/c x SJA F1 mice, clearly showed that Ig-1^b antibody production only occurred when recipients had been reconstituted with T cells from an animal heterozygous for the IgG2a allotype. TH cells from the homozygous BALB/c x SJA F1 could only help B cells to make an IgG2a response of the Ig-1^a allotype. This inability to help B cells to make antibody of the Ig-1^b allotype was not due to T suppressor cells, since their addition to limiting numbers of T cells from the heterozygous F1 did not affect the amount of Ig-1^b made.

The BALB/c x SJL F1 mouse is peculiarly susceptible to chronic allotype suppression of the paternal allotype which is mediated, as will be described later, by allotype-specific suppressor cells. Studies utilizing irradiated recipients reconstituted with hapten-primed B cells and carrier-primed T cells from a suppressed animal, demonstrated an absence of help for the Ig-1^b allotype. Deletion of Ts by treatment of the T cells with anti-Ly2 and complement allowed these T cells to help B cells make antibody of the Ig-1^b allotype. Further experiments by these workers demonstrated that, although memory B cells bearing the paternal Ig-1^b allotype were present in suppressed animals, there was no increase in the avidity of these B cells following antigen boost. In contrast, the avidity of B cells making the non-suppressed allotype increased 100-fold. The conclusion from these studies is, therefore, that allotype-specific TH cells are the target of allotype-specific Ts cells, and that these TH cells play a role in avidity maturation.

Idiotype-specific T helper cells. It has been suggested that an optimal antibody response is produced when two types of TH cell interact with B cell and antigen: one recognizing the carrier determinant on the antigen, and the other recognizing the idiotype of the B cell product. This latter TH cell has been alternatively called TH2 or TH anti-Id. Several lines of evidence indicated that a TH population was present which was not carrier-specific. The early experiments of Janeway and colleagues demonstrated that two populations of T cells synergized to produce an optimal T dependent antibody response. This second population of T cells, which was not a conventional carrier-specific set, was only generated when idiotype was produced. Thus, B cell-depleted (anti-μ treated) animals did not generate TH anti-Id, and CBA/N mice (carrying the Xid gene) failed to develop the TH anti-Id directed towards the T15 idiotype. T15 is a dominant idiotype associated with the response to phosphoryl choline, and since CBA/N mice are genetically incapable of making a response to this antigen, they never make any circulating T15. A particularly compelling observation has been provided by Rohrer and colleagues, showing that a subpopulation of T helper cells (Ly1$^+$,2$^-$,Qa1$^+$), recognizing idiotypic determinants on an IgA plasmacytoma, acts in concert with carrier-specific TH (TH1) to increase secretion of the plasmacytoma IgA.

It has been shown that administration of idiotype or anti-idiotype can result in an increase in production of this idiotype following subsequent challenge with the antigen. The generation of idiotype-specific TH cells could account for these observations, but other mechanisms, such as direct triggering of Id$^+$ B cells or blocking anti-idiotypic suppression, must also be considered (see also Chapter 13).

T CELLS CAN SUPPRESS THE IMMUNE RESPONSE

There is now a considerable body of evidence suggesting that T cells, as well as providing help for B cells and other T cells, can also suppress the activity of these effector populations. This is currently regarded as a rather controversial area by some immunologists, therefore an attempt will be made to review the evidence for the existence of T cell-mediated suppression. The first experimental data suggesting the presence of T cells which could mediate suppression came from the studies of Gershon and Kondo. These workers showed that spleen cells from mice immunized with high doses of SRBC contained T cells which, on transfer to irradiated recipients reconstituted with normal spleen cells, could suppress the subsequent induction of SRBC-specific responses in

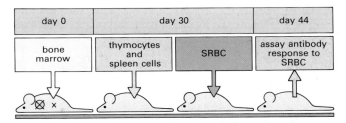

Spleen cells		Log$_2$ antibody response
1	8 × 10^7 SRBC-primed splenocytes	6
2	—	4
3	8 × 10^7 SRBC-tolerized splenocytes	0

Fig.10.14 Suppressor cells in immunological tolerance.
Mice were thymectomized, irradiated and reconstituted with bone marrow cells. After 30 days they were recolonized with thymocytes and spleen cells, and challenged with SRBC. Recipients given splenocytes primed with an immunogenic dose of SRBC make a strong response (1). Animals receiving no spleen cells have a moderate response (2), but animals which received cells from mice tolerized to SRBC (with a high dose of antigen) do not respond (3), indicating that cells from tolerized animals actively suppress the response in the recipient. Based on data of Gershon and Kondo, 1972.

the recipients (Fig.10.14). This was termed 'infectious immunological tolerance', and the cells transferring this tolerant state were called T suppressor (Ts) cells.

This observation was followed by several others ascribing a regulatory influence to Ts cells. Some of the evidence was indirect. For example, experiments were carried out which showed that treatment of mice with anti-lymphocyte serum (ALS) enhanced the response to T independent antigens such as pneumococcal polysaccharide SIII; injection of normal T cells depressed the immune response.

The IgE response in experimental animals is usually of short duration, as the major response to antigen is IgG. Tada and his colleagues, in their early studies on the regulation of IgE responses in the rat, demonstrated that the IgE response could be augmented by various kinds of treatment including anti-thymocyte serum (ATS), sublethal irradiation, adult thymectomy and splenectomy. This enhanced IgE response could be suppressed by the transfer of immune T cells. In those studies, dinitrophenylated *Ascaris suum* extract (DNP-Asc) was used as antigen, since it proved, when administered with *B. pertussis,* to be a very powerful inducer of IgE responses. Passive transfer of spleen cells or thymocytes from rats hyperimmunized with the carrier (but not the hapten) suppressed the augmented IgE anti-DNP response of irradiated rats immunized with DNP-Asc. This suppression was shown to be specific in that carrier-primed spleen cells could only suppress the response to hapten on the same carrier. The cell mediating the suppression appeared to be a T cell, since treatment of the carrier-primed spleen cell population with ATS and complement abolished the suppression (Fig.10.15 overpage).

Herzenberg and colleagues have extensively studied a different system in which carrier-primed T cells suppress the induced anti-hapten response. This involved priming animals with KLH and then challenging them with

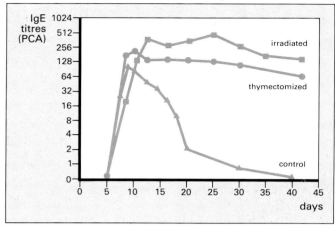

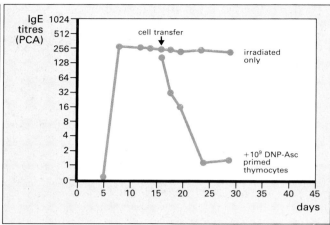

Fig.10.15   Isotype-specific suppression mediated by T cells.
Rats immunized with DNP-Asc in pertussis adjuvant develop a short-lived IgE response after five days, which wanes by day 35 (control). If the animals are irradiated or thymectomized, the IgE response persists (left). In a second experiment (right), thymocytes from an animal immunized with DNP-Asc in complete Freund's adjuvant were transferred to irradiated Asc-DNP/pertussis-primed animals, and were able to turn off the IgE response. The degree of turn-off depends on the number of cells transferred. In additional experiments, splenocytes were shown to be as effective as thymocytes. Based on data of Okumura and Tada, 1971.

Fig.10.16   Suppression of anti-hapten response by carrier priming. Adult mice were immunized at 0, 6 and 12 weeks to various antigens, and the IgG2 response to hapten (DNP) or carriers (KLH or CGG) was measured two weeks later. Mice immunized with DNP-KLH make a strong response to DNP (3), but if the animals were primed beforehand with KLH, the anti-DNP response was reduced even though the anti-KLH response was increased (2). KLH alone produced a weak response to itself (1). The second series of experiments showed that the effect was epitope-specific: if the DNP was linked to another carrier (DNP-CGG), the suppression did not occur (4). However, the suppression is maintained when the suppressive schedule precedes an otherwise immunogenic stimulation with DNP-CGG (5). If the initial carrier priming is omitted, the suppression does not develop (6). Data of Herzenberg et al., 1983.

	Immunization week			week 14 IgG2a antibody response to		
	0	6	12	DNP (µg/ml)	KLH %	CGG %
1	KLH	–	–	3	20	
2	KLH	DNP - KLH	–	5	170	
3	–	DNP - KLH	–	35	15	
4	KLH	DNP - CGG	–	20		21
5	KLH	DNP - KLH	DNP - CGG	6		8
6	–	DNP - KLH	DNP - CGG	60		9

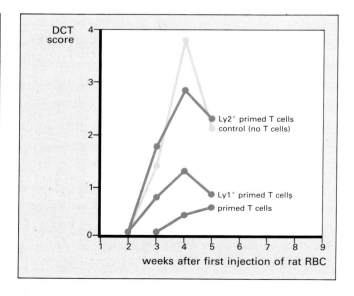

Fig.10.17   Autoantibody suppression by Ly1⁺ T cells. Mice immunized with rat red blood cells (RBC) are induced to make autoantibodies which react with cross-reactive determinants on mouse and rat red cells. T cells from such animals were transferred into recipients, which then received four weekly injections of rat RBC. The antibody response to mouse RBC was then measured by direct Coombs' test (DCT). Animals receiving no T cells made a strong autoantibody response. Unfractionated T cells and Ly1⁺ cells suppressed the response, whereas Ly2⁺ cells did not. Based on data of Hutchings et al., 1985.

DNP-KLH. They showed that there was carrier-specific suppression of the IgG anti-hapten response, but the response to the carrier itself was not affected. This suppression could be demonstrated both *in situ* and by transfer studies (Fig. 10.16).

Ts cells can also be shown to play a role in regulating the induction of autoantibodies. In Chapter 12, experiments are described in which erythrocyte autoantibodies were induced in mice following hyperimmunization with rat red blood cells (RBC). Transfer of splenic Ly1[+] cells from such primed mice suppresses the induction of autoantibodies in naive recipients (Fig. 10.17). The suppression appears to be epitope-specific, since only the response to determinants shared between mouse and rat RBC (autoantigens) is suppressed (the response to non-cross-reacting determinants on rat RBC is not suppressed). This would appear, therefore, to be another example of carrier-specific induction of hapten-specific suppression.

Herzenberg and colleagues identified another suppressor system in the mouse: allotype suppression. This is a particularly interesting model, illustrating clearly the effect of the maternal immune response on the observed responsiveness of the offspring. Jacobsen and Herzenberg generated chronic allotype suppression in F1 mice by either neonatal or *in utero* administration of antibody of the paternal allotype. Thus, when male SJL mice were mated to female BALB/c mice (with the IgG2a allotype Ig-1[a]) which had been previously immunized with SJL IgG2a (allotype

	GAT-(responder×non-responder) spleen cells	GAT-pulsed macrophages	Anti-GAT response
1	normal	responder	+
2	normal	non-responder	+
3	GAT-primed	responder	+
4	GAT-primed	non-responder	−
5	GAT-primed + normal	responder	+
6	GAT-primed + normal	non-responder	−

Fig. 10.19 Non-responsiveness due to Ts generation.
Mice of H-2[p,q] haplotypes fail to respond to GAT, but do respond to GAT coupled to methylated BSA (GAT-MBSA). Priming with GAT before GAT-MBSA challenge decreases the anti-GAT response in non-responder strains, but not in responders. The basis of this was examined *in vitro*, using (responder x non-responder) F1 spleen cells stimulated by responder or non-responder GAT-pulsed macrophages. F1 spleen cells could respond to GAT on responder and non-responder macrophages (1,2), indicating that non-responder macrophages can present GAT. However, if the spleen cells were primed previously with GAT, there was only an anti-GAT response in the presence of responder macrophages (3,4). It could be shown that the failure to respond was due to active suppression, since GAT-primed T cells would suppress the response of normally reactive unprimed cells (5,6). This implies that suppressor cells are generated from GAT-primed cells cultured in the presence of non-responder macrophages. Based on data of Pierce *et al.*, 1977.

Ig-1[b]), the offspring were suppressed with regard to production of Ig-1[b] IgG2a. In an adoptive transfer system and also *in vitro* it was shown that T cells (Ly2[+]) were present in the spleens of suppressed animals which specifically suppressed the Ig-1[b] antibody response (Fig. 10.18). However, the exact mechanism of suppression is still unclear. There has been a suggestion that suppression resulted from the action of the Ts on an allotype-specific TH cell, but the studies of Jacobsen demonstrating that these cells could suppress the Ig-1[b] response in nude mice also argued for a direct effect of the Ts on B cells.

The generation of suppressor cells in response to some antigens has been shown to be MHC-associated. For example, the non-responsiveness of H-2[q] mice to the synthetic polypeptide GAT has been shown to be circumvented by linking this polypeptide to methylated BSA (GAT:MBSA) as a carrier, thus demonstrating that B cells were present which were capable of responding. However, preimmunization of H-2[q] mice with GAT rendered them unable to respond to GAT:MBSA, and it was shown that Ts had been generated in response to presentation of GAT in association with non-responder Ia (Fig. 10.19). Mice which were non-responders to GAT (H-2 [p,q,s]) were also non-responders to GT, but could respond to GA. When GA was modified by attaching oligotyrosines to the C-terminal ([G,A]−T), non-responsiveness was observed suggesting that suppression in this system arises when Ts cells are presented with tyrosine residues. TH cells in these mice are therefore responding to determinants encoded by glutamic acid and alanine.

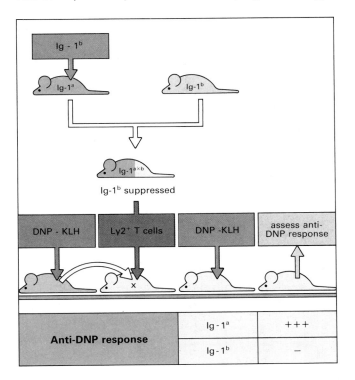

Fig. 10.18 Allotype-specific suppression. Female BALB/c mice of immunoglobulin allotype Ig-1[a] were immunized with Ig-1[b] antibody, and mated with an SJL Ig-1[b] male. The offspring could theoretically express both allotypes, but their Ig-1[b] expression was suppressed by the transfer of maternal antibody to Ig-1[b]. Ly2[+] cells from these mice were used to repopulate irradiated recipients, along with DNP-KLH-primed spleen cells and DNP-KLH antigen. The anti-DNP response in these animals was of the Ig-1[a] allotype, indicating that Ig-1[b] was actively suppressed by Ly2[+] suppressor cells. Based on data of Herzenberg *et al.*, 1973.

Fig. 10.20   Suppressor determinants.
Hen egg white lysozyme (HEL) can be cleaved by cyanogen bromide or acid hydrolysis to produce fragments including the LII peptide and the N-C peptide. The LII peptide is recognized by T$_H$ cells, while the N-C peptide is seen by B cells and, in non-responder strains, also by Ts cells. Using different species of lysozyme which differ in their amino acid sequences, it was shown that species with phenylalanine at position 3 generated suppressors, while species with tyrosine did not. This demonstrates the importance of this amino acid in suppressor cell generation. Based on data of Sercarz et al., 1978.

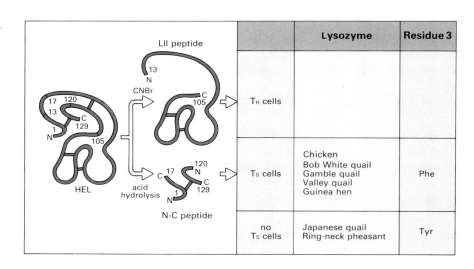

		Lysozyme	Residue 3
T$_H$ cells			
Ts cells		Chicken Bob White quail Gamble quail Valley quail Guinea hen	Phe
no Ts cells		Japanese quail Ring-neck pheasant	Tyr

This finding of specific suppressor epitopes on the antigen GAT is also seen in the response to the protein antigen hen egg white lysozyme (HEL). The response to HEL is under Ir gene control, with H-2^b mice being poor responders and H-2^q or H-2^a mice being high responders. Low responsiveness to HEL was clearly shown to be due to the generation of suppressor cells in H-2^b mice. Cleavage of HEL with cyanogen bromide gives rise to two fragments: the

N-C peptide (comprising the amino terminal residues 1-17 disulphide bonded to a carboxyterminal peptide composed of residues 120-129) and the LII peptide (residues 13-105). The LII peptide was consistently shown to induce T$_H$ cells in low responder strains, whereas the N-C peptide induced Ts cells. Thus, priming non-responder mice with either the N-C peptide or HEL induces Ts which block the response of T$_H$ to the LII peptide. So HEL generates suppression in low

Fig.10.21   Ts cells in regulation of the response to LDHβ. Studies of the proliferative response of lymph node T cells from different congenic mouse strains to LDHβ showed that B10.A (2R) mice (E$_β^k$:E$_α^k$) did not respond. Pretreatment of the cell populations with different antisera showed that the B10.A (2R) mouse could develop a proliferative response to LDHβ, but that it was held in check by an Ly1$^+$2$^+$ Ts which was I-E-restricted. The proliferative response was I-A-restricted (upper panel). The specificity of the Ly1$^+$2$^+$ Ts was shown in an experiment (lower panel) in which T cells were initially depleted of alloreactive cells by incubating with alloantigen and bromodeoxyuridine and light to remove proliferating cells. These depleted T cells were primed with LDHβ on syngeneic or

I-E		Treatment and effect on LDHβ reponse				
		none	αLy2+c'	αI-E	αI-A	αI-A+αI-E
B10.	E$_β^b$:E$_α^k$	+	+	+	−	−
B10.A (4R)	none	+	+	+	−	−
B10.A (5R)	E$_β^b$:E$_α^k$	+	+	+	−	−
B10.A (2R)	E$_β^k$:E$_α^k$	−	+	+		

allogeneic APCs, and a proliferative response was only observed on rechallenge if LDHβ was presented on the APC type used in the priming step. Thus, the proliferating T cell was restricted to the Ia of the APC initially employed to present LDHβ. The Ly1$^+$2$^+$

Ts from B10.A (2R) mice could only suppress the response of B10.S T cells primed with LDHβ on B10.A (2R) antigen-presenting cells, and could not suppress the response of B.10A (2R) T cells primed with LDHβ on B.10.S antigen-presenting cells. Data of Baxevanis et al., 1981.

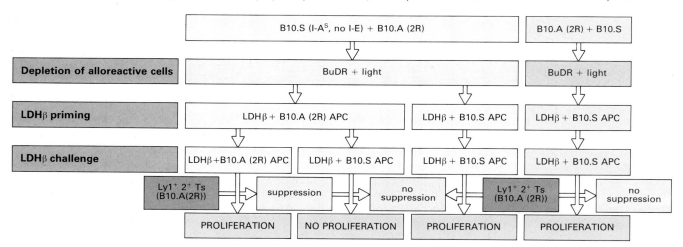

responder animals because it contains the suppressor epitope N-C (Fig.10.20). Using lysozymes from different, but closely related, avian species which differed in only a few amino acids, the suppressor epitope was shown to depend on the presence of a phenylalanine at position 3 in the amino terminus of lysozyme. The suppressor cells in this system, which are N-C-specific, appear to directly suppress the TH cells that recognize LII (see Chapter 8).

With regard to the influence of the MHC on the generation of Ts cells, an interesting series of experiments has been carried out by Baxevanis and colleagues in studies of the response to lactate dehydrogenase β (LDHβ). The response to this antigen is under Ir gene control; B10.A(2R) mice are non-responders, whereas B10, B10.A(4R) and B10.A(5R), which differ only in the MHC, are responders to LDHβ. Non-responder T cells are unable to proliferate *in vitro* in response to LDHβ. However, if pretreated with either anti-Ly2 and complement or anti-I-E antibodies, a proliferative response can be seen. In this system TH see LDHβ in association with the product of the I-A locus, since proliferative responses of both responder and Ts-depleted non-responder T cells to this antigen are inhibited by anti-I-A antibody. Further *in vitro* experiments showed that Ly1$^+$2$^-$ cells proliferate in response to LDHβ and addition of Ly1$^+$2$^+$ cells inhibited this proliferation. The proliferative response was inhibited by anti-I-A antibody, and this Ly1$^+$2$^+$-mediated inhibition of response was abrogated by anti-I-E antibody (Fig.10.21). Further analyses showed that the TH cells from a responder B10.S animal were only suppressed by Ts if they were of the same MHC as the APC used to present LDHβ in the initial priming culture. This has led to the suggestion that the Ts inhibits by means of a receptor or production of a factor which acts as an internal image of the determinant initially recognized by the TH cell on the APC (see Chapter 5).

The above are a selection of the many clear examples in which the phenomenon of specific suppression of the immune response has been demonstrated. In some cases, a complex interacting network of cells seems to be involved in producing the observed suppression, and there has been some evidence suggesting that suppressor factors play a role in these circuits. Some of the suppressor cells and corresponding suppressor factors were found to carry a determinant (I-J), originally thought to be coded by genes within the MHC. This is now known not to be the case, and although the possibility remains that anti-I-J antibodies in fact recognize some idiotypic determinant on an Ia-recognition element on the Ts cell, clarification is awaited as regards the significance of these markers on subpopulations of T cells interacting within the suppressor circuit.

Feedback Suppression
In vitro studies, such as those of Eardley, Gershon and their associates, demonstrated that the response to SRBC was subject to feedback suppression utilizing a complex circuit of cells interacting through a series of factors (Fig.10.22). The first cell in the circuit has been termed the 'suppressor inducer'; it was an Ly1$^+$, I-J$^+$, Qa1$^+$ T cell which produced a suppressor factor (TsiF), which in turn acted on an Ly1$^+$23$^+$, I-J$^+$, Qa$^+$T cell (transducer cell). This interaction was not MHC-restricted, despite the presence of I-J determinants on the factor, but it was restricted by immunoglobulin V$_H$. The transducer cell triggered an Ly23$^+$ effector suppressor cell which mediated its suppressor effect in an antigen-specific, MHC-restricted manner on the antigen-specific TH cell. Whether such

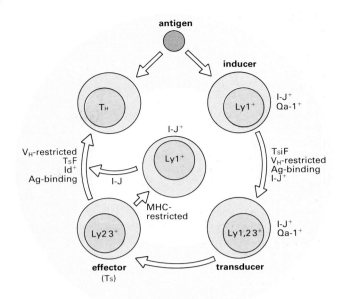

Fig.10.22 Feedback suppression. Gershon and colleagues noted that antigen *in vitro* could lead to suppression by activating a cascade of interactions. They thought that an inducer Ly1$^+$ cell, distinguishable from a TH cell, produced a suppressor inducer factor (TsiF) which was antigen-specific and restricted by Ig heavy chain V genes. This acted on a transducer cell which transmits the suppression from the inducer to the Ly2 3$^+$ Ts cell, and is assisted in this function by another Ly1$^+$ cell. It has been suggested that the Ts cell produces one chain of a T suppressor factor while the other is produced by the Ly1$^+$ cell. The factor acts on the TH cell in a Ig V$_H$ chain-restricted fashion. These cells express the various surface markers indicated. Based on data of Eardley *et al.*, 1978.

circuits have a relevance *in vivo* remains to be established.

Perhaps one of the best examples of a suppressor circuit in which suppressor factors have been reported to play a role has been provided by studies on the regulation of the response to the hapten azobenzenearsonate (ABA). Injection of spleen cells derivatized with this hapten into mice generates suppressor cells (Ts1) which can bind antigen and appear to carry a cross-reactive idiotype associated with anti-ABA antibodies. The activity of these cells is mediated by factors (TsF1) which appear to be Ig$_H$-restricted and elicit the development of another suppressor cell, Ts2, which is anti-idiotypic and makes a corresponding factor, TsF2. TsF2 appears to function in an MHC-restricted manner, and in turn it activates an idiotype-positive Ts cell (Ts3). This linear array of suppressor cells, which are thought to regulate DTH responses to ABA, are thus linked via idiotype/anti-idiotype interactions (Fig.10.23 overpage). Since the T cell receptor does not utilize Ig V$_H$ region genes, this finding was surprising. One explanation for the presence of the antibody cross-reactive idiotype (CRI) on the Ts1 (and indeed for those Ts systems in which V$_H$ region restriction is observed) is that of molecular mimicry at the receptor level. Exposure to B cell idiotypes during ontogeny could result in the setting up of complementary idiotypic networks, not only between B cells but also between T cells (see Chapter 13). Evidence that this may play a role in establishing suppressor circuits has been provided by the experiments of Benacerraf and colleagues

Fig. 10.23 Suppressor pathways. A suppressor pathway using azobenzene arsonate (ABA) as the antigen, utilizes an antigen-specific suppressor cell (Ts1) which releases a factor (TsF1) interacting with an idiotype-specific suppressor (Ts2). This in turn releases an idiotype-specific factor to act on a non-specific suppressor (Ts3). The cells and factors express the determinants indicated. Modified from Benacerraf *et al.*, 1980.

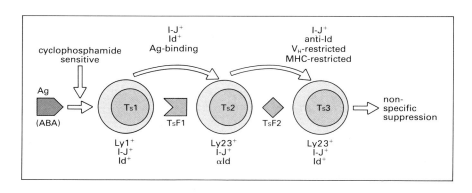

in which it was shown that μ-suppressed mice, which do not make immunoglobulin, did not appear to generate Ts1-derived suppressor factors. A further series of experiments revealed that μ-suppressed mice could, in fact, make Ts1 cells as well as the corresponding factor, but the factor bore an idiotype which was not normally expressed in that mouse strain. For example, antibodies to ABA in C.AL-20 mice normally express the dominant idiotype CRI_A, whereas those in BALB/c mice express CRI_C. TsF1 isolated from these mice normally express the dominant idiotype of the ABA antibodies, but those isolated from μ-suppressed animals expressed the usually silent idiotype for that strain (that is to say, TsF1 from μ-suppressed BALB/c mice expressed the CRI_A idiotype). This implies that the expressed B cell repertoire influences the composition of the Ts repertoire. Exposure of Ts cells to a new B cell repertoire can be shown to result in the generation of new patterns of TsF1 restriction (Fig. 10.24).

This last section has outlined a number of systems which suggest that immune responses may be regulated by a series of cellular interactions in which the cells are either linked by some form of antigen-bridging mechanism, or via complementary idiotypic interactions. In some cases it has also been asserted that soluble factors may play a role in these regulatory interactions. Whilst there is no doubt that the phenomenon of suppression exists, the means by which it is executed at a molecular level remains unclear. For example, it is not known if suppressor cells use the same form of T cell receptor as T_H and T_C cells, therefore their recognition mechanisms are not known. Thus, until these cells are cloned and fully characterized, suppressor networks, however intuitively attractive, must remain in the realms of speculation. This proviso also applies to the various suppressor factors outlined above. Attempts are being made to resolve the issue, and there are a few recent reports of T cell hybridomas which make suppressor factors. Clarification of this problematical area should be possible within the next few years.

Antigen-Non-Specific Suppression

This can arise in a variety of circumstances, such as following polyclonal T cell activation, allogeneic stimulation (MLC) and graft-versus-host (GvH) reactions. The ability of such activated T cells to suppress is often demonstrated as a suppression of *in vitro* antibody responses or of an MLR or MLC response. In many cases, it is not clear whether true suppression of the immune response or a cytotoxicity is really what is being observed. Many *in vitro* systems in which suppressor cells are generated also produce cytotoxic effectors which are capable of killing syngeneic cells (so-called 'promiscuous' cytotoxicity). Ts and Tc cells carry the same surface markers and thus cannot be differentiated on the basis of phenotype. Therefore, the interpretaton of such data requires caution.

Fig. 10.24 Ig determines Ts factor restriction. Mice of haplotype Ig-1^b were sublethally irradiated and repopulated with splenic T cells from mice of the Ig-1^n haplotype. After five days they were immunized with ABA coupled to spleen cells (ABA-SC), and spleen cells were taken seven days later. By treating the spleen cells with anti-Thy 1.1 and complement, only the Thy 1.2-bearing cells derived from the original donor were isolated. These cells were used to generate TsF1 which was tested *in vivo* for its ability to suppress the activity of CTL of different strains. Normally, TsF1 from Ig-1^n mice will only suppress cells from mice of the Ig-1^n haplotype, i.e. it is V_H-restricted (1,2). However, if the Ig-1^n-derived T cells are passaged through an irradiated host of a different allotype (Ig-1^b), they will acquire the ability to produce TsF1 which suppresses CTL derived from that allotype also (3,4), but they still do not interact with cells

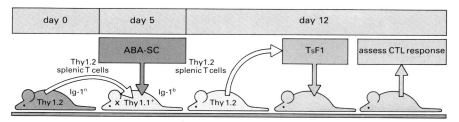

	Donor T cells	Transferred to host	Suppression of CTL response by TsF1 in mice of allotype	
1	Ig-1^n	–	Ig-1^n	+++
2	Ig-1^n	–	Ig-1^b	–
3	Ig-1^n	Ig-1^b	Ig-1^n	+++
4	Ig-1^n	Ig-1^b	Ig-1^b	+++
5	Ig-1^n	Ig-1^b	Ig-1^a	–

from mice of other allotypes (5). The T cells generate TsF1 restricted to the haplotype of B cells with which they mature. Data of Hayglass *et al.*, 1986.

When normal mouse spleen cells are cultured in supraoptimal concentrations of Con A, Ts cells are generated which can suppress an *in vitro* antibody response in a secondary culture. Using this system, Rich and Pierce showed that Con A stimulated T cells to produce a soluble immune response suppressor substance (SIRS). This suppression is not MHC-restricted, and it acts via macrophages. Activated T cells produce a variety of lymphokines (see Chapter 11), some of which (LTN and IFN$_\gamma$) can act on macrophages. Since it is known that activated macrophages produce PGE2 which can suppress the immune response, this would be one possible mechanism of suppression. IFN$_\gamma$ is itself antiproliferative and, if present at the beginning of a B cell response, it is inhibitory. There is, therefore, the additional possibility that IFN$_\gamma$ acts directly on a B cell. A T cell line producing SIRS has recently been characterized, therefore its identity should soon be revealed.

There has been suggestion that non-specific suppressor cells may function by consuming IL-2, thus blocking T$_H$ function and the development of Tc cells. However, this cannot be the whole explanation, since Cooke and Marshall-Clarke demonstrated that Ts generated by supraoptimal Con A could directly suppress hybridoma antibody production. Abbas and colleagues additionally showed that, while idiotype-specific Ts cells selectively inhibited the corresponding idiotype in a hybrid myeloma, non-specific Ts cells suppressed the production of both idiotypes produced by this hybrid. With regard to both these studies, a direct effect of the Ts is manifest on a factor-independent cell line.

Contrasuppression

Suppressor cells have been shown to regulate both cell-mediated as well as antibody responses. In some cases the Ts appear to act directly on B cells, but in others they appear to act on T$_H$ cells necessary for the immune response. Recently, Gershon and Greene described a mechanism by which T$_H$ cells can be protected from the effects of suppressor cells. The cell mediating this protection was called a 'contrasuppressor' cell. Since the initial description of this cell type, several other workers have provided supportive evidence for its existence, both in mouse and in man.

The early studies on contrasuppression utilized an *in vitro* culture system in which the immune response to SRBC was suppressed by Ts cells. It was shown that the activity of these Ts cells could be abolished if another cell type was added. These contrasuppressor cells (Tcs) were found to carry some distinctive surface antigens which allowed enrichment protocols to be developed. The Tcs were shown to be Ly1$^+$, I-J$^+$ cells which bound to the lectin from *Vicia villosa*. The selective binding of Tcs to *Vicia villosa* has been used to enrich these cells and study their characteristics. These cells can be demonstrated in a variety of situations. They are found in the spleens of hyperimmune animals, and in populations of neonatal spleen cells cultured *in vitro*. These cells can also be revealed in splenic populations depleted of Ts, and in mice in which autoimmunity has been induced by thymectomy and polyclonal activation. A complex circuitry has been proposed involving inducers, transducers and effectors of contrasuppression, which is analogous and complementary to the circuitry described for suppressor cells (Fig.10.25). As with suppressor cells, cloning and molecular characterization of contrasuppressor cells is required before their activity can be fully accepted.

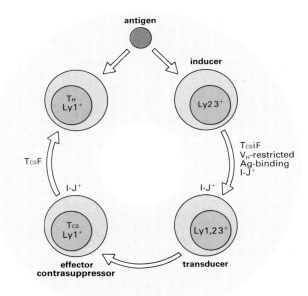

Fig.10.25 Contrasuppression. A cellular circuit was identified which counteracted the activity of the feedback suppressor circuit. Contrasuppressor cells prevented the T$_H$ cell from being suppressed. A number of cells were identified as members of this contrasuppression circuit; they appear to be analogues of those cells within the feedback suppression loop, but are differentiated by phenotype. A distinguishing feature of the Ly1$^+$, I-J$^+$ contrasuppressor cell is that it binds to the lectin *Vicia villosa*. This provides a convenient enrichment procedure. From Gershon *et al.*, 1981.

REGULATION OF THE IMMUNE RESPONSE BY IMMUNOGLOBULIN

Enhancement of the Immune Response by IgM

In 1968, Henry and Jerne showed that administration of rabbit IgM antibody to SRBC enhanced the immune response of mice to subimmunogenic doses of SRBC, whereas IgG antibody specifically suppressed this response. Enhancement by specific IgM antibodies is now well documented and can successfully be achieved with monoclonal antibodies (Fig.10.26 overpage). However, the underlying mechanism is still poorly understood. It has been reported that enhancement can be obtained in the absence of exogenous antigen, thus implicating the idiotype network (see Chapter 13). However, this may only apply to some monoclonals, since many workers have found that antigen is essential in order to observe IgM-mediated enhancement. Furthermore, the finding that the antibody response to TNP is enhanced by monoclonal IgM antibody to SRBC when TNP-SRBC is used as the immunogen, suggests that the idiotype network does not play a role in this enhancement.

When spleen cells are isolated from an animal primed with SRBC and monoclonal IgM antibody to SRBC, the observed *in vivo* enhancement can also be demonstrated *in vitro*. Both B and T cells from such animals appear to be more active *in vitro* than control cells derived from animals primed with SRBC alone. This suggests that IgM promotes priming of both T and B cells, perhaps by enhancing antigen presentation or by increasing localization of antigen to the spleen. This phenomenon of IgM-mediated enhancement

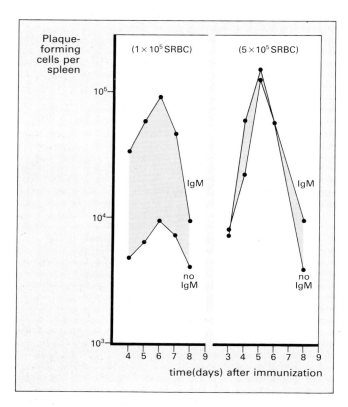

Fig.10.26 IgM-mediated immunological enhancement.
Mice received monoclonal IgM to SRBC (upper lines) two hours prior to immunization with SRBC. The antibody response (PFC) to SRBC was measured over the following eight days. By comparison with animals which received no IgM (lower lines) the response is enhanced, and this is also dependent on the antigen dose used. Data of Lehner *et al.*, 1980.

of the immune response was utilized by Harte and colleagues, to counteract the suppressive effect of maternal antibody on the immune response of offspring. Studies in murine malaria have shown that vaccination of offspring of immune mothers is ineffective for up to eight weeks after birth, due to the presence of maternal IgG in the colostrum. However, successful vaccination in the presence of such powerful suppression can be accomplished if IgM monoclonal antibody to the parasite (*P. yoelii*) is given together with formalin-fixed parasite vaccine. Thus, monoclonal IgM can act as an adjuvant to specifically, and perhaps physiologically, overcome maternal inhibition of malaria vaccination. These workers could find no evidence for the participation of the idiotype network (it was antigen-dependent), or for increased localization of antigen to the spleen. Thus the mechanism of the adjuvant effect is still unclear. It is, however, known that suppressor cells may play a role in the inhibited response of the offspring, and it is suggested that IgM somehow circumvents this suppression.

Enhancement through the Idiotype Network
This area has been extensively covered in Chapter 13, and therefore only a few instances will be discussed here. Suppression of the immune response by maternal IgG has been documented previously, but there are some situations where maternal IgG has been shown to play a beneficial role. The response to some T_{ind} antigens (polysaccharides) develops relatively late in ontogeny, in both mice and man.

Neonatal mice cannot be vaccinated against *E. coli* K13, even when this polysaccharide capsule antigen is made into a T dependent antigen by coupling it to an immunogenic carrier. Stein and Soderstrom performed a series of particularly interesting experiments on the response of mice to *E. coli*. These workers raised an IgG1 monoclonal anti-idiotype to an IgM monoclonal antibody which was known to be capable of conferring passive protective immunity. Treatment of neonates with either the IgM antibody or its IgG1 anti-idiotype enabled them to resist a lethal *E. coli* infection. In this context, the anti-idiotype (which was known to have paratopic specificity) was able to act as internal image of the antigen (surrogate antigen) under conditions in which the antigen itself was not efficacious. Furthermore, injection of mothers with the anti-idiotype immediately after birth resulted in the transmission of the anti-idiotype, and hence protective immunity, via the milk to the suckling (Fig.10.27). Such observations emphasize the unique potential of anti-idiotype vaccines:
1. An anti-idiotype can mimic carbohydrates or glyco-lipoproteins, antigens which cannot be gene-cloned.
2. The antigen itself does not even need to be isolated; all that is needed is a protective antibody.
3. Anti-idiotype can vaccinate under conditions where antigen is not effective, probably because of its immunoglobulin nature.

Although in the above case the anti-idiotype induced a protective B cell response, anti-idiotype reagents can also increase cell-mediated responses, such as DTH, which may also play a role in protective immunity.

	Treatment at birth	Immunization at 4 weeks	Percent survival
1	Id, 1μg	K13 vaccine	87
2	anti-Id, 50ng	K13 vaccine	93
3	anti-Id 10μg given to mothers	K13 vaccine	83
4	K13 polysaccharide, 2.5μg	K13 vaccine	33
5	none	K13 vaccine	44
6	none	none	0

Fig.10.27 Neonatal immunization by Id or anti-Id. Neonatal mice were given either IgM antibody to *E. coli* polysaccharide K13 (Id) or an IgG1 anti-Id to this antibody. They were immunized with K13 vaccine at 4 weeks and later infected with *E. coli*. Unvaccinated mice are unprotected (6), and vaccinated mice are only partly protected (4,5), but both priming with Id or anti-Id gave protection in association with the K13 vaccine (1,2). Anti-Id given to the mothers within 24 hours of delivery was transmitted to the offspring via the milk, and also allowed them to develop protective immunity when vaccinated (3). Hence, maternal antibody can have major effects on the development of immunity in neonates. Modified from Stein and Soderstrom, 1984.

Suppression by IgG
While IgM antibodies enhance the antibody response, IgG monoclonal antibodies may specifically suppress the immune response if administered just prior to, or at the time of, immunization. This suppression is also observed *in vitro*

following IgG and antigen administration *in vivo*. Again, the mechanism of suppression is poorly understood. It has been claimed that IgG may act by masking antigenic determinants, but it is difficult to reconcile this with the total suppression of the response to a complex antigen by an antibody reacting with only one determinant. Induction of Ts cells has also been suggested, but no evidence has been found for the activity of these cells in this system. It is possible that the monoclonal antibody simply acts by aiding opsonization and clearance of the antigen.

Suppression via the Idiotype Network
This has also been covered in detail in Chapter 13. It is clear that administration of idiotype or anti-idiotype can profoundly influence the subsequently expressed B cell repertoire. Suppressor T cells, acting within an interacting idiotypic network of cells (see above), can suppress both antibody and cell-mediated immune responses. In addition, some direct effect on B cell responsiveness has been observed.

Idiotype-specific regulation has been extensively studied using the plasmacytoma MOPC-315 as a model system. This plasmacytoma is an IgAλ2 anti-TNP, immunoglobulin-secreting, transplantable tumour of BALB/c mice. Rohrer, Lynch and their colleagues have shown that when BALB/c mice are immunized with the MOPC-315 immunoglobulin, subsequent growth of the tumour and secretion of immunoglobulin are selectively impaired. This may be accomplished by a variety of mechanisms. Idiotype-specific T cells are involved in the cytostasis of the tumour, but anti-idiotypic antibodies and idiotype-specific suppressor cells have also been identified. The mechanism of action of this $Ly1^-2^+$ Ts cell has been analysed, and it has been

found to be specific for an idiotope on V_H of 315 immunoglobulin and to act via a soluble factor. The effect of this suppression on the plasmacytoma is to selectively inhibit production of λ light chain by selective inhibition of mRNA for light chain. The mRNA for heavy chain and J chain can still be found in normal amounts, and can be shown to be functional in cell-free translation systems, suggesting that the light chain plays a regulatory role in heavy chain production. Using a hybrid myeloma cell line (MPC-11 × MOPC-315), Abbas and colleagues found that idiotype-specific Ts cells could selectively regulate the production of the corresponding idiotype (Fig.10.28). This provides a useful system for dissecting the mechanism of specific suppression.

SUMMARY

The maintenance of a given immune response is ultimately controlled by the availability of antigen. Following stimulation by antigen, T and B cells move from a resting state (G0) into G1, produce a variety of interleukins, and express receptors for these growth factors which allow them to progress to cell division and, in the case of the B cell, immunoglobulin secretion. Once antigen is removed, the cells gradually return to a quiescent state.

Genetic factors also influence the immune response. Differences in APC function can clearly affect the ability of different strains of animals to respond effectively to antigen. Inability of a given antigenic determinant to associate with a particular MHC antigen would render strains with that haplotype unresponsive to that epitope. Some animals also develop Ts cells in response to antigen presented to them in association with MHC, and they are therefore non-responders to the antigen. Ts cells can be demonstrated in a variety of situations, and may play a role in down-regulating an immune response as well as in maintaining states of tolerance. Several kinds of Ts have been described: antigen-specific, idiotype-specific and antigen-non-specific. The exact way in which suppression is accomplished remains to be clarified in most systems. Antigen-specific suppressor factors have been described, but definitive molecular characterization must be available before those factors can be assigned a role in immunoregulation. Immunoglobulin itself can both enhance or suppress B cell and cell-mediated immune responses. This can also be accomplished by a variety of mechanisms including antigen clearance, more efficient antigen localization, the generation of sub-populations of TH or Ts cells, or anti-idiotypic antibodies.

Another mode of T cell-mediated regulation has recently been described: contrasuppression. Contrasuppressor T cells (Tcs) apparently protect TH cells from suppressive influences. As with many of the complex immunoregulatory circuits, the fine molecular details remain to be characterized in order that their validity and *in vivo* role can be assessed.

Ts		IgA PFC/10^3cells	IgG PFC/10^3cells
1	none	459 ± 27	486 ± 26
2	MOPC 315 Ts	241 ± 41	518 ± 34
3	MPC 11 Ts	481 ± 50	360 ± 21

Fig.10.28   Effect of Id-specific Ts cells on hybridomas. A hybrid cell line was derived by fusing two myelomas, MOPC-315 (IgA λ2 anti-DNP) and MPC-11 (IgG2^{b,k}). Idiotype-specific Ts cells were prepared by immunizing BALB/c mice with spleen cells coupled to the respective myeloma Ids. Purified Ts cells were cocultured with the hybrid, and the effect on antibody production by the hybrid was measured. The hybrid normally makes both IgG and IgA (1). Ts cells specific for MOPC-315 selectively suppress the IgA response (2), while Ts cells specific for MPC-11 selectively suppress the IgG response. Thus, the idiotype-specific Ts cells selectively suppress synthesis of the antibody which they recognize, but not of other antibodies produced by the same cell. Data of Abbas *et al.*, 1980.

FURTHER READING

Abbas A.K. Burakoff S.J. Gefter M.L. & Greene M.I. (1980) *T lymphocyte-mediated suppression of myeloma function in vitro. III. Regulation of antibody production in hybrid myeloma cells by T lymphocytes.* J. Exp. Med. **152**, 969.

Asherson G.L. (1986) *An overview of T suppressor circuits.* Ann. Rev. Immunol. **4**, 37.

Baxevanis C.N. Nagy Z.A. & Klein J. (1981) *A novel type of T-T cell interaction removes the requirement for 1-B region in the H-2 complex.* Proc. Natl. Acad. Sci. U.S.A. **78**, 3809.

Benacerraf B. (1980) *Genetic control of the specificity of T lymphocytes and their regulatory products.* Prog. Immunol. **4**, 420.

Biozzi G., Mouton D., Sant'Anna O.A., Passos H.C., Gennari M., Reis M.H., Ferreira V.C.A., Heumann A.M., Bouthillier V., Ibanex O.M., Stiffel C. & Siqueira M. (1979) *Genetics of immunoresponsiveness to natural antigens in the mouse.* Curr. Top. Microbiol. Immunol. **85**, 31.

Blackwell J.M., Ulczak O.M., & Channon J.V. (1983) *Immunogenetics and immunoregulation of parasitic infection in mice with specific reference to Leishmaniasis.* In Experimental Bacterial and Parasitic Infections, Keusch and Wadstrom (Eds). Elsevier Science Publishing Co., Inc.

Bottomly K., Janeway C.A., Mathieson B.J. & Mosier D..E. (1980) *Absence of an antigen-specific helper T cell required for the expression of the T15 idiotype in mice treated with anti-μ antibody.* Eur. J. Immunol. **10**, 159.

Cooke A. & Marshall-Clarke S. (1981) *Action of Con A induced suppressor cells on a B-cell hybridoma.* Cell Immunology **61**, 300.

Dorf M.E. & Benacerraf B. (1984) *Suppressor cells and immunoregulation.* Ann. Rev. Immunol. **2**, 127.

Dutton R.W. (1973) *Inhibitory and stimulatory effects of Concanavalin A on the response of mouse spleen cells to antigen. II. Evidence for separate stimulatory and inhibitory cells.* J. Exp. Med. **138**, 1496.

Eardley D.D., Hugenberger J., McVay-Boudreau L., Shen F.K., Gershon R.K. & Cantor H. (1978) *Immunoregulatory circuits among T-cell sets. I. T-helper cells induce other T-cell sets to exert feedback inhibition.* J. Exp. Med. **147**, 1106.

Erb P., Vogt P., Matsunaga T., Rosenthal A. & Feldmann M. (1980) *Nature of T cell-macrophage interaction in helper cell induction in vitro. III. Responsiveness of T cells differentiating in irradiation or allophenic chimeras depends on the genotype of the host.* J. Immunol. **124**, 2656.

Gershon R.K., Eardley D.D., Durum S., Green D.R., Shen F.W., Yamauchi K., Cantor H. & Murphy D.B., (1981) *Contra-suppression = a novel immunoregulatory activity.* J. Exp. Med. **153**, 1533.

Gershon R.K. & Kondo K. (1972) *Infectious Immunological Tolerance.* Immunology **21**, 903.

Gershwin L.J. & Gershwin M.E. (1986) *The regulation of the IgE response.* Immunology Today **7**, 328.

Green D.R., Flood P.M. & Gershon R.K. (1983) *Immunoregulatory T cell pathways.* Ann. Rev. Immunol. **1**, 439

Green D.R. & Gershon R.K. (1984) *Contrasuppression: the second law of thermodynamics revisited.* Adv. Cancer Research **12**, 277.

Hanley-Hyde J.M. & Lynch R.G. (1986) *The physiology of B cells as studied with tumour models.* Ann. Rev. Immunol. **4**, 621

Harte P.G., Cooke A. & Playfair J.H.L. (1983) *Specific monoclonal IgM a potent adjuvant in murine malaria vaccination.* Nature **302**, 256.

Harte P.G., de Souza J.B. & Playfair J.H.L. (1982) *Failure of malaria vaccination in mice born to immune mothers.* Clin. Exp. Immunol. **49**, 509.

Hayglass K.T., Benacerraf B. & Sy. M.-S. (1986) *The influence of B cell idiotypes in the repertoire of suppressor T cells.* Immunology Today **7**, 179.

Hedrick S.M. & Watson J. (1979) *Genetic control of the immune response to collagen. II. Antibody responses produced in fetal liver restored radiation chimeras and thymus reconstituted F1 hybrid nude mice.* J. Exp Med. **150**, 646.

Henry C. & Jerne N. (1968) *Competition of 19S and 7S antigen receptors in the regulation of primary immune response.* J. Exp. Med. **128**, 133.

Herzenberg L.A., Chan E.L., Ravitch M.M., Riblet R.J. & Herzenberg L.A. (1973) *Active suppression of immunoglobulin allotype synthesis. III. Identification of T cells as responsible for suppression by cells from spleen, thymus, lymph node and bone marrow.* J. Exp. Med. **137**, 1311.

Herzenberg L.A., Okumura K., Cantor H., Sato V.L., Shen F.W., Boyse E.A. & Herzenberg L.A. (1976) *T-cell regulation of antibody responses: demonstration of allotype specific helper T cells and their specific removal by suppressor T cells.* J. Exp. Med. **144**, 330.

Herzenberg L.A., Tokuhisa T. & Hayakawa K. (1983) *Epitope-specific regulation..* Ann. Rev. Immunol. **1**, 609.

Heyman B., Andrighetto G. & Wigzell H. (1982) *Antigen-dependent IgM-mediated enhancement of the sheep erythrocyte response in mice: evidence for induction of B cells with specificities other than that of the injected antibodies.* J. Exp. Med. **155**, 994.

Howard J.G., Hale C. & Liew F.Y. (1982) *Genetically determined response mechanisms to cutaneous Leishmaniasis.* Trans. R. Soc. Trop. Med. & Hygiene **76**, 152.

Hutchings P., Marshall-Clarke S. & Cooke A. (1985) *Suppression of induced erythrocyte autoantibodies is dependent on Lyt 1+ T cells.* Immunology **56**, 269.

Isakov N., Scholz W. & Altman A. (1986) *Signal transduction and intracellular events in T-lymphocyte activation.* Immunology Today **7**, 271.

Ishizaka K. (1984) *Regulation of IgE synthesis.* Ann. Rev. Immunol. **2**, 159.

Jacobsen E.B., Herzenberg L.A., Riblet R.J. & Herzenberg L.A. (1972) *Active suppression of immunoglobulin allotype synthesis. I. Chronic supression following prenatal exposure to maternal antibody to paternal allotype of (SJL x BALB/c) F1 mice* J. Exp. Med. **135**, 1163.

Janeway C.A., Murgita T.A., Weinbaum F.I., Asofsky R. & Wigzell H. (1977) *Evidence for an immunoglobulin dependent antigen-specific helper T cell.* Proc. Natl. Acad. Sci. USA. **74**, 4582.

Krco C.J. & David C.S. (1981) *Genetics of Immune Response: a survey.* CRC Critical Reviews in Immunology **1**, 211.

Lehner P., Hutchings P., Lydyard P.M. & Cooke A. (1983) *Regulation of the immune response by antibody. II. IgM-mediated enhancement: dependency on antigen dose, T cell requirement and lack of evidence for an idiotype-regulated mechanism.* Immunology **50**, 503.

Longo D.L. & Schwarz R.H. (1981) *Inhibition of antigen induced proliferation of T cells from radiation induced bone marrow chimeras by monoclonal antibody directed against an Ia determinant on the antigen-presenting cell.* Proc. Natl. Acad. Sci. USA **78**, 514.

Marrack P. & Kappler J.W. (1978) *The role of H-2 linked genes in helper T-cell function. III. Expression of immune response genes for trinitrophenyl conjugates of Poly-L (Tyr, Gln) -Poly-D, L-Ala-Poly-L-Lys in B cells and macrophages.* J. Exp. Med. **147**, 1596.

Miller R.G. (1986) *The veto phenomenon and T cell regulation.* Immunology Today **7**, 112.

Mitchison N.A. (1971) *The carrier effect in the secondary response to hapten-protein conjugates. II. Cellular cooperation.* Eur. J. Immunol. **1**, 18.

Okumura K., Metzler C.M., Tsu T.T., Herzenberg L.A. & Herzenberg L.A. (1976) *Two stages of B-cell memory development with different T-cell requirements.* J. Exp. Med. **144**, 345.

Okumura K. & Tada T. (1971) *Regulation of homocytotropic antibody formation in the rat. VI. Inhibitory effect of thymocytes on the homocytotropic antibody response.* J. Immunol. **106**, 1019.

Pierce C.W., Germain R.N., Kapp J.A. & Benacerraf B. (1977) *Secondary antibody responses in vitro to L-glutamic acid60-L-Alanine30-L-tyrosine10 (GAT) by (Responder x Non responder) F1 spleen cells stimulated by parental GAT-macrophages.* J. Exp. Med. **146**, 1827.

Rich S.A. & Rich R.R. (1974) *Regulatory mechanisms in cell mediated immune response. I. Regulation of mixed lymphocyte reactions by alloantigen-activated thymus-derived lymphocytes.* J. Exp. Med. **140**, 1588.

Rohrer J.W. & Lynch R.G. (1978) *Antigen-specific regulation of myeloma cell differentiation in vivo by carrier-specific T cell factors and macrophages.* J. Immunol. **121**, 1066.

Schwartz R.H. (1968) *Immune response (Ir) genes of the murine major histocompatibility complex.* Advances in Immunology **38**, 31.

Sercarz E.E., Yowell R.L., Turkin D., Miller A., Araneo B.A. & Adorini (1978) *Different functional specificity repertoires for suppressor and helper T cells.* Immunol. Rev. **39**, 108.

Shevach E.M., Paul W.E. & Green I. (1972) *Histocompatibility-linked immune response gene functions in guinea pigs. Specific inhibition of antigen induced lymphocyte proliferation by alloantisera.* J. Exp. Med. **136**, 1207.

Shevach E.M. & Rosenthal A.S. (1973) *Function of macrophages in antigen recognition by guinea pig T lymphocytes. II. Role of the macrophage in the regulation of genetic control of the immune response.* J. Exp. Med. **138**, 1213.

Skamene E., Gros P., Forger A., Kongshavn P.A.L., St. Charles C. & Taylor B.A. (1982) *Genetic regulation in resistance to intracellular pathogens.* Nature **297**, 506.

Staeheli P. & Haller O. (1985) *An interferon-induced human protein with homology to protein Mx of influenza virus-resistant mice.* Mol. Cell. Biol. **5**, 2150.

Staeheli P., Haller O. & Boll W. (1986) *Mx protein: constitutive expression in 3T3 cells transformed with cloned M DNA confers selective resistance to influenza virus.* Cell **44**, 147.

Staeheli P., Pravtcheva D., Lundin L-G., Aclin M., Ruddle F., Lindenmann J. & Haller O. (1986) *Interferon-regulated influenza virus resistance gene Mx is localized on mouse-chromosome 16.* J. Virol. **58**, 967.

Stein K.E. & Soderstrom T. (1984) *Neonatal administration of idiotype or anti-idiotype primes for protection against Escherichia coli K13 infection in mice.* J. Exp. Med. **160**, 1001.

Tada T. (1984) *Help, suppression and specific factors.* Chapter 18 in Fundamental Immunology. W.E. Paul (Ed.) Raven Press, New York.

Tada T., Taniguchi M. & Okumura K. (1971) *Regulation of homocytotropic antibody formation in the rat. II. Effect of x irradiation.* J. Immunol. **106**, 1012.

Tadakuma T. & Pierce C.W. (1978) *Mode of action of immune response suppressor (SIRS) produced by Concanavalin A-activated spleen cells.* J. Immunol. **120**, 481.

Waldmann H., Lefkovitz I. & Feinstein A. (1976) *Restriction in the functions of single helper T cells.* Immunology **31**, 353.

Waldmann H., Pope H. & Lefkovitz I. (1976) *Limiting dilution analysis of helper T cell function. III. An approach to the study of the function of single helper T cells.* Immunology **31**, 343.

11 Lymphokines

The simplest definition of a lymphokine is that given by Gillis of a water-soluble regulatory peptide which is produced by a lymphocyte or acts on a lymphocyte. The existence of lymphokines has been recognized for over twenty years. It was known that the inflammatory process was dependent on the release of soluble factors from activated T cells and macrophages which would recruit other cells to the site of inflammation. Factors, such as macrophage activation factor (MAF), were known to be produced by T cells and to make macrophages more efficient at phagocytosing invading microorganisms. Much progress has recently been made in identifying those factors which provide relatively short range communication between the cells of the immune system. These factors, called interleukins, will be the main concern of this chapter. Interleukins have been indentified which act on B cells, T cells and macrophages. Some of the interleukins have marked biological effects on other cells, for example endothelial cells, epithelial cells and fibroblasts. The observation that the production and activity of interleukins can be regulated by glucocorticoids points to a means by which the immune system can be interlinked with the pituitary-hypothalamic axis.

There are several reasons for the recent progress in identifying the interleukins. Firstly, cell lines have been isolated which are dependent on certain interleukins for their growth. This provides a bioassay essential for any purification procedure. Secondly, clones of cells have become available which produce large amounts of interleukin following lectin challenge, thus providing a source of material both for gene cloning and for straightforward biochemical analysis. Finally, the application of gene cloning technology to this area of research has been fruitful. Several of the interleukins (IL-1, IL-2, IL-3, IFNs and lymphotoxins) have now been gene-cloned.

INTERLEUKIN-1 (IL-1)

This peptide of 15kD was originally thought to be produced only by cells of the monocyte/macrophage series. It is, however, becoming apparent that IL-1 may belong to a family of related molecules which can be produced by a variety of cell types, including skin keratinocytes, endothelial cells, kidney mesangial cells, astrocytes, glial cells, NK cells, corneal epithelium, macrophages and dendritic cells. IL-1 is produced by macrophages/monocytes in response to a variety of stimuli ranging from bacterial products and adjuvants to crystals of urate or silica (Fig.11.1). IL-1 also manifests a range of activities, as shown in Figure 11.2, overpage. A few of these activities were initially attributed to distinct entities and were given suitable acronyms (Fig.11.3 overpage). However, the availability of recombinant IL-1 and antibodies to IL-1 has established that all these activities are due to IL-1.

It is thought that IL-1 is synthesized as a larger molecular weight product (35kD) which is subsequently subjected to post-translational modification, such as proteolytic cleavage. Some of the size heterogeneity seen in IL-1 preparations may be due to incomplete post-translational modification, but in addition there may be multiple genes coding for an IL-1 family. In support of the latter, two distinct human cDNA clones have recently been produced, whose coded products are termed IL-1$_\alpha$ and IL-1$_\beta$.

IL-1 is an interesting lymphokine in that it functions as both a short range and a long range messenger. For example, in its latter capacity as a circulating hormone it is thought to act directly or indirectly on hepatocytes, causing production of acute phase proteins (such as C-reactive protein), or on the hypothalamus, inducing fever. Owing

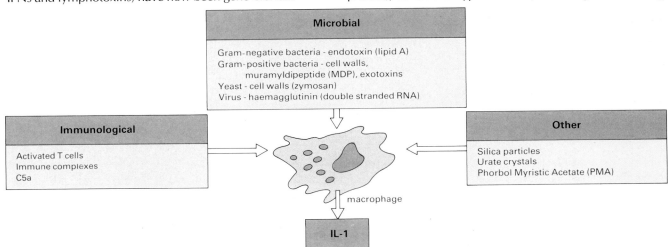

Fig.11.1 Stimuli of IL-1 release. From the immunologist's viewpoint, cells of the monocyte/macrophage system and other antigen-presenting cells are the most important sources of IL-1. The stimuli listed above stimulate IL-1 release from macrophages.

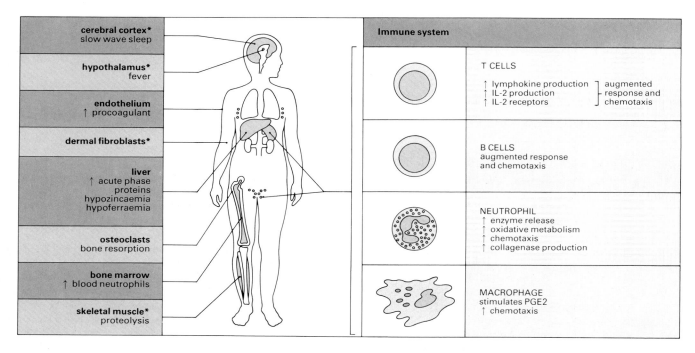

Fig.11.2 Effects of IL-1. IL-1 is a mediator produced by numerous cell types, whose effects are not limited to the immune system. IL-1 has been recognized in many different assays by its action on different cell types. Some of the main activities are listed in the diagram. * indicates that IL-1 stimulates PGE2 synthesis in these cells, partly accounting for its actions.

| Lymphocyte Activating Factor (LAF) |
| Endogenous Pyrogen (EP) |
| Mononuclear Cell Factor (MCF) |
| Leucocyte Endogenous Mediator (LEM) |
| Epidermal cell-derived Thymocyte Activating Factor (ETAF) |
| Proteolysis Inducing Factor (PIF) |
| Synovial Factor (SF) |
| Catabolin |
| Fibroblast Proliferating Factor |
| Osteoclast Activating Factor (OAF) |

Fig.11.3 Activities of IL-1. IL-1 has been discovered and rediscovered on several occasions acting in different systems. It is only recently that biologists have realized that the various factors listed above are all IL-1.

to this ability of IL-1 to induce fever, it was originally identified as an 'endogenous pyrogen'. Since it has been shown that T cell activity can be enhanced at febrile temperature, this action of the monocyte on the central nervous system may have important immunological consequences (Fig.11.4).

As a short range mediator in the immune response, IL-1 can evoke a variety of responses. If IL-1 is added with PHA or Con A (T cell mitogens) to thymocytes, marked proliferation is induced. IL-1 in conjunction with antigen or mitogen stimulates the release of IL-2 from peripheral T

cells, and it has also been shown to enhance the expression of the IL-2 receptor. IL-1 may not even need to be released from the cell to participate in accessory cell-dependent T cell activation, since there is some evidence that macrophages 'fixed' with paraformaldehyde can present antigen, and that they have membrane-bound interleukin-1. Interleukin-1 potentiates T helper cell activity, possibly through several pathways. It affects T helper cells by:
1. Increasing interleukin-2 release and interleukin-2 receptor expression.
2. Raising bodily temperature, thus enhancing the T cell response.
3. Protecting T helper from T suppressor cells. IL-1 can act as a contrasuppressive agent antagonising the effect of T suppressor factor (TsF).

B cells can also respond to interleukin-1. IL-1 has been shown to both drive maturation of B cell responses and to act synergistically with other lymphokines to stimulate B cell proliferation.

Macrophages themselves can respond to interleukin-1 by releasing prostaglandin E2 (PGE2) and producing tumour necrosis factor (TNF). In most cases it is not clear whether the cells which respond to interleukin-1 also produce it. Since prostaglandin E2 can inhibit interleukin-1 production by macrophages and decrease Ia expression, the process of interleukin-1 production may be self-limiting.

As a variety of cells outside the immune system can also produce this lymphokine, it is of interest whether some of these cells, for example, endothelial cells and astrocytes, also act as antigen-presenting cells when they produce IL-1 and express class II MHC molecules. B cells have been shown to be capable of presenting antigen to T cells and, recently, membrane-bound IL-1 has been located on these cells.

IL-1 has been implicated in pathological changes associated with tissue destruction in joint diseases, including rheumatoid arthritis. IL-1 has been shown to

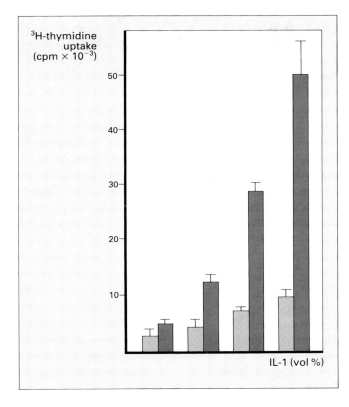

Fig.11.4 Effect of temperature on T cell proliferation.
Thymocytes from C3H/HeJ mice were stimulated with IL-1 and Con A (1 µg/ml) and maintained at either 37°C (pink) or 39°C (brown). The proliferation was measured by uptake of ^{3}H-thymidine on day 3. IL-1 induces thymocyte proliferation, but the effect is greatly enhanced at febrile temperatures. Data of Duff and Durum (1983).

inhibit sulphate incorporation into proteoglycan and the synthesis of collagen. Osteoclast activating factor (OAF) shows N-terminal sequence homology with IL-1$_\beta$, and shares many of the biochemical characteristics of this molecule (pI 6.8, 17.4 kD). This strongly suggests that OAF is in fact IL-1$_\beta$. Chondrocytes can be induced to resorb cartilage proteoglycan by IL-1, and bone resorption can be stimulated by IL-1 acting on osteoclasts, possibly through an initial interaction with osteoblasts. This ability of IL-1 to cause cartilage and bone resorption gave rise to the name 'catabolin', and identity with catabolin has only been established recently.

IL-1 production and activity is modulated by a variety of agents. An inhibitor of IL-1 has been isolated which may play a physiological role since serum levels of this inhibitor are elevated during fever. Aspirin and indomethacin are inhibitors of the cyclooxygenase pathway of arachidonate metabolism, and they have been shown to block the activity of IL-1 on the hypothalamus, implying that arachidonic acid metabolites modulate IL-1 effects. Corticosteroids, which are known anti-inflammatory agents and immuno-suppressants, also block IL-1 production. Antimalarial drugs (mepacrine and chloroquine) and gold components (for example, auranofin) which are used to treat rheumatoid arthritis, have been shown to affect IL-1 production. Interferons α and γ appear to positively stimulate IL-1 production, and since these agents can also enhance class II MHC expression, better antigen presentation would be a consequence.

INTERLEUKIN-2 (IL-2)

Interleukin-2 was previously called T cell growth factor (TCGF), adescriptive term providing a functional definition. This mitogenic lymphokine induces T cell proliferation and provides a means by which antigen-triggered T cells can be clonally expanded *in vitro*. The nucleotide sequence coding for IL-2, the genomic structure and the amino acid sequence giving rise to IL-2 activity have all been established. IL-2 is a single peptide of 15.4 kD, produced by T cells within hours of stimulation by antigen. IL-2 is sialylated and glycosylated; however, the carbohydrate component appears to play no part in the activity of the peptide, since recombinant IL-2 is equally effective at stimulating T cell proliferation as glycosylated IL-2. IL-2 can also be made by NK cells or large granular lymphocytes. In fact, NK cells produce a large variety of cytokines including IL-2, IL-1, BCGF and IFN, following stimulation with lectin or antigen.

Use of biosynthetically labelled IL-2 has allowed the identification of a specific membrane receptor for IL-2. This receptor has a high affinity for IL-2 ($Kd = 0.5$-2.0×10^{-12}M). More recently, evidence has emerged showing that a low affinity receptor is also present on activated T cells, and may constitute the major proportion of the IL-2 receptors. Since the two forms of the receptor are antigenically similar, this suggests that a single protein can be expressed in functionally distinct forms. Monoclonal antibodies have been generated which react with rat and mouse IL-2 receptors, and a monoclonal antibody with specificity for activated human T cells (anti-Tac) blocks binding of IL-2 to the receptor on human T cells. These monoclonal antibodies have been used to isolate and characterize the IL-2 receptor, which has recently been cloned and sequenced and appears to be a membrane glycoprotein of 55 kD. The gene for the human IL-2 receptor has been localized on chromosome 10. There is just one copy, and cDNA probes to the gene also hybridize at low stringency to the equivalent gene in the mouse. Details of IL-2 and its receptor are outlined in Figure 11.5, overpage.

The IL-2 receptor is only transiently expressed on T cells following antigen activation and there is some suggestion that, after cell division, antigen triggering must occur again before the IL-2 receptors are reexpressed at high density (see Chapter 4). Therefore, the response to IL-2 is restricted by the availability of IL-2 receptors, and since the density of IL-2 receptor expression is dependent on stimulation of the responding cells by antigen, the process remains antigen-specific although IL-2 is in itself a non-specific effector molecule. All three functional T cell subsets (T$_H$, Tc and Ts) can be induced to develop IL-2 receptors and will proliferate in the presence of IL-2, but it is not clear whether a given T cell can both produce and respond to IL-2 at the same time, or whether production and response to this lymphokine is restricted to certain phases of the cell cycle (Fig. 11.6 overpage). IL-2 also acts on other lymphoid cells. For example, NK activity is augmented by IL-2. This effect may in part be due to IL-2 stimulating production of IFN$_\gamma$ which is known to enhance NK cytolytic activity. B cells have been shown to express IL-2 receptors following antigenic stimulation, and proliferation and antibody production by B cells are increased by IL-2.

IL-2 synthesis is inhibited by glucocorticoids and by cyclosporine. IL-1 increases IL-2 production, and the glucocorticoid effect on IL-2 may be primarily attributable

Fig.11.5 IL-2 and the IL-2 receptor. The gene structure of human IL-2 (top) and the IL-2 receptor (bottom) are illustrated. The IL-2 gene lies on chromosome 4, and has four exons (numbered boxes), of which the first includes a leader peptide (L) which is required for translation but is cleaved before the protein is secreted. There are untranslated (UT) sections at both the 5' and 3' ends. The secreted protein has a single chain with a molecular weight of approximately 15.5 kD. The IL-2 receptor is encoded on chromosome 10, and is formed by eight exons, of which the seventh has the characteristics of a transmembrane segment (TM). Exons 2 and 3 have some homologies with 4 and 5, and have probably arisen by a gene duplication. The receptor molecule consists of a single peptide which has potential glycolsylation sites, and it is the target for a monoclonal antibody (anti-Tac).

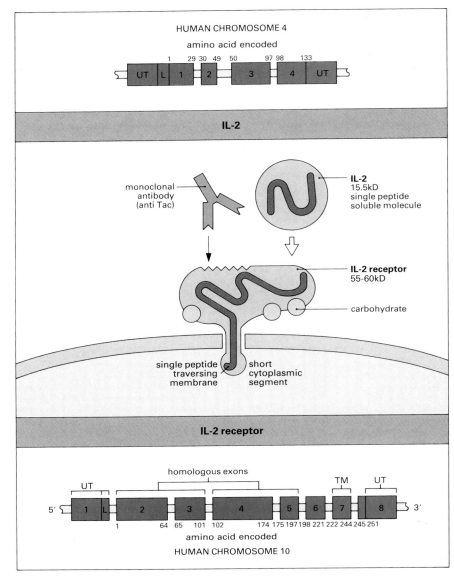

Fig.11.6 TH, Tc and Ts respond to IL-2 and proliferate in its presence.
Antigen-presenting cells process and present antigen to TH cells in the context of class II MHC antigens. IL-1 produced by antigen-presenting cells augments the response of some T cells. In response to these stimuli, TH cells produce IL-2 which allows those T cells with IL-2 receptors to proliferate. IL-2 receptor expression is increased following antigen presentation (shown here for class II-restricted T cells), and it is therefore probable that the same cell can both produce and respond to IL-2 (an autocrine pathway) as well as trigger other cells.

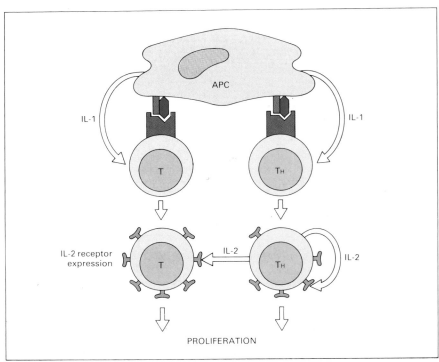

to an inhibition of IL-1 production. One way in which cyclosporine has been shown to act on the immune system is by affecting transcription of mRNA for IL-2. In some systems cyclosporine has also been shown to affect the expression of the IL-2 receptor. Inhibitors of IL-2 have been identified in murine sera, which may explain the rapid removal of activity of injected IL-2, and may be a means of controlling the immune response. Interleukin-2 has been shown to be able to break tolerance perhaps by affecting T suppressor activity. This will be discussed more fully in Chapter 12.

INTERFERON

Interferons (IFNs) were originally identified by their ability to prevent viral replication, and were isolated following stimulation of non-immune cells with virus. Interferons are an extremely heterogeneous family of proteins which were originally subdivided into Type I and Type II. Type I interferons (IFN$_\alpha$ and IFN$_\beta$) are produced following viral infections of leucocytes and fibroblasts respectively. Type II, or IFN$_\gamma$, is produced by mitogen- or antigen-activated T lymphocytes. The characteristics of interferons are outlined in Figure 11.7. Interferon γ is functionally similar in some respects to interferon α and interferon β, but it also has several distinct effects on cells of the immune system and of the myelomonocytic series. Furthermore, although some of these functions can also be mediated by IFN$_\alpha$, IFN$_\gamma$ is operative at much lower concentrations. Interferon γ is therefore a very important regulator of the immune response. As with many other lymphokines, the availability of recombinant IFN$_\gamma$ and antibodies specific for the interferon α subtypes, and for interferon β and γ, has made it easier to define this regulatory role of interferon in the immune system.

Interferon γ is a glycosylated protein of 20 or 25 kD depending on the extent of glycosylation. From the cloned cDNAs and genes of α, β and γ interferons it appears that there are at least twenty genes in the human interferon α gene family and a separate gene for interferon β and γ. There is no sequence homology between α, β and γ genes. Interferon γ acts on a variety of cells within the lymphoid system via interaction with a specific receptor, and some of its activities are discussed below (see also Figs. 11.8 and 11.9).

Macrophages and Monocytes

So-called macrophage activating factor (MAF) was one of the first lymphokine activities to be demonstrated. Using monoclonal antibodies to IFN$_\gamma$ it has been possible to prove the need for IFN$_\gamma$ in some MAF preparations. IFN$_\gamma$ has been shown to increase the number of high affinity Fc receptors for IgG on monocytes and macrophages. This has important consequences in terms of clearance of immune complexes, phagocytosis and antibody-dependent cellular cytotoxicity (ADCC). IFN$_\gamma$ has also been shown to activate oxidative metabolism in monocytes or macrophages, leading to loss of their ability to kill intracellular microbial or protozoan pathogens and tumour cells in vitro.

Class I and II MHC antigen expression can be induced or enhanced in various cell types by IFN$_\gamma$. IFN$_\gamma$ induces class II expression not only on macrophages, but also on Langerhans cells, vascular endothelial cells, keratinocytes, melanoma cells and some epithelial cells (for example, thyroid). When a macrophage cell line is cultured with IFN$_\gamma$, there is a ten-fold increase in the level of mRNA derived from the I region. This increase in membrane Ia would lead to an increase in the efficiency and number of cells acting as antigen-presenting cells. The increase in IL-1 production which follows IFN$_\gamma$ treatment of monocytes will also aid T cell activation.

T Cells

There is some evidence suggesting that interleukin-2 can cause T cells to produce interferon γ, which can in turn augment T cell expression of interleukin-2 receptors. This perhaps explains the enhanced cytotoxic T cell activity when treated with interferon γ. Interestingly, IFN$_\gamma$ has been shown to increase the susceptibility of the target to T cell killing, possibly through an effect on MHC antigen expression.

B Cells

Interferon has been shown to either suppress or enhance antibody production in vivo and in vitro. The outcome appears to depend on the dose and timing of administration of the interferon.

There are several reports suggesting that IFN$_\gamma$ can function as a late acting B cell growth factor inducing terminal maturation in activated B cells. If recombinant murine IFN$_\gamma$ is added to the murine B cell line 70 Z/3, it can cause the cell line to express surface immunoglobulin. T cell replacing factor (TRF) activity has been shown to involve IFN$_\gamma$, since

Interferon	Cell source (stimulus)	Physicochemical characteristics	Chromosome location (human)	No. of genes	Effects on targets
α	T,B macrophages (mitogen, viral)	peptides 18-20 kD acid stable	9	20	antiviral, antiproliferative ↑ class I MHC antigens synergizes with other lymphokines
β	fibroblasts epithelial cells (viral)	glycoproteins 23kD acid stable	9	1	antiviral, antiproliferative ↑ class I MHC antigens
γ	T$_H$, T$_C$, T$_S$ NK (antigen, mitogen viral)	glycoproteins 20-25kD acid (pH 2.0) labile	12	1	antiviral, antiproliferative ↑ class I, induce or ↑ class II MHC antigens B cell growth factor synergizes with other lymphokines

Fig.11.7 Interferons. Three groups of interferons have been identified by their ability to inhibit viral proliferation. (Type I: IFN$_\alpha$ and IFN$_\beta$; Type II: IFNγ). IFNγ also has numerous immunological functions. There are two distinct types of IFN receptor: type I receptor for IFN$_\alpha$ and IFN$_\beta$, and type II receptor for IFN$_\gamma$. Each receptor type is specific for its own interferon(s).

this activity is inhibitable by antibody specific for this mediator (see Fig.11.8).

Several workers have shown that the IFN$_\gamma$ can almost act like an adjuvant: if administered together with antigen, the response to some antigens can often be enhanced. This may not be a direct effect on the B cell, but may be attributable to increased MHC class II expression by macrophages causing enhanced antigen presentation. IFN$_\gamma$ has been shown to

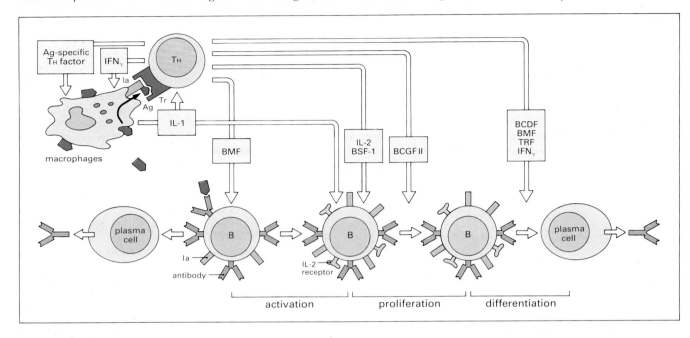

Fig.11.8 Role of lymphokines in B cell activation and differentiation. IL-1 produced by macrophages helps not only T cells to respond to antigen, but also B cells. IL-2 and BSF-1 (IL-4) produced by activated T$_H$ cells are also early acting B cell growth factors. BCGF II causes clonal expansion of B cells, and maturation of the response arises as a result of the action of T cell products BCDF, BMF, IFN$_\gamma$ and TRF. One kind of BMF described by Sidman and his colleagues causes resting B cells to progress to immunoglobulin secretion. Once the B cells are pushed into the cell cycle, they require continuous stimulation with B cell growth and differentiation factors to continue division and terminal differentiation into antibody-secreting plasma cells.

Fig.11.9 Multiple activities of IFN$_\gamma$.
IFN$_\gamma$ is produced by T helper cells following antigen/MHC-specific stimulation. It enhances MHC class II expression on antigen-presenting cells, and can induce class II expression on some facultative antigen-presenting cells which do not normally carry class II. It acts synergistically with other B cell stimulating factors, causing B cell proliferation and differentiation as well as direct macrophage activation. It also synergizes with tumour necrosis factor (TNF) and enhances the susceptibility of target cells to cytotoxic T and K cells. Its antiviral action is reflected in its ability to inhibit protein synthesis, which also appears as a seemingly paradoxical inhibition of B and T cell proliferation in some systems.

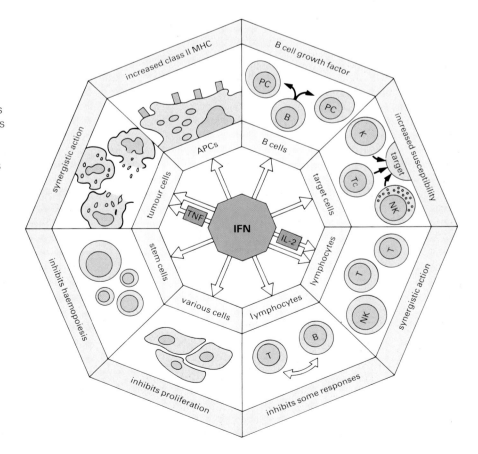

be capable of inhibiting some T independent antibody responses. Again, this may not be due to a primary action of IFN$_\gamma$ on the B cell, but may be induced by an effect on macrophage prostaglandin production. In this context it has been suggested that a soluble immune response suppressor (SIRS) factor, produced by Con A-activated T cells, may indeed be IFN$_\gamma$.

NK Cells

NK cells are large granular lymphocytes constituting about 1-3% of the total mononuclear cells. IFNs (α, β and γ) together with IL-2 have been shown to augment the function of NK cells. IFN$_\gamma$ appears to increase NK activity not only by recruiting pre-NK cells to become mature cytotoxic cells, but also by increasing the range of cells lysed. *In vivo* administration of IFNs can also lead to increased NK activity, although the results of such experiments are not always consistent.

Bone Marrow

Myelopoiesis has been shown to be inhibitable by interferons. Interferon α and γ has been shown to profoundly depress haemopoietic colony formation *in vitro*. This may be attributable not only to a direct antiproliferative effect of IFN on the progenitor cell, but also to the activation of macrophages and NK cells in this context. For example, the suppression of haemopoiesis observed in aplastic anaemia has been attributed to the activity of suppressor cells. The ability to abrogate this suppression *in vitro* by the use of antibodies to IFNγ suggests that this may be produced by the activated T cells in these patients.

LYMPHOTOXINS AND TUMOUR NECROSIS FACTOR

Lymphotoxin was one of the earliest lymphokines to be studied. It was shown in 1967 that stimulated lymphoid cells could produce a factor(s) that could be cytotoxic or cytostatic for a variety of cell types. The stimuli employed were either non-specific, such as mitogens, or specific, such as antigen. One of the toxic agents has been termed 'tumour necrosis factor' (TNF); this is macrophage-derived. The other toxic agent is called 'lymphotoxin' and is lymphocyte-derived. There are two terminologies for these cytotoxins: the lymphocyte-derived cytotoxin is called both lymphotoxin (LTN$_\alpha$) and tumour necrosis factor (TNF$_\beta$). The macrophage-derived cytotoxin is called both tumour necrosis factor (TNF$_\alpha$) and lymphotoxin (LTN$_\beta$). Here, these agents will both be described as TNF$_\alpha$ and TNF$_\beta$. The cytotoxic factor which was initially described as TNF was found in the sera of animals injected with LPS and BCG. This factor was shown to be produced by monocytes, and to be cytotoxic or cytostatic for several tumour cell lines. TNF can also kill some tumours *in vivo*. However, there is now considerable evidence demonstrating that TNF activity is not restricted to transformed cells, but that normal cells are affected in a variety of ways by this monokine. TNFs may be important mediators of tissue destruction (seen in auto-allergic responses), and may represent a means by which non-antibody-mediated cytotoxity is carried out.

TNF$_\beta$ is produced by OKT4$^+$ and 8$^+$ T cells in the human. The gene for TNF$_\beta$ has been cloned and it has been established that the gene product is 25 kD and subject to subsequent glycosylation. In the human, the TNF$_\beta$ gene is located on chromosome 6 as is the gene for TNF$_\alpha$.

Interestingly, both TNF$_\alpha$ and TNF$_\beta$ are cytotoxic proteins with 30% amino acid sequence homology.

Several types of cells can be affected by TNF, including fibroblasts, LPS-stimulated B cells, lymphoid tumour lines and some T cell clones. Little species specificity is exhibited by these cytotoxic factors, and the apparent ability of TNF to kill some transformed but not non-transformed lines led to some speculations that these factors may be of therapeutic value. However, not all transformed cell lines are susceptible to TNF, and susceptibility probably reflects the presence of a receptor on the cell (see below).

Recombinant IL-2 induces not only IFN$_\gamma$ production by peripheral blood lymphocytes, but also TNF$_\beta$. There appears to be synergy between IL-2 and IFN$_\gamma$ in the induction of TNF release; in addition, IFNγ acts synergistically with TNF to kill target cells. The mechanism of this may be through an effect of IFN on target cell susceptibility. One consequence of such synergistic activities may be that, when viral particles stimulate T cells to produce IL-2 and IFN, effective removal of virally infected cells is guaranteed.

Cachexia is a condition characterized by weight loss which is found in patients with certain infections and malignancy. This condition is associated with a mobilization of triglycerides and plasma elevation of very low density lipoprotein due to a loss of lipoprotein lipase activity in the peripheral tissue. Cachectin is a monokine of 17kD, produced when macrophages are stimulated with endotoxin. Cachectin has currently been shown to suppress the activity of the enzyme lipoprotein lipase in an adipocyte cell line, by specifically inhibiting transcription of those genes coding for the lipogenic enzymes in this line. The effects can also be demonstrated in these cells using recombinant TNF$_\alpha$. This finding and the N-terminal sequence similarity with cachectin suggest that cachectin is TNF$_\alpha$. Since it has been shown that muscle and liver cells, as well as adipocytes, have receptors for cachectin and respond with an increase in catabolism, it is possible to understand how a wasting syndrome can develop: during the course of certain diseases, macrophages are activated, TNF$_\alpha$ is produced in large amounts, and cachexia results.

Eosinophils play a number of roles in combating infection, and are also often involved in allergic responses, and have been shown to kill parasitic helminths. Factors produced by T cells and by activated macrophages will in turn promote eosinophil killing of schistosomulae of *S. mansoni* in the presence or absence of antibody. One of the factors known to activate eosinophils is a 17kD polypeptide which has been termed 'eosinophil cytotoxicity enhancing factor' (M-ECEF), recently identified as being TNF$_\alpha$.

Neutrophils have also been shown to be capable of mediating cytotoxic effects on virally infected or tumour cells. This may occur by antibody-dependent cell cytotoxicity (ADCC), or via the production of oxygen-derived metabolic products (superoxides). Both TNF$_\alpha$ and TNF$_\beta$ have been shown to increase the phagocytic activity of human neutrophils, and a marked synergy was observed between TNF$_\beta$ and IFN$_\gamma$ in eliciting this effect.

NK cells have been found to inhibit the development of haemopoietic colonies *in vitro*, and it may be that they play this role *in vivo*. Two activities have been identified in the culture fluids of NK cells: one factor, called 'NK cell-derived colony-inhibiting activator' (NK-CIA), is responsible for the inhibition of haemopoiesis. On the other hand, the 'NK cell-derived cytotoxic factor' (NKCF) is thought to be involved in the killing of NK-susceptible targets. NKCF appears to be released from NK cells when they come in contact with the target cell. Both factors have recently been shown to be identical molecules, and IFN$_\gamma$ plays a significant role in their activities. That is, synergy of IFN$_\gamma$ with NK-CIA results in mediation of IFN$_\gamma$ effects on growth of haemopoietic colonies as well as enhancement of NKCF cytotoxicity. NK-CIA and NKCF have been shown to be identical to TNF$_\alpha$. Production of TNF$_\alpha$ and TNF$_\beta$ is enhanced by recombinant IL-2 (rIL-2), probably through an effect on gene transcription. Although rIFN$_\gamma$ does not directly enhance TNF production, a marked synergy is seen between rIL-2 and rIFN$_\gamma$ in the induction of these cytotoxic factors. The presence of receptors for TNF on a variety of non-transformed cells and the synergistic interactions between the TNFs and IFN$_\gamma$ or IL-2 suggest that these molecules may play an important role in the regulation of cell interactions and perhaps in autoimmune pathology.

B CELL GROWTH AND DIFFERENTIATION FACTORS

Using *in vitro* systems for antibody synthesis, it has been possible to show that T dependent antibody responses could be maintained *in vitro*, provided a source of T cell replacing factor (TRF) activity is present. TRF activity is generally found in Con A or allogeneically stimulated spleen cell supernatants. Further analysis of such supernatants in conjunction with the isolation and purification of lymphokines such as IFN$_\gamma$, IL-1 and IL-2 has allowed further definition of distinct B cell growth and maturation factors. Several systems have been employed to analyse the separate stages in the process of B cell differentiation. Initial triggering of the B cell can be accomplished by crosslinking of the Ig receptors on the surface of the cell (antigen, anti-immunoglobulin or anti-idiotype can be used). However, such activated cells cannot proliferate or

Name	Molecular weight	PI	Comment
BSF-1 (IL-4)	18kD	6.7	early acting ↑ Ia on B cell
IL-1	15kD	5.0-6.8	↑ proliferation antibody production
IL-2	15kD	4.4	↑ proliferation antibody production
TRF	18kD	4.9-5.1	causes differentiation to antibody secretion
BCGF II	55kD	5.4	factor determining magnitude of response causes proliferation
BCDF$_\mu$	30-60kD		↑ IgM secretion
BCDF$_\gamma$	20kD 30kD	5.5-6.0	causes isotype switch IgG3-IgG1
IFN$_\gamma$	20-25kD		acts late induces differentiation to antibody secretion
BMF	16kD	4.1-4.5	induces antibody secretion

Fig. 11.10 Characteristics of murine B cell growth and differentiation factors.

differentiate in the absence of T cell-derived factors. The latter can be found in mitogen-activated supernatants, in supernatants from thymoma cells stimulated with the tumour promoter phorbol myristic acetate (PMA), as well as in the supernatants of antigen- or mitogen-activated T cell clones or hybridomas. These supernatants have been fractionated by a variety of techniques, and several factors have been identified (Fig.11.10).

B Cell Stimulation Factor I (BSF-I) (IL-4)

BSF-I (BCGF 1 according to the old terminology) was identified using a costimulator assay employing anti-μ to trigger resting murine B cells. Stimulation of the B cell was augmented when the B cell growth factor was present. This factor was shown to be present in T cell supernatants such as those obtained when EL4 cells are stimulated with PMA. BSF-1 is 15-20 kD, with a pI value of 6-7. A similar factor of 20 kD has been found in cultures of mitogen-activated human peripheral blood lymphocytes. Receptors for BSF-1 are found on stimulated B cells shortly after cultivation with antigen, mitogen or anti-immunoglobulin, but not on resting B cells or on B cells at a late stage of maturation. BSF-1 receptors are also not normally expressed on T cells. BSF-1 functions at an early stage of B cell activation, inducing a B cell to proliferate but not to secrete Ig.

B Cell Growth Factor II

A growth factor (BCGF II) has been isolated from murine T cell culture supernatants which will drive activated B cells through to maturation and secretion of immunoglobulin. BCGF II is 50-55 kD with a pI value of 5.5; it can be conveniently assayed by its ability to cause a murine B cell line, BCL1, to proliferate. A comparable human factor has been isolated from HTLV-transformed T cell lines.

B Cell Differentiation Factor

B cell differentiation factors (BCDF) carry the cell to high rates of immunoglobulin secretion. For example, BCDF$_\mu$ causes a B cell to secrete IgM. This activity has been demonstrated in the mouse using the BCL1 tumour which can be induced to proliferate in the presence of BCGF II and to secrete IgM in the presence of BCDF$_\mu$ which is 20-60 kD. Using the human B cell lymphoblastoid cell line CESS it has been possible to show that, in the presence of human BCDF, CESS cells show an increase in mRNA specific for secretory IgG. This BCDF activity is found to be 20 kD or 30-35 kD, depending on the source, and to have pI values in the range of 5.5-6. Murine BCDF$_\gamma$ activity has been shown to cause isotype switching in which the dominant IgG3 response to LPS is diverted to IgG1 in the presence of the factor. Factors have been described which appear to be capable of taking the resting B cell through to a fully mature immunoglobulin-secreting cell; they have been called B cell maturation factors (BMF). It is interesting to note that T cells from the enlarged lymph nodes of the autoimmune mouse strain MRL/lpr secrete a factor (L-BCDF) which induces terminal differentiation in B cells. These animals suffer from a generalized polyclonal B cell activation. IL-1, IL-2 and IFN$_\gamma$ have been shown to act in concert with all the previously described B cell growth factors (see Fig.11.8). To ensure maximum high rate immunoglobulin secretion, B cells express IL-2 receptors following activation; therefore IL-2 acts as a growth factor, whereas IFN$_\gamma$ has been shown to be a differentiation or late-acting growth factor. The characteristics of B cell growth and differentiation factors are listed in Figure 11.10.

COLONY-STIMULATING FACTORS

It has been known for some time that multipotential stem cells can give rise to all the cell types in the lymphoid and erythroid series. With the use of media conditioned in different ways, cell biologists were able to stimulate selective growth of various progenitor cells. Cells of the granulocytic/monocytic series are preferentially selected for when stem cells are cultured in the presence of the growth factor termed GM-CSF. This growth factor is produced by mouse lung tissue and T cell lines. GM-CSF is a 23 kD glycoprotein, and has recently been gene-cloned.

Multi-CSF is produced by lymphocytes and has alternately been called IL-3, burst promoting activity (BPA), P cell-stimulating factor (PCSF), haemopoietic cell growth factor (HCGF), mast cell growth factor (MCGF), erythroid, megakaryocyte and eosinophil-stimulating factor (E-CSF, MEG-CSF and EO-CSF respectively). Therefore, IL-3 acts on a wide variety of cell types promoting the growth and differentiation of various myeloid progenitor cells. IL-3 (24 kD) stimulates the proliferation of eosinophils, mast cells, megakaryocytes, granulocytes, macrophages and erythroid cells. Like GM-CSF, IL-3 can stimulate the growth of macrophage and granulocyte colonies from progenitor cells. This might suggest that they share some amino acid sequence homology; however, IL-3 and GM-CSF have both been gene-cloned and comparison of sequences has revealed little homology. Gene cloning will allow production of large quantities of homogeneous growth factors, which in turn will facilitate a detailed analysis of their different activities. IL-3, because it is multifunctional like IL-1, is particularly intriguing. It will soon be possible to know whether its diverse activities are mediated by a single site or different sites on the molecule.

ANTIGEN-SPECIFIC FACTORS

Various factors have been isolated from lymphoid cells or tissue culture supernatants which are shown to be capable of providing antigen-specific help or suppression. It is thought that the antigen-specific TH factor might act on the macrophage to increase the efficacy of antigen presentation. This factor has not been gene-cloned, despite the presence of TH cell clones. Some of the characteristics of this factor are presented in Figure 11.11.

T suppressor factors are also produced by activated T cells, but the cells producing these antigen-specific factors are of the Ly23 phenotype, whereas antigen-specific helper factors are produced by Ly1 cells. Cloning of genes for an antigen-specific suppressor factor has recently been demonstrated. This factor does not bear any resemblance to the T cell receptor. The characteristics of antigen-specific suppressor factors are also listed in Figure 11.11.

	Helper factor	Suppressor factor
Source	Ly1+ T cell	Ly23+ T cell
Target	macrophage B cell	T cell
Effect	induces B cell	suppresses T cells
Ag specificity	+	+
Mol. wt.	55-80kD	55-80kD
Serology V/C	+	+
MHC determinants	I-A (I-J)	I-J
MHC restriction	+ or −	+ or −

Fig.11.11 Antigen-specific factors. Antigen-specific helper and suppressor factors have been described, although they are less well characterized than the antigen-non-specific factors. They appear to have variable (V) and constant (C) portions, recognizable with specific antibodies, although this finding does not specifically refer to antibody or T cell receptor variable and constant regions. Major histocompatibility complex-related determinants have been identified in some cases by adsorption of the factors on anti-Ia or anti-IJ columns, and in some systems these factors act in an MHC-restricted fashion.

SUMMARY

Interactions between cells of the immune system are effected by a combination of direct cell/cell contacts, and by the release of various mediators. In recent years these factors have been characterized and their effects documented. The main antigen-non-specific factors fall into three groups: the interleukins (IL-1, IL-2 and IL-3), the interferons (IFN$_\alpha$, IFN$_\beta$ and IFN$_\gamma$) and B cell stimulating factors (B Cell Stimulation Factor I [BSF-1], B Cell Growth Factor II [BCGF II] and B Cell Differentiation Factor [BCDF]). These factors act in concert to control cell proliferation and differentiation during the development of an immune response, each having particular target cells which are only receptive to the factors at specific stages of their differentiation. Interleukin-1 and the interferons also have a number of effector functions on cells other than those of the immune system. Antigen-specific factors have also been described which can substitute for direct cell/cell interactions in some systems. *In vivo* the range of the factors is usually limited to cells in the immediate vicinity of the cell producing the mediator. Since antigen-specific cells will cluster around antigen-presenting cells, even the non-specific mediators will preferentially modulate antigen-specific interactions.

FURTHER READING

Beutler B. & Cerami A. (1986) *Cachectin and tumour necrosis factor as two sides of the same biological coin.* Nature **320,** 584.

Beutler B., Greenwald D., Hulmes J.D., Chang M., Pan Y.-C.E., Mathison J., Ulevitch R. & Cerami A. (1985) *Identity of tumour necrosis factor and the macrophage-secreted factor cachectin.* Nature **316,** 552.

Dijkema R., van der Meide P.H., Powels P.H., Caspers M., Dubbeld M. & Schellekens H. (1985) *Cloning and expression of the immune interferon gene of the rat.* EMBO J. **4,** 761.

Duff G.W. & Durum S.K. (1983) *The pyrogenic and mitogenic activities of interleukin-1 are related.* Nature **304,** 449.

Durum S.K., Schmidt J.A. & Oppenheim J.J. (1985) *Interleukin 1: an immunological perspective.* Ann. Rev. Immunol. **3,** 263.

Fung M.C., Hapel A.J., Ymer S., Cohen D.R., Johnson R.M., Campbell H.D. & Young I.G. (1983) *Molecular cloning of cDNA for murine interleukin-3.* Nature **307,** 222.

Gough N.M., Gough J., Metcalf D., Kelso A., Grail P., Nicola N.A., Burgess A.W. & Dunn A.R. (1984) *Molecular cloning of cDNA encoding a murine haemopoietic growth regulator granulocyte-macrophage colony stimulating factor.* Nature **309,** 763.

Gray P.W., Aggarwal B.B., Benton C.V., Bringman T.S., Henzel W.J., Jarret J.A., Leung D.W., Moffat B., Ng P., Svederesky L.P., Palladino M.A. & Nedwin G.E. (1984) *Cloning and expression of cDNA for human lymphotoxin, a lymphokine with tumour necrosis activity.* Nature **312,** 721.

Greene W.C. & Leonard W.J. (1986) *The human interleukin-2 receptor.* Ann. Rev. Immunol. **4,** 69.

Hanaoka T. & Ono S. (1986) *Regulation of B-cell differentiation: interaction of factors and corresponding receptors.* Ann. Rev. Immunol. **4,** 167.

Kashima N., Takaoka N.C., Fujita T., Taki S., Yamada G., Hamuro J. & Taniguchi T. (1985) *Unique structure of murine interleukin-2 as deduced from cloned cDNAs.* Nature **313,** 402.

Kishimoto T. (1985) *Factors affecting B cell growth and differentiation.* Ann. Rev. Immunol. **3,** 133.

March C.J., Mosley B., Larsen A., Cerretti D.P., Braedt G., Price V., Gillis S., Henney C.S., Kronheim S.R., Grabstein K., Conlon P.J., Hopp T.R. & Cosman D. (1985) *Cloning, sequence and expression of two distinct human interleukin 1-complementary DNAs.* Nature **315,** 641.

Melchers F. & Andersson J. (1986) *Factors controlling the B cell cycle.* Ann. Rev. Immunol. **4,** 13.

Oppenheim J.J., Kovacs E.J., Matsushima K. & Durum S.K. (1986) *There is more than one interleukin 1.* Immunology Today **7,** 45.

Ruddle N.H. (1985) *Lymphotoxin Redux.* Immunology Today **6,** 156.

Schrader J.W. (1986) *The panspecific haemopoietin of activated T lymphocytes (Interleukin-3).* Ann. Rev. Immunol. **4,** 205.

Sidman C.L., Paige C.J. & Schrier M.H. (1985) *B cell maturation factors.* Lymphokines **10,** 187.

Smith K.A. (1984) *Interleukin 2.* Ann. Rev. Immunol. **2,** 319.

Swain S.L., Wetzel G.D. & Dutton R.W. (1985) *B cell growth and differentiation factors.* Lymphokines **10,** 1.

Taya Y., Devos R., Tavernier J., Cheroutre H., Engler G. & Fiers W. (1982) *Cloning and structure of the human immune interferon-γ chromosomal gene.* EMBO J. **1,** 953.

Watson J.D. & Prestidge R.L. (1983) *Interleukin 3 and colony stimulating factors.* Immunology Today, **4,** 278.

12   Tolerance and Autoimmunity

The term 'tolerance' defines a state of specific immunological unresponsiveness to an antigen which arises after an initial encounter with the antigen. This is a purely functional definition of a state which may be achieved in a variety of ways, including clonal deletion of specific T or B cells, activation of idiotype- or antigen-specific T suppressor cells, effector cell blockade and/or antibody-mediated specific immunosuppression. These possible mechanisms, which are not mutually exclusive, will be discussed in detail later on. Immunological unresponsiveness arising as a result of administration of exogenous antigen is termed 'acquired immunological tolerance', whereas the unresponsiveness to endogenous antigens is termed 'natural immunological tolerance' or 'self tolerance'. The exact relationship between natural and induced states of tolerance is unclear, but several systems have been described in which self tolerance is broken and autoimmune responses are induced. These autoimmune states can often be regulated by the induction of a state of acquired immunological unresponsiveness.

Perhaps the first demonstration of tolerance induction was that of Wells and Osborne, who showed that an anaphylactic response of guinea-pigs to antigen could be diminished by orally administering a large quantity of antigen to the animals. Subsequent experiments by Chase and colleagues showed that when picryl chloride (trinitrophenol TNP) is fed to guinea-pigs, the delayed hypersensitivity and antibody responses to TNP conjugates are depressed. Numerous experiments followed, describing the induction of specifically unresponsive states. One particularly interesting observation was made by Owen in 1945, namely that dizygotic twin cattle which share a common placenta (Freemartins) are frequently chimaeric as a result of sharing blood cells during embryonic life. Such cattle are capable of accepting skin grafts from one another, manifesting a state of naturally induced tolerance. These observations led to the development of a theory by Burnet and Fenner in 1949, expounding the necessity of the discrimination of self from non-self, and postulating that such capability is learnt by the immune system during ontogeny. Since the immune system could, in theory, respond against a whole universe of antigens, it is necessary to prevent development of responses against self antigens (and hence autoimmunity). A classic experiment carried out by Triplett illustrates this point (Fig. 12.1): complete removal of the pituitary from the tree frog during early life resulted in the animal being capable of rejecting grafted pituitary tissue, whereas if only part of the pituitary was removed, these frogs tolerated the grafted tissue. This suggested that self antigens were recognized during ontogeny, and that tolerance to them was established as a result.

Other observations are consistent with this proposition. Reichlin's finding that rabbits can only make antibody to those determinants on haemoglobin which are not on rabbit haemoglobin suggests that functional deletion of the B cell repertoire has occurred. Also, studies carried out on C5-deficient animals show that animals genetically

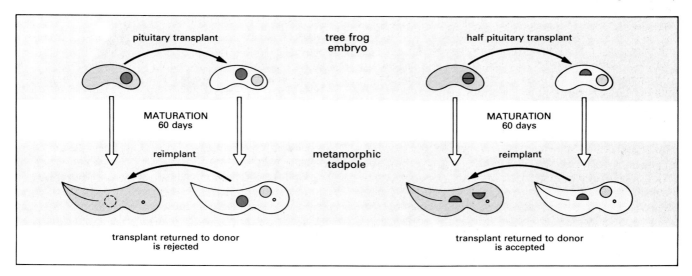

Fig. 12.1 Tolerance to self antigens is 'learnt' during ontogeny. The buccal component of the pituitary gland of tree frog embryos was removed and implanted in the dermis of other animals. Metamorphosis was allowed to continue by supplementing the diet of the operated animals with thyroid extract. At sixty days, the explanted hypophyses were removed and reimplanted in the dermis of the original donor.

These animals rejected the graft within forty days on average. However, when only half of the hypophysis was initially removed, the reimplanted half hypophyseal graft was accepted, suggesting that the ability to recognize antigen as self was acquired by contact with these antigens during the period of development in which immunological competence is acquired.

incapable of producing this serum protein (normally present in serum at 50-85 mg/ml) are not tolerant to C5, whereas normal animals are tolerant to this self antigen. C5-deficient animals will produce antibody to C5 if exposed to it.

In some cases, states of incomplete or partial tolerance are induced. This simply means that only some arms of the immune response against an antigen are affected, for example delayed hypersensivity while the antibody response remains intact, or it may be that only some subclasses of immunoglobulin are affected. Isotype shifts are frequently observed in states of partial tolerance. IgE responses are more sensitive to tolerance induction than IgG, and in turn IgG is more sensitive than IgM in response to T independent antigens. High affinity antibody production may also be affected, leaving the response restricted to only low affinity antibody production.

FACTORS AFFECTING TOLERANCE INDUCTION

Age of the Animal
Following on from the studies of Owen and Traub demonstrating that exposure to antigen *in utero* results in tolerance to that antigen, Billingham, Brent and Medawar induced tolerance to allografts by injecting allogeneic spleen and bone marrow cells into embryonic or neonatal mice. Similar observations were made by Hasek and colleagues in the chicken in which chimaerism was obtained by embryonic parabiosis. Many other investigators have confirmed the observation that tolerance is more readily induced in immature animals than it is in adults, and it also appears to be of longer duration.

These ontogenic differences probably reflect the differential sensivity of immature and mature B and T cells to tolerizing signals transduced via their membrane antigen-specific receptors. This is seen in the experiments of Nossal and colleagues, in which the ability of anti-μchain antibody to induce tolerance of adult and newborn splenic B cells was investigated. It was found that thirty times more antibody was required to inhibit B cell mitogenesis or antibody formation by mature B cells. Detailed studies have been carried out using isolating antigen-specific immature B cells or adult splenic B cells to determine the conditions that induce tolerance. B cells were tolerized for 24 hours with a hapten/carrier conjugate (FLU/HGG) and then challenged with the immunogen (FLU/POL). Using these conditions with different antigens, it was found that immature B cells were more readily tolerized than adult B cells.

Genetic Background
Recent experiments by Matzinger and colleagues, and Rammensee and Bevan, have indicated that self tolerance, at least for cytotoxic T cells, is MHC-restricted. Strain differences have been observed in the ease and maintenance of tolerance induction in mice. The autoimmune mouse strains (NZB×NZW)F1 were difficult to tolerize, and the tolerance that was induced was found to be of short duration. All murine strains which develop symptoms similar to human systemic lupus erythematosus (SLE) have been shown to be resistant to tolerance induction with hapten-substituted or deaggregated immunoglobulin. This, however, may not be universally true for other antigens; for example, one of the

autoimmune strains (MRL/lpr) can be tolerized by haptenated, syngeneic spleen cells. Cinader and colleagues have shown that SJL mice are also resistant to tolerance induction; this is of particular interest, since the SJL strain is highly susceptible to the induction of experimentally induced autoimmune diseases. Indeed, antigen-specific suppressor cells which can regulate the experimental induction of autoantibodies to red blood cells are not generated in this strain. The genetic basis of these observations is not yet clear.

Composition of the Antigen
The physical properties of the antigen are critical in determining its efficacy as a tolerogen. In general, agents which are poorly degraded are good tolerogens. For example, supraimmunogenic doses of polysaccharides or polymers composed of D-amino acids are slowly catabolized, hence they persist and maintain the state of tolerance. The experiments of Dresser were extremely important in the history of tolerance: they showed that if complexed or macromolecular antigen was removed by ultracentrifugation, the soluble antigen (in minute amounts) could induce tolerance in adult animals. The aggregated fraction, on the other hand, was a powerful immunogen. *In vivo* or *in vitro* fractionation of antigen into tolerogenic or immunogenic pools can be achieved by a process of 'biological filtration'. In general, materials which are readily phagocytosed are powerful immunogens, whereas those that are poorly phagocytosed are highly tolerogenic. It therefore seems likely that 'biological filtration' by the antigen-processing cells performs the equivalent function of ultracentrifugation in Dresser's experiments, with the monomeric antigen being poorly phagocytosed.

Alteration of the degree of substitution of an antigen with a hapten can influence the induction of tolerance as can the nature of the carrier. In the experiments of Pike and Nossal, different amounts of FLU were coupled onto either HGG or the $F(ab')_2$ fragment of HGG or BSA, and these conjugates were tested for their efficacy as tolerogens. The results clearly showed that the greater the degree of substitution with the hapten (FLU), the less antigen was required to achieve a given state of tolerance. It is generally found that highly derivatized material is a more powerful tolerogen than sparsely derivatized conjugates.

Another interesting aspect of these experiments was the observation that FLU-HGG, at any given substitution ratio, was a more effective tolerogen than FLU coupled to the $F(ab')_2$ of HGG. Both sets of conjugates were better tolerogens than FLU-BSA. It seems that the Fc region of the HGG may play a role in the generation of tolerance, perhaps by binding to the Fc receptor on the B cells. When haptens are coupled to autologous immunoglobulin, a powerful tolerogen is created which is capable of acting directly on adult B cells. However, the way in which Fc receptor binding of antigen could influence the signal delivered to the B cell is not clear. Isolated Fc has been shown to act as a polyclonal B cell activator; B cells, by virtue of bearing class II MHC molecules and having immunoglobulin receptors, have been shown to act as efficient antigen-presenting cells (see Chapter 6). Perhaps occupancy of an Fc receptor with haptenated immunoglobulin could result in the hapten being presented to the antigen-specific B cell as a multivalent array of haptenic determinants, resulting in tolerance (Fig. 12.2).

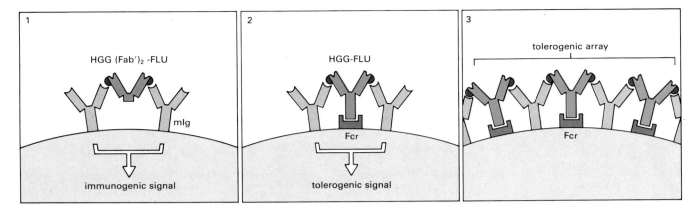

Fig. 12.2 Tolerization of B cells. Normal IgG is an efficient tolerogen, while the F(ab')₂ is a poor tolerogen. This implies that Fc receptors (Fcr) on B cells could be involved in tolerance induction, as proposed above. HGG F(ab')₂-FLU provides an immunogenic signal to the B cell, by binding to the B cell's membrane Ig (mIg). The antigen may be internalized and represented in association with class II MHC molecules (1). HGG-FLU can crosslink the Fc receptor and membrane Ig, producing a tolerogenic signal (2). Alternatively, the concentration of antigen on the cell by the Fc receptors creates a dense array of hapten on the cell surface, interfering with normal processing and producing tolerance.

Haptenated spleen cells or erythrocytes are also able to induce hapten-specific tolerance. Again, the higher the degree of substitution, the more effective the induction of tolerance.

Dose of the Antigen
Early studies demonstrated that the dose of the antigen could influence the degree and duration of tolerance. In general, it was found that supraimmunogenic doses of antigen could sometimes induce immunological unresponsiveness; detailed dose curves were carried out by Mitchison, clearly demonstrating that for some T dependent antigens tolerance could be induced at two dose ranges, one lower and one higher than that employed for optimal immunization (Fig. 12.3). In the case of T independent antigens, such a biphasic response was not observed. Cell transfer studies showed that at low antigen doses the T cells were tolerized, whereas at higher doses B as well as T cells could be tolerized. This was called low and high zone tolerance respectively. The dose of antigen required to tolerize mature T cells is many-fold lower (sometimes a thousand-fold) than that required to tolerize mature B cells. The amount of antigen required to cause B cell tolerance depends on the affinity of the B cell immunoglobulin receptor for the antigen. High affinity B cells can be tolerized at lower concentrations of antigen than low affinity B cells. This observation may explain why in some cases of incomplete tolerance only low affinity antibody is found.

Similar considerations are probably also true for T cells, although in this case the affinity of the cells for the appropriate combination of antigen and MHC molecule may also be important. Factors such as antigen processing (see Chapter 6) which influence the association of antigen and MHC molecules might, therefore, play a role in establishing a state of tolerance.

Route of Antigen Administration
The outcome of the immune response often depends on the route of antigen administration. Subcutaneous or intramuscular injection is usually immunogenic, whereas oral administration is often very efficient in inducing tolerance. Injecting antigen intravenously has also been shown to be a way of providing a tolerogenic signal. As stated earlier, 'biological filtration' can remove immunogenic material from an antigen preparation, leaving the non-processed, tolerizing portion unaffected. This may be the case when antigen is administered by these latter two routes.

Manipulations Facilitating Tolerance Induction
Tolerance induction is facilitated by measures which can decrease the amount of available T cell help. Therefore, treatment of an animal with total lymphoid irradiation (TLI), anti-lymphocyte antibody (ALS), anti-L3T4 or cyclosporine appears to favour the development of tolerance and/or the generation of T suppressor cells. This result may occur because these agents will prevent interleukin-2 (IL-2) production, the presence of which is known to interfere with the generation of a state of tolerance.

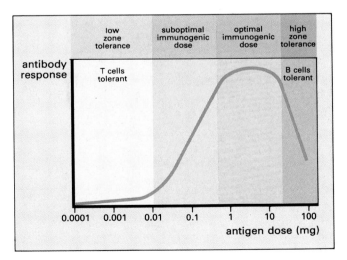

Fig. 12.3 High and low zone tolerance. Immunization of animals (for example the rabbit) with a T dependent antigen produces a characteristic dose response curve of antibody levels. In the supraimmunogenic region (high zone) B cells are tolerant, while T cells may be tolerized in the subimmunogenic (low zone) region.

Fig. 12.4 Neonatal tolerance is not developed in the presence of IL-2.
Tolerance to allogeneic stimuli can be developed if neonates are given large numbers of semi-allogeneic cells. For example, CBA mice are tolerized to C57Bl/10 ScSn alloantigen, by neonatal administration of semi-allogeneic (CBAxC57Bl/10 ScSn)F1 bone marrow. Such tolerized animals retain skin grafts from C57Bl/10 mice longer than normal mice. This is shown by the skin graft survival time for normal compared to tolerized animals. Control animals which were tolerized and received medium without IL-2 developed tolerance and did not show accelerated graft rejection. However, if IL-2 is

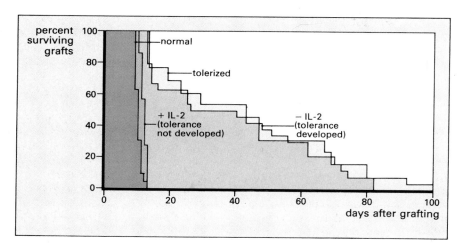

administered immediately after tolerization, tolerance is not developed.

Based on data by Malkovsky and Medawar.

The ability of IL-2 to modulate tolerance induction is particularly interesting, since it may provide an additional explanation other than the state of the B or T cell. Several convincing experiments have been performed, supporting this suggestion: it has been shown that neonatal spleen cells do not produce IL-2 following Con A stimulation. This age-related ability to secrete IL-2 may play a role in tolerance induction. Administration of a normally tolerogenic signal in the presence of IL-2 abrogates the induction of tolerance (Fig. 12.4). In summary:
1. Stimuli known to trigger IL-2 production (the lectin Con A, graft-versus-host reactions) block tolerance induction;
2. Drugs (for example cyclosporine, glucocorticoids), which suppress IL-2 production, favour tolerance induction;
3. Deletion *in vivo* of cells making IL-2 (for example by treatment of mice with anti-L3T4) allows tolerance to be developed to some antigens;
4. *In vivo* administration of IL-2 blocks the development of tolerance to alloantigens and the generation of antigen-specific T suppressor cells by haptenated cells.
Whereas induction of tolerance in adult animals often requires the antigen to be administered in a deaggregated

form, such measures are not necessary for induction of tolerance in neonates. Administration of antigen to neonates often results in specific and long-lasting tolerance to the antigen. It has been found, however, that total lymphoid irradiation renders a treated adult animal or individual more susceptible to tolerance induction and makes it behave more like a neonatal animal. Total lymphoid irradiation is a treatment in which fractionated doses of irradiation are administered and the cumulated dose is very high. This is accomplished by shielding the marrow, lungs and other vital non-lymphoid organs with lead during irradiation, thereby allowing doses as high as 4000rads to be given without severe side effects. Such treatment has been shown to create a window of time during which long-lasting tolerance can be induced to a variety of antigens, including transplantation antigens (Fig. 12.5). This allows allogeneic bone marrow chimaeras to be established without the development of graft-versus-host disease. Tolerance in this situation appears to be maintained by the generation of specific suppressor cells. These cells, called natural suppressor cells, are found in the spleens of both neonatal and irradiated animals, and they do not bear any conventional T cell markers. They appear to resemble NK cells

Fig. 12.5 Parallels between neonatal and adult tolerization by total lymphoid irradiation (TLI).
The diagram depicts the prelymphocyte and lymphocyte populations of primary and secondary lymphoid organs. In the neonate, there is a period during which tolerance is readily induced. This period follows the initial colonization of the thymus and secondary lymphoid tissues, when the immature cells have developed the antigen receptors, but before cell maturation. Total lymphoid irradiation in the adult denudes the thymus and secondary lymphoid organs of mature lymphocytes, and therefore creates a window of tolerizability before the secondary lymphoid

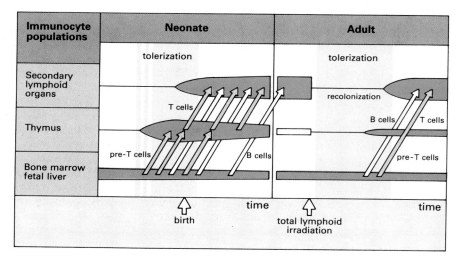

organs are recolonized from bone marrow stem cells. The bone marrow

stem cells are shielded from the lymphoid irradiation.

phenotypically but not functionally, since they do not kill NK-sensitive targets.

Cyclophosphamide is known to act on both T and B cells: at concentrations of 20mg/kg it has been shown to block the generation of Ts cells in the mouse, and at higher concentrations (200-300mg/kg) it can affect B cell function. When cyclophosphamide is given to an animal just prior to immunization with a T independent antigen, tolerance to this antigen is developed. In this case, as the antigen is T independent, any effect is not due to an interference with T cell help. Although other antimitotic drugs, such as cytosine arabinoside, 6-mercaptopurine and amethopterine, also facilitate tolerance induction, cyclophosphamide is the most effective in inducing tolerance to antigen. Its efficacy may be related to its ability to prevent regeneration of Ig receptors on B cells; in this regard, the B cell becomes like a neonatal B cell.

MECHANISMS OF TOLERANCE INDUCTION

Clonal Deletion of B Cells
One mechanism that has been proposed to explain B cell tolerance is exhaustive terminal differentiation, which would effectively result in clonal deletion of the B cell. One way to test for B cell clonal deletion would be by assessing the ability of polyclonal B cell activators to produce tolerance. If the ability to respond is not restored upon transfer into a naïve irradiated recipient, then tolerance is due to clonal deletion of responding cells and not to T suppressor cells in the donor. It is also possible to establish whether clonal deletion has occurred, by comparing the frequency of B cells for a particular antibody response in a non-tolerized population with that in a tolerized population. This has been carried out by Klinman and colleagues using murine B cells and the autoantigen cytochrome c. They established that many more precursors for a response against a particular cytochrome c peptide were present in the pre-B cell pool, than were present in the mature B cell pool. This could be interpreted as indicating that these autoreactive cells were purged from the B cell repertoire during ontogeny.

Effector Cell Blockage
In 1974, Schrader and Nossal demonstrated that specific antibody production could be down-regulated by the binding of multivalent antigen to the membrane Ig receptors on the B cell. Further experiments by other workers using a plasmacytoma as a clonal B cell source have shown that immune complexes may be particularly effective in this role. Using a hybridoma specific for FLU, Nossal and colleagues have shown that immunoglobulin synthesis is specifically and markedly reduced in the presence of multivalent FLU conjugates, while total protein synthesis is unaffected. The FLU conjugate could be seen on the surface of the cells, and following its enzymatic removal immunoglobulin synthesis was recovered. D-isomers of polypeptide antigens can also block the immunoglobulin receptors in an almost irreversible manner, since animals do not possess proteases to degrade these polypeptides.

Treadmill Tolerance
High concentrations of a poorly degraded antigen can lead to this apparent form of tolerance in which antibody is bound to the antigen, the immune complex is phagocytosed, and the non-degraded antigen is released to bind another antibody. Thus, although a response occurs, no free antibody is found in the circulation.

T Suppressor Cells
T suppressor cells have been shown to play an immunoregulatory role in many arms of the immune response. One of the first experiments demonstrating suppressor T cell activity was part of an investigation of the mechanism of immunological tolerance. In 1971, Gershon and Kondo found that when animals were given a large dose of sheep red blood cells they became tolerant or unresponsive to this antigen. Furthermore, splenic T cells could transfer this unresponsive state to other mice. This phenomenon was called infectious immunological tolerance, and was said to be mediated by T suppressor cells. Subsequently, many investigators demonstrated similar findings with different antigens; transfer of Ts cells will block the induction of immune responses, including those against self. An experiment demonstrating this is shown in Figure 12.6 overpage; Ts cells maintain tolerance and/or prevent immune responses to:
1. Thyroglobulin;
2. Myelin basic protein;
3. Erythrocytes;
4. Transplantation antigens;
5. Human gamma globulin;
6. Bovine serum albumin;
7. Haptens.

Interesting experiments have been carried out by Basten and colleagues, which have shown that memory Ts cells exist. Tolerance was established to HGG by using a large dose of antigen (100 mg), but very low doses were required (1 mg) to induce Ts cell memory. This means that tolerogenic doses of antigen could induce Ts cells, and their maintained activity could be guaranteed by the development of memory Ts cells following subsequent exposure to low doses of the tolerogen. Therefore, it is possible that tolerance could be achieved by a combination of clonal deletion and Ts cell activity. High doses of antigen could delete specific B cells from the repertoire, and also induce antigen-specific Ts cells which would block the induction of any future responses against this antigen. In the case of tolerance to self antigen and the acceptance of organ grafts, the same scenario could apply with the addition perhaps of memory Ts cells which would be developed by continual exposure to antigen.

Suppressor T cells have also been found which are idiotype-specific. They specifically suppress the production of a particular idiotype, presumably by direct interaction with B cells producing this idiotype. This form of immune regulation is discussed in greater detail in Chapter 10, but in the context of tolerance it can be seen that if an immune response is dominated by expression of a particular idiotype, idiotype-specific Ts cells could play an important role in maintaining an apparent state of tolerance to an antigen.

Mice can be protected against malaria by vaccination with parasite antigens. In 1985, Harte and Playfair showed that if animals are given specific IgG prior to vaccination no protection is manifest. This has been attributed to the generation of Ts cells (possibly idiotype-specific) in animals injected with specific immunoglobulin which can suppress the production of protective antibody in vaccinated animals.

Fig. 12.6 Splenic suppressor cells regulate the induction of RBC autoantibodies in mice.

Autoantibody present on the mouse red cells is measured in the weeks following the first injection of rat RBCs. Spleen cells transferred from animals primed with rat RBCs into naïve recipients suppress the induction of mouse red cell autoantibodies by rat red cells. This suppression is antigen-specific; only the autoantibody response is suppressed by these cells. CBA mice were compared with the spontaneously autoimmune strain (NZBxBALB/c)F1. Following a secondary course of rat RBCs, the autoantibody titre rises rapidly in CBA, but also falls rapidly, suggesting that the autoimmune response is turned off by T suppressors in this strain. The autoimmune strain does not show this switch-off (bottom left). The effect of suppressor cells is demonstrated (bottom right) by transferring splenocytes from primed CBA mice to recipients and challenging them with rat RBCs. Normal CBAs (2) develop autoantibody, as do recipients of normal splenocytes (1), but recipients of splenocytes from animals primed six months (3) or three weeks (4) before transfer suppress the auto-antibody response in the recipients.

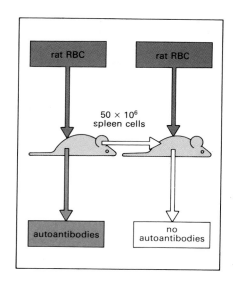

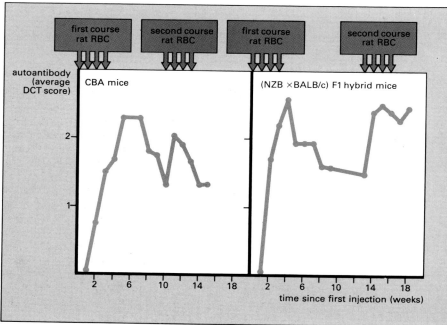

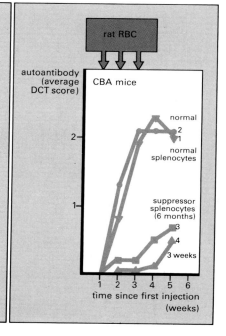

B Cell-mediated Tolerance

It is clear that antibody can enhance or suppress the immune response. Several workers have been able to show that if IgM antibodies to a particular antigen are given to an animal before the antigen, an enhanced immune response against this antigen is seen. On the other hand, when specific IgG antibodies are given to the animal, specific suppression of the immune response results. The way in which this suppression is effected is not completely understood, but certainly simple clearance of antigen or covering of antigenic determinants plays a role. However, it is also known that the immune complexes are good inducers of an anti-idiotypic response, and perhaps this provides another layer of control to block the specific immune response against an antigen. Such idiotypic control would be expected to act on both T and B cells, and is discussed in Chapters 10 and 13.

The IgE response is known to be depressed by specific IgG. This knowledge is utilized in desensitization programmes, in which an IgG response is specifically elicited against the allergen. In this case, IgG may be competing with IgE for the antigen, T suppressor cells may be induced, and there is also some evidence suggesting that an anti-idiotype can be induced suppressing the IgE response.

It is important in these cases to distinguish the effects of tolerance from those caused by competition between epitopes on the antigen (internal antigenic competition). It is clear that some regions of antigens are more immunogenic than others. The immunodominance of some epitopes is partly dependent on the species and the responder status of the strain. The failure to respond to weakly immunogenic determinants is not necessarily due to tolerance, but rather due to poorer processing and presentation of those determinants.

In situations where there are limited quantities of antigen present, high affinity B cells will selectively deplete the antigen pool and subsequently be able to interact with T helper cells, while low affinity cells will not be stimulated. This too can lead to a variety of responses to different epitopes on one antigen. In fact, it is possible to independently tolerize an animal to different epitopes on a single antigen. This is a condition which disturbs the immune response specificity profile against the antigen, leading to new epitopes becoming immunogenic.

Serum blocking factors have been demonstrated which will block the immune response against a tumour target. In some cases, these blocking factors have been identified as antibodies which may prevent an effective immune response against the tumour by masking antigenic determinants (see Fig. 12.7). Similar effects are seen in the responses to some bacteria, where inappropriate immune effector systems interfere with appropriate defensive reactions. The effects are not necessarily due to tolerance to the target, but due to the deviation of the immune response away from the correct target structure.

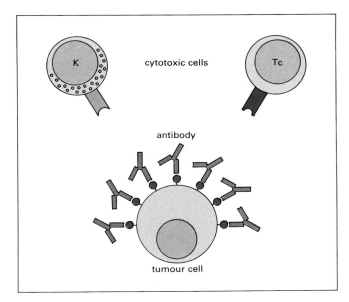

Fig. 12.7 Immunological enhancement. In some cases, antibody can actually promote tumour growth: this is called immunological enhancement. Antibody at high concentrations can block the binding of K cells or shield the determinants recognized by cytotoxic T cells.

T Cell Tolerance

It has been shown that many states of unresponsiveness arise due to a lack of T cell help. This form of tolerance can arise through any of the mechanisms described for B cells. Experiments have been carried out showing clonal deletion or abortion of specific T cells. In 1981, Nossal and Pike tolerized CBA (H-2^k) mice to BALB/c (H-2^d) antigens by neonatal injections of (CBA×BALB/c)F1 spleen cells. The frequency of anti-H-2^d cytotoxic T cell precursors (CTL-P), estimated by limiting dilution analysis, was found to be reduced by ninety percent, compared to normal mice.

Similar experiments have been carried out in which the numbers of hapten-reactive cytotoxic T lymphocyte precursors have been estimated in tolerant and normal mice. Adult mice are readily made tolerant to hapten by injecting them with haptenated syngeneic spleen cells, a finding which has been exploited to analyse the kinetics and basis of this tolerance. The animals were injected intravenously with reactive hapten which coupled *in situ* to autologous cells, and it was found that within twenty-four hours tolerance to the hapten was detectable. Limiting dilution analysis established that hapten-specific CTL-P were reduced in these tolerant animals.

Another example of tolerance being due to functional T and not B cell deletion is the cellular basis of tolerance to C5. As stated earlier, congenitally C5-deficient animals are not tolerant to this complement component, whereas C5-sufficient animals are tolerant. Congenic strains of mice exist such that one strain is deficient in C5. Cell transfer studies carried out between these strains revealed that only the T cells of the C5-sufficient animal were tolerant, since T cells from C5-deficient mice could help the B cells from either strain to make antibody against C5. There was no clonal deletion of the autoreactive B cells in the C5-sufficient mouse strain.

Fully allogeneic kidney grafts can be accepted and survive if recipients are subjected to immunological enhancement or immunosuppressive chemotherapy. In the case of immunological enhancement, antibody to donor alloantigens is generated in the animal by injection of donor strain spleen cells prior to transplantation. Passive enhancement is achieved when antibody specific for the allogeneic spleen cells is passively administered. Long-term graft acceptance can be obtained in animals if recipients are pretreated with allogeneic spleen cells, and are given antibody to the donor alloantigens prior to and also twenty-four hours after transplantation.

Several mechanisms have been proposed to explain this state of specific tolerance. These mechanisms include the destruction of Ia antigen-bearing passenger leucocytes in the graft, thus preventing them from sensitizing the recipient, as well as hindering the subsequent development and action of T suppressor cells. Rejection of kidney grafts can be delayed or abrogated if recipients are given spleen cells form tolerant animals, which implies the presence of T suppressor cells. This graft acceptance is specific for the tolerizing alloantigen. Recent experiments in rats have shown that the T suppressor cells which are generated in grafted animals appear to recognize T cell receptor idiotypes on alloreactive T cells, and to suppress their function. These suppressor cells are also generated in animals which are treated with the immunosuppressive drug cyclosporine to achieve graft survival, and this may explain why it has been found that patients require diminishing amounts of the drug during the later post-transplantation period. Thus, it may be that tolerance is maintained in these patients by idiotype-specific suppressor cells.

TERMINATION OF TOLERANCE AND METHODS OF INDUCING AUTOIMMUNITY

Tolerance is not established to antigens which are normally sequestered from the immune system, such as sperm antigen and lens crystallin. Autoantibodies can often be detected following trauma, which allows contact of those antigens with the immune system.

T cell tolerance can be bypassed by immunization with a cross-reacting antigen. For example, Weigle and colleagues showed that animals rendered tolerant to human gamma globulin (HGG) could produce antibodies to it if they were primed with bovine gamma globulin (BGG). Bovine gamma globulin shares some epitopes with human gamma globulin, but it also has some antigenic differences. These differences give rise to T helper cells which can provide support for those B cells reacting specifically with bovine gamma globulin, and

Fig. 12.8 Termination of tolerance by cross-reacting antigens. Human IgG (HGG) and bovine IgG (BGG) share some antigenic determinants, but differ in others. When animals tolerized to HGG are injected with the cross-reacting antigen BGG, TH cells are generated which recognize determinants on BGG. These TH cells provide help for B cells so that antibody is made which recognizes both BGG and HGG.

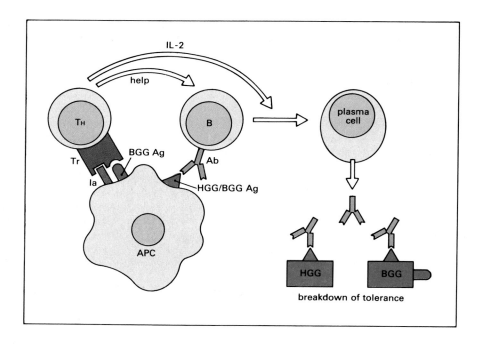

also for those responding against cross-reacting determinants (Fig. 12.8). The antibody produced to HGG is entirely cross-reactive with BGG.

Tolerance to self can also be broken in this way. As seen earlier, it is generally assumed that tolerance to self antigens is acquired during ontogeny, but if animals are injected with a cross-reacting thyroglobulin or red blood cells (RBC), autoantibodies against self thyroglobulin or self RBC (Fig. 12.9) can be detected. Before the use of synthetic insulins, this ability of antigenically cross-reacting antigens to induce autoantibodies led to complications in the therapy of patients with type I or insulin-dependent diabetes mellitus, since the use of

porcine or bovine insulin provoked autoantibody responses in some individuals. Insulin is a polypeptide with an A and B chain. Bovine insulin differs from human insulin by three amino acids, while porcine insulin differs by only one amino acid. These differences, however, are enough to allow these proteins to provoke the development of antibodies against porcine or bovine insulin, some of which cross-react with human insulin (i.e. autoantibodies). A further complication followed the use of insulin preparations which were contaminated with proinsulin. Insulin is synthesized in the β cell as preproinsulin which, compared to proinsulin, has an additional twenty amino acids at the N-terminal end. When this

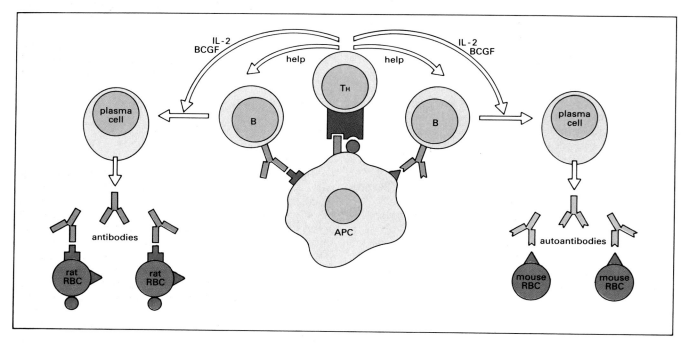

Fig. 12.9 Termination of self tolerance by cross-reacting antigens. Rat RBCs and mouse RBCs share some antigenic determinants but differ in others. TH cells are generated which recognize those foreign determinants and provide help for B

cells specific for both cross-reacting antigens and foreign antigens. This produces autoantibodies to mouse RBCs. light pink : autoantibodies (recognizing both rat RBCs and mouse RBCs); dark pink : antibodies to rat RBCs.

presequence is removed, proinsulin remains as a single chain polypeptide with positions A1 and B30 joined by a connecting peptide called the C peptide. This appears to assist in correct alignment for pairing disulphide bridges and folding of the protein (Fig. 12.10). Proinsulin is enzymatically converted to insulin which is stored in granules prior to release into the circulation. Hence, proinsulin is not normally found in the circulation, and tolerance to this precursor protein would not be developed. Proinsulin administration can, therefore, result in the development of insulin autoantibodies due to the activation of TH cells specific for the C peptide.

This provision of a so-called 'T cell bypass' can aid not only autoantibody production, but also cell-mediated autoimmune destruction such as that seen in experimental allergic encephalomyelitis where demyelination is T cell-mediated. It is also probable that, in thyroiditis, the destruction of the thyroid is not only mediated by antibody but by T cells, since pathology in this experimentally induced autoimmune state can also be mediated by T cell lines in the absence of autoantibody production.

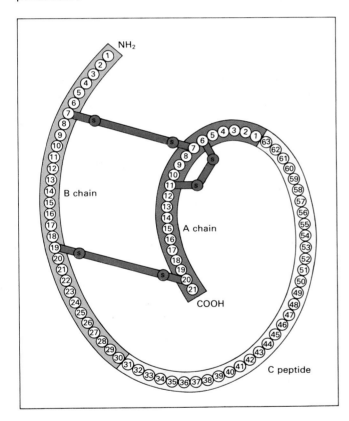

Fig. 12.10 The primary structure of proinsulin. Insulin is formed from proinsulin following enzymatic removal of the C peptide. Proinsulin is usually sequestered from the immune system, but if it is released into the circulation TH cells specific for the C peptide may develop, and can help B cells to produce antibody specific for the secreted insulin molecule. In the diagram, insulin A and B chains are depicted in orange and are crosslinked by disulphide bonds.

In the case of T cell tolerance, direct stimulation of the B cell by polyclonal B cell activators such as LPS can result in autoantibody production. When normal animals are injected with LPS, antibodies can be readily detected

which can react against self IgG (rheumatoid factors), DNA, or enzyme-modified self red blood cells. In addition, administration of a self antigen (such as mouse thyroglobulin) with LPS results in the generation of specific autoantibodies.

An alternative mode of B cell stimulation could be via the idiotype network (see Chapter 13). The ways in which network interactions could give rise to autoimmunity are outlined in Figure 12.11, overpage. In the first case, anti-idiotype to an antimicrobial antibody is anti-self. This could occur, for example, following a viral infection in which the possibility arises that some antiviral antibodies 'look like' the receptor for the virus on the cell; such an anti-idiotype would be an autoantibody.

It has been shown that anti-idiotypic antibody can, under certain conditions, augment production of all immunoglobulin molecules bearing this idiotype, some of which do not recognize the original antigen used to elicit the idiotype but may recognize autoantigen. Antibody production by B cells can be helped not only by carrier- but also by idiotype-specific TH cells. It is therefore possible for T cells to be generated following an infection, which recognize the idiotype on antimicrobial antibody and could help all B cells carrying this idiotype to secrete antibody. Some of these antibodies which constitute the so-called non-specific parallel set may be autoantibodies (see Fig. 12.11). It is notable in this context that a single point mutation in an antibody to phosphoryl choline (and hence against pneumococci) causes it to become reactive to polynucleotides (autoantigens). Since idiotype-specific TH cells can be generated to T15$^+$ anti-phosphoryl choline B cells, these may also regulate autoreactive mutants derived from the T15 idiotype-bearing cells.

A third possibility is that microbial antibody is itself an anti-idiotype to an autoantibody (see Fig. 12.11). Finally, it is possible that if an antigen on a microbe resembles an idiotype on an antibody, antimicrobial antibody could act as an anti-idiotype to the autoantibody and stimulate autoantibody production.

Allogeneic stimulation is also capable of breaking self tolerance, and a variety of autoantibodies can be detected in the sera of animals undergoing a graft-verus-host interaction. Autoantibodies are formed against:

1. Epithelial cells;
2. Erythrocytes;
3. Thymocytes;
4. Nuclear antigens;
5. Double-stranded DNA.

In this case, excessive IL-2 production could give rise to abrogation of suppression. Contrasuppressor cells are a subpopulation of T cells which appear to be able to prevent the action of Ts on TH cells. Any situation which favours the generation of contrasuppressor cells will prevent tolerance maintenance by Ts cells. Experiments have been carried out by Green and colleagues demonstrating the occurrence of autoantibodies in animals in which contrasuppressor cells are generated. There is increasing evidence that some diseases which have autoimmune components (for example multiple sclerosis) can be triggered by viral infections. This has led to the idea that co-processing of virus and self antigens could lead to the breakdown of self tolerance (Fig. 12.12 overpage). Additional functions would be required to produce autoimmune disease, otherwise autoimmune disease could develop frequently after many viral infections.

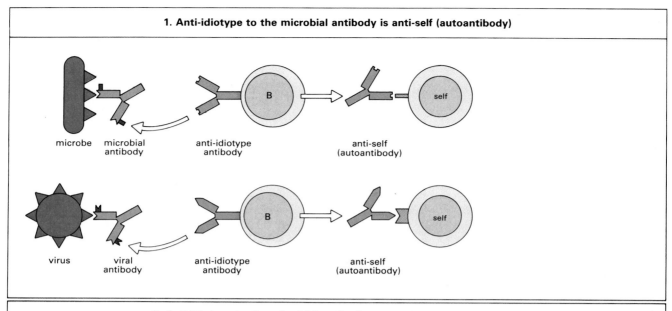

1. Anti-idiotype to the microbial antibody is anti-self (autoantibody)

microbe   microbial antibody   anti-idiotype antibody   anti-self (autoantibody)

virus   viral antibody   anti-idiotype antibody   anti-self (autoantibody)

2. Anti-idiotype to the microbial antibody up-regulates the parallel sets

parallel sets

help

microbe   microbial antibody   anti-idiotype   help   auto-reactive B cell   autoantibody   self

help

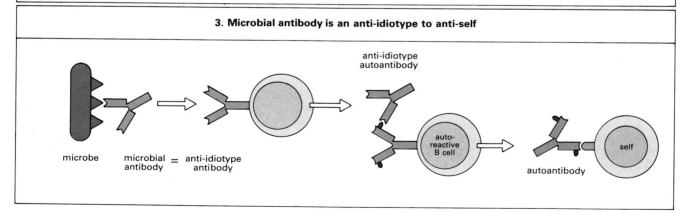

3. Microbial antibody is an anti-idiotype to anti-self

anti-idiotype autoantibody

microbe   microbial antibody = anti-idiotype antibody   auto-reactive B cell   autoantibody   self

Fig. 12.11 Development of autoimmunity by idiotypic interaction. Autoimmunity may develop via fortuitous cross-reactivity within sets of idiotypically regulating cells. (1) Antibody to a pathogenic microbe or virus carries a determinant resembling a self epitope. Anti-idiotypic antibody stimulated by the first antibody is self-reactive. (2) Antibody to a microbe is regulated by an idiotype-specific T helper cell (TH/B). If the idiotope is shared by a parallel set of autoreactive B cells, these will be concomitantly up-regulated. B cells producing cross-reactive anti-idiotype could also stimulate autoantibody in a similar way. (3) The microbe itself may express an epitope which resembles an idiotope on an autoantibody. In this case, antibody to that epitope will stimulate idiotope-bearing autoreactive B cells.

Fig. 12.12 Virus induction of autoimmunity. Enveloped viruses bud from the membrane of an infected cell and may incorporate host cell proteins into the envelope. Such viruses, rendered non-infectious by antiviral antibody, are taken up by phagocytes via their Fc receptors (Fcr). The virus or viral fragments are internalized and processed, resulting in the expression of viral antigen in association with MHC class II molecules. If the self proteins are processed similarly, they can then stimulate autoreactive T cells.

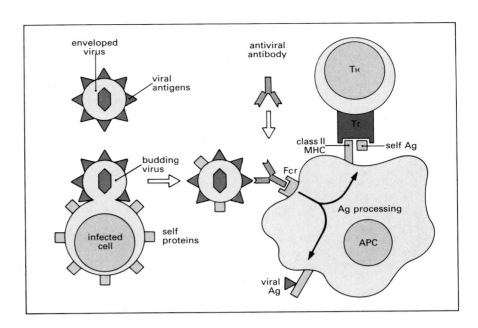

AUTOIMMUNE DISEASE

Tolerance to self antigens can be broken in a variety of ways as described in the previous sections, but it should be emphasized that, although all individuals can be induced to manifest autoreactive responses, few develop autoimmune disease. This is probably because normal individuals can regulate autoreactive cells. The ability of several workers to isolate T cell clones from immunized animals which recognize self antigen suggests that T cells specific for self antigen are not clonally deleted, but are normally held in check by some suppressor mechanism. The finding that organ-specific or non-organ-specific autoimmune states were generated following depletion of particular T cell subsets, supports this hypothesis.

In those studies, T cells were clearly necessary for the development of autoimmunity, but removal of Ly1+ (for organ-specific) or Ly2+ (for non-organ-specific) T cells led to autoantibody production and the development of autoimmune pathology. There have been reports demonstrating that there appears to be a lack of Ts cells in autoimmune individuals, or that there are abnormalities in the TH/Ts ratios in the peripheral blood of affected individuals. Additionally, it has been shown in some patients and in animal models of autoimmunity that an anti-idiotype specific for the autoantibody is only found during patient remission or in non-affected animals, suggesting that the idiotype network may play a role in the regulation of autoimmune processes.

Many studies have been carried out in order to establish factors contributing to the generation of autoimmune pathology. One approach has been to analyse the changes in the target organ undergoing autoimmune attack in diseases such as autoimmune thyroid disease (Hashimoto's and Graves') or insulin-dependent diabetes mellitus (IDDM). In the course of such an investigation, an interesting observation was made by Bottazzo and his colleagues, showing that target endocrine cells in a diseased individual were expressing class II MHC antigens (see Fig. 12.13 overpage). Since such MHC expression does not occur in normal individuals, these

researchers described this phenomenon as 'aberrant' class II MHC expression and suggested that this might be a means by which autoimmune pathology might be initiated. It was proposed that T cells could be triggered by self antigen in the context of MHC class II antigens, and that this would lead to autoimmune pathology. As many cells which do not normally express class II MHC antigens do so following normal physiological triggering (for example, lactating mammary epithelium), or following infection or exposure to interferon γ (gut epithelium, thyroid epithelial cells, astrocytes, endothelial cells), such expression reflects a differentiation or physiological change in the cell.

In an attempt to understand whether class II MHC antigen expression on an endocrine cell is a primary initiating event of autoimmune pathology or a secondary consequence of lymphocytic infiltration (and concomitant local interferon γ production), longitudinal studies have been carried out using spontaneous animal models of the human autoimmune endocrine diseases. In the BB rat, which is a model of human IDDM, animals spontaneously develop the disease at about ninety-six days of age. Detailed analyses of the pancreas, both by cohort studies and by sequential pancreatic biopsy, revealed that class II expression on the insulin containing beta cell (the target of autoimmune attack) could be observed before the animal developed overt diabetes, but was only observed when there also was a lymphocytic infiltration suggesting that such expression was a secondary feature of the disease. Studies carried out on the obese strain chicken (an animal model of Hashimoto's disease) also showed that class II MHC antigen expression on the thyroid epithelial cells never arose in the absence of a lymphocytic infiltrate. However, although class II MHC antigen expression does not seem to play a role in initiating the autoreactive process, it may do so in exacerbating or perpetuating the disease.

Figure 12.14 depicts those cells which are known to be present in the autoimmune pancreas. This picture is seen in man and also in the two spontaneous animal models of the human disease, the BB rat and the NOD (non-obese diabetic) mouse. Using antibodies specific for different lymphocyte subsets it has been possible to identify T

Fig. 12.13 Breakdown of self tolerance by class II induction.
Class II MHC expression occurs on endocrine cells in both IDDM and thyroid autoimmune disease. This may be induced by IFN$_\gamma$ released by activated T$_H$ cells. T$_H$ cells recognize autoantigen on the endocrine target and can help B cells to make autoantibody. The antibody may produce complement-mediated damage to the cells and arm K cells for antibody-dependent cytotoxicity. NK cells and cytotoxic T cells are induced by IL-2 and IFN$_\gamma$. The former release tumour necrosis factor (TNF) and lymphotoxin (LTN), while cytotoxic T cells recognize surface antigens on the target cell. Release of antigen from damaged cells allows macrophages to take up antigen and potentiate the process.

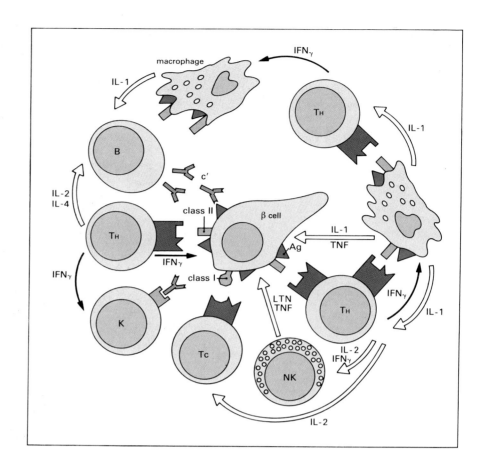

helper, cytotoxic and suppressor cells, natural killer (NK) cells, B cells and macrophages in the pancreatic infiltrates (see Fig. 12.14). Cells possessing Fc receptors, for instance macrophages, NK cells and cells of the monocyte lineage, can potentially kill the beta cell if armed with antibody directed against this target. Of course, the B cell product (immunoglobulin) may be able to fix complement and directly kill the cell. Class II MHC antigen-restricted T cells have been shown to be capable of cytotoxicity, therefore it is possible that cells phenotypically designated as T$_H$ may actually be functioning as

Tc cells in this situation. These killing mechanisms and the role of monokines and lymphokines in this process have been discussed in detail in Chapters 7 and 11. It seems, therefore, that there are a variety of ways in which the beta cell could theoretically be selectively destroyed, but how this actually happens remains to be seen. We know from the animal models of organ-specific autoimmune disease that T cells are necessary for the development of pathology, and that immunosuppressive drugs which affect T cells suppress the onset of the disease. Administration of antibody to class II MHC antigens is also known to prevent the onset of both organ-specific and non-organ-specific autoimmune diseases, but this could be via an effect on any class II-bearing cell, including B cells. Interestingly, in the case of diabetes, the drug Desferal (which is an iron chelator) and nicotinamide prevent the onset of the disease; it is supposed that Desferal prevents the formation of free radicals, and nicotinamide allows the β cell to repair DNA strand breaks. In summary, agents known to delay or depress the onset of diabetes are:

1. ALS – affecting mainly T cells;
2. Thymectomy – affecting T cells;
3. Anti-Thy 1.2 – affecting T cells;
4. Cyclosporine – affecting T, some B, and antigen-presenting cells (APC);
5. Anti- (I-E) – affecting APC;
6. Desferal, nicotinamide, silica – affecting oxidative metabolism, free radicals, phagocytosis, NAD.

This suggests that antigen-presenting cells and T cells are involved in autoimmune pathology.

Interferon γ is known to be able to readily induce class II MHC antigens on thyroid epithelial cells and β cells from diabetes-prone rats. T cells produce IFN$_\gamma$ following

Cell type	Diabetic	Prediabetic	
	Human	NOD	BB
NK cell	+	+	+
macrophage	+	++	++
T$_H$ cell	+	+	+
Tc/s cell	++	+	+
B cell	+	+	+

Fig. 12.14 Cells present in autoimmune pancreas. The table indicates that a variety of immunocytes and accessory cells are seen in the autoimmune pancreas, but these are also present in the prediabetic phase of the autoimmune mouse (NOD) and rat (BB) strains. This shows that penetration of the islets by immunologically competent cells precedes the development of the disease.

Fig. 12.15 Effects of IFN$_\gamma$ in the development of immune reactions. IFN$_\gamma$ is thought to play an important role in autoimmunity, by its effects both on cells of the immune system and on the local tissues.

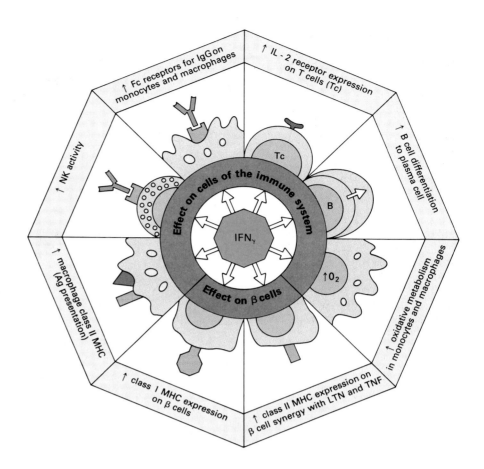

antigenic challenge, and it is probable that this is produced locally in the target organ during an autoimmune attack. The possible consequences of this are summarized in Figure 12.15, and have been described in detail in Chapter 11.

Autoimmune reactions can arise in a variety of ways but disease only develops in a few individuals. Genetic predisposition clearly plays an important role, and autoimmune diseases show an association with MHC. Other genes are also known to be involved, but the genetic basis of autoimmunity is poorly understood. Breeding studies carried out in the animal models have revealed that the diseases are under polygenic control (at least three genes in the case of diabetes in the non-obese diabetic mouse), but the exact contribution of each of these genes to the genesis of an autoimmune state is not known. It seems likely that individuals who develop autoimmune disease have a defect in regulating the immune response.

SUMMARY

Tolerance or specific immunological unresponsiveness can arise and be maintained in a variety of ways, from clonal deletion to activation of T suppressor cells. The exact relationship of experimentally induced tolerance to self tolerance is not completely understood, but it is often assumed that comparable mechanisms are employed in maintaining the body in a state of self tolerance. Tolerance to self antigens can be broken in a variety of ways. Since most normal individuals can be induced to develop autoreactive cells, with a few of them progressing to develop autoimmune disease, it is clear that complete clonal deletion of autoreactive cells does not occur, but that these cells are subject to some form of immunoregulation.

FURTHER READING

Allison A.C. (1971) *Unresponsiveness to self antigens.* Lancet. **ii**, 1401.

Bottazzo G.F., Dean B.M., McNally J.M., MacKay E.M., Swift P.G.F. & Gamble D.R (1985) *In situ characterisation of autoimmune phenomena and expression of HLA molecules in the pancreas of diabetic insulitis.* New Engl. J. Med. **313**, 353.

Burnet F.M. & Fenner F. The production of Antibodies. 2nd Ed. (1949) Macmillan, London.

Cooke A., Lydyard P.M. & Roitt I.M. (1983) *Mechanism of auto-immunity: a role for cross-reactive idiotypes.* Immunol. Today. **4**, 170.

Cooke A., Lydyard P.M. & Roitt I.M. (1984) *Autoimmunity and idiotypes.* Lancet **ii** 723.

Daar A.S., Fuggle S.V., Fabre J.W., Ting A. & Morris P.J. (1984) *The detailed distribution of MHC class II antigens in normal human organs.* Transplantation **38**, 293.

Dean B.M., Walker R., Bone A.J., Baird J.D. & Cooke A. (1985) *Pre-diabetes in the spontaneously diabetic BB/E rat: lymphocyte subpopulations in the pancreatic infiltrate and expression of rat MHC class II molecules in endocrine cells.* Diabetologia **28**, 464.

Dresser D.W. (1962) *Specific inhibition of antibody production. II. Paralysis induced in adult mice by small quantities of protein antigen.* Immunology **5**, 378.

Dresser D.W. (1976) *Tolerance induction as a model for cell differentiation.* British Medical Bulletin **32**, 147.

Fujiwara M. & Cinader B. (1974) *Cellular aspects of tolerance. VII. Inheritance of the resistance to tolerance induction.* Cell Immunol. **12**, 214.

Gleichmann E., Pals S.T., Rolink A.G., Radaszkiewicz T. & Gleichmann H. (1984) *Graft-versus-host reactions: clues to the etiopathology of a spectrum of immunological diseases.* Immunol. Today **5**, **11**, 324.

Green D.R., Flood P.M. & Gershon R.K. (1983) *Immunoregulatory T-cell pathways.* Ann. Rev. Immunol. **1**, 439.

Hanafusa T., Pujol-Borrell R., Chiovato L., Russell R.C.G., Doniach D. & Bottazzo G.F. (1983) *Aberrant expression of HLA-DR antigen on thyrocytes in Graves' disease: Relevance to autoimmunity.* Lancet **ii**, 1111.

Harris D.E., Cairns L., Rosen F.S. & Borel Y. (1982) *A natural model of immunological tolerance: tolerance to murine C5 is mediated by T cells and antigen is required to maintain unresponsiveness.* J. Exp. Med **156**, 567.

Hasek M., Holan V. & Hraba T. (1986) *From Immunological Tolerance to Immunoregulation.* Concepts Immunopathol. **3**, 158 (Karger, Basel).

Jemmerson R., Morrow P. & Klinman N. (1982) *Antibody responses to synthetic peptides corresponding to antigenic determinants on mouse cytochrome c.* Fed. Proc. **41**, 420.

Jerne N.K. (1974) *Towards a network theory of the immune system.* Ann. Immunol. Paris **125c**, 373.

Klareskog L., Forsum U., Wigren A. & Wigzell H. (1982) *Relationships between HLA-DR expressing cells and T lymphocytes of different subsets in rheumatoid synovial tissue.* Scand. J. Immunol. **15**, 501.

Lindstrom J. (1985) *Immunobiology of Myasthenia Gravis, Experimental Autoimmune Myasthenia Gravis, and Lambert-Eaton Syndrome.* Ann. Rev. Imm. **3**, 109.

Loblay R.H., Fazekas de St Groth B., Pritchard - Briscoe H. & Basten A. (1983) *Suppressor T cell memory. II. The role of memory suppressor T cells in tolerance to human gamma globulin.* J. Exp. Med. **157**, 957.

Looms L.M., K-Uemura, Childs R.A., Paulson J.C., Rogers G.N., Scudder P.R., Michalski J.C., Hounsell E.F., Taylor-Robinson D. & Feizi T. (1984) *Erythrocyte receptors for Mycoplasma pneumoniae are sialylated oligosaccharides of Ii antigen type.* Nature **307**, 560.

Malkovsky M. & Medawar P.B. (1984) *Is immunological tolerance (non-responsiveness) a consequence of interleukin 2 deficit during the recognition of antigen?* Imm. Today. **5**, 340.

Mandrup-Poulsen T., Bendtzen K., Nerup J., Dinarello C.A., Svenson M. & Nielson J.H. (1986) *Affinity purified human IL-1 is cytotoxic to isolated islets of Langerhans.* Diabetologia **29**, 63.

Maron R., Elias D., de Jongh B.M., Bruining G.J., van Rood J.J., Schechter Y. & Cohen I.R. (1983) *Autoantibodies to the insulin receptor in juvenile onset insulin-dependent diabetes.* Nature **303**, 817.

Nossal G.J.V. & Pike B.L. (1981) *Functional clonal delection in immunological tolerance to major histocompatibility complex antigens.* Proc. Natl. Acad. Sci. USA **78**, 3844.

Plotz P. (1983) *Autoantibodies are anti-idiotype antibodies to antiviral antibodies.* Lancet **ii**, 824.

Reichlen M. (1972) *Localising antigenic determinants in human haemoglobin with mutants: molecular correlations of immunologic tolerance.* J. Mol. Biol. **64**, 485.

Schrader J.W. & Nossal G.J.V. (1974) *Effector cell blockade. A new mechanism of immune hyporeactivity induced by multivalent antigens.* J. Exp. Med. **139**, 1582.

Spencer J., Pugh S. & Isaacson P.G. (1986) *HLA-D region antigen expression in stomach epithelium in the absence of autoantibodies.* Lancet **ii**, 983.

Triplett E.L. (1962) *On the mechanism of immunogenic self-recognition.* J. Immunol. **89**, 505.

Walker R., Cooke A., Bone A.J., Dean B.M., Van der Meide P. & Baird J.D. (1986) *Induction of class II MHC antigens in vitro on pancreatic β cells isolated from BB/E rats.* Diabetologia **29**, 749.

Wasserman N.H., Renn A.S., Freimults P.I., Treptow N., Wentzel S., Cleveland W.L. & Erlanger B.F. (1982) *Anti-idiotypic route to anti-acetyl choline receptor antibodies and experimental myasthenia gravis.* Proc. Natl. Acad. Sci. **79**, 4810.

Weigle W.O. (1971) *Recent observations and concepts in immunological unresponsiveness and autoimmunity.* Clin. Exp. Immunol. **9**, 437.

Wong G.H.W. & Schrader J.W. (1986) *Regulation of H-2, Ia, TL and Qa Antigen expression by interferon γ.* Lymphokines **11**, 47.

13 Idiotype Networks

During the first half of this century, the reactions of the immune system were seen in terms of the ability to recognize antigens which originated outside the individual. With the discovery of autoantibodies to the body's own molecules in a number of diseases, it was realized that the immune system is also potentially capable of recognizing self antigens. In 1963, Oudin and Kunkel described the presence of epitopes (idiotopes) on human and rabbit antibodies which were specific for the individual and for the antigen-specific set within that individual. These two observations paved the way for the network theory of immune reactions, proposed by Jerne.

In its simplest form this theory states that, since antibodies express antigenic determinants and can apparently recognize any antigen which they encounter, there is the possibility that antibodies and B cells interact specifically with each other by recognition of their idiotypes. Moreover, these interactions could lead to physiological consequences including immunoregulation of cells via their idiotype-bearing antigen receptors.

Although the theory was originally proposed in terms of antibody and B cell interactions, it now encompasses T cells which also express idiotypes on their antigen receptors. The theory does not make any predictions as to the nature of interaction between cells expressing or recognizing particular idiotypes, and there is evidence that both idiotype-specific help or suppression can occur in different circumstances.

It is now fully accepted that T cells, B cells and antibodies can interact with each other as proposed above; however, the physiological significance of their reaction is still debated, as many of the experiments used to investigate idiotype networks are distinctly unphysiological. Despite this, network interactions are important in some immune reactions, and although idiotype network regulation of the immune system is of lesser importance than that exerted by antigen and antigen-specific T cells, it enables immunologists to specifically manipulate immune reactions.

TERMS DESCRIBING NETWORK INTERACTIONS

Idiotypes (Ids) are the specific set of epitopes (idiotopes) expressed by antigen receptor molecules of B cells and T cells. They can be present in the germline V domain genes, or they may be generated by the processes of recombination and mutation involved in the production of V region genes. Some require the presence of two associated V domains of the right specificity (for example, heavy and light chains of specific subgroups). The relationship of Ids to the immunoglobulin genes is discussed in Chapter 2.

When examining network interactions (Fig. 13.1), it is often useful to describe where in the chain a particular antibody or receptor lies. Therefore, antibodies which are directed to an external antigen are called Ab1, antibodies

which are generated by Ab1 are Ab2, antibodies generated by Ab2 are Ab3, and so on. The Ab1 antibodies express a particular set of Ids, and thus the Ab2 population which recognize them are anti-idiotypic antibodies (anti-Id). Similarly, the Ab3 population are anti-anti-Id. If two different antibodies express the same idiotope (cross-reactive idiotope) but react to different antigens, they are

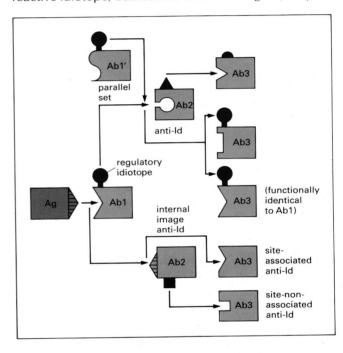

Fig.13.1 Idiotype networks. Antigen (Ag) induces a population of antigen-specific molecules, e.g. antibody (Ab1) expressing a number of site-associated and site-non-associated idiotopes. These idiotopes are recognized by a set of anti-Ids (Ab2) which in turn can stimulate anti-anti-Ids (Ab3). When each antibody expresses many idiotopes recognized by different anti-Ids, the network is said to be 'highly branched'. As the interactions between the antibodies may involve paratope/paratope, paratope/non-paratope and non-paratope/non-paratope interactions, it is not meaningful to describe one member of the pair as the 'antibody' and the other as the 'antigen', except in experiments where deliberate immunization has occurred. In this diagram, one of the Ab2 molecules mimics the epitope on the antigen and is, therefore, its internal image. Ab1 shares an idiotope with Ab1', but not the paratope, and may be corregulated via cells expressing Ab2. It is, therefore, termed a 'parallel set'. Note also that some of the induced antibodies in the Ab3 population may be functionally identical to Ab1, although this similarity occurs more often between Ab2 and Ab4 populations. Where particular idiotopes recur at different levels through an idiotype network, they are often of particular importance in immunoregulation and are termed 'regulatory idiotopes'.

said to belong to parallel sets. In cases where the antigen which binds to one of them is known and the specificity of the other is not, the latter is referred to as a 'non-specific parallel set'.

Since both antigen and anti-Id bind to Id, sometimes they will have structural similarities with each other. In other words, the anti-Id partly mimics the antigen in its structure, and in these circumstances it is effectively an image of the antigen. This is referred to as the 'internal image', since it is generated by the immune system itself as opposed to the antigen which is external. Anti-Ids can often mimic the funtions of antigen because both can crosslink antigen receptors of lymphocytes; however, internal image anti-Ids go beyond funtional mimicry of antigen and structurally resemble that part of the antigen which binds to the Id.

THE STRUCTURE OF IDIOTYPE NETWORKS

When considering how cells and antibodies can interact via their idiotypes, the first question is how many different cells can form a regulatory network. There are two extreme possibilities:

A. Each Id-bearing cell interacts with a large number of different anti-Id-bearing cells, each recognizing different idiotopes on the first cell. In turn, each of the anti-Id-bearing cells is recognized by several anti-anti-Id-bearing cells, as well as by the Id+cell.
B. Each Id-bearing cell interacts with only one specificity of anti-Id-bearing cell, and this in turn is recognized by only the Id-bearing cells.

In the first case, the network interactions are analogous to a ripple in a pond spreading outwards from the initial idiotype. Each part of the immune system is regulated by many other cells, and the network is said to be 'highly branched'. In the second case, each cell is regulated by very few other cells, hence the network is not branched. An analogy for this would be a seesaw, where the immune system consists of several mini-networks acting independently of each other. Immunoregulation through such small networks could occur in one of two ways: a) the activity of the cells could settle into a temporarily stable state ('eigen state') in which Id+ are active and anti-Id+ inactive or vice versa; b) if the Id+ cells stimulate anti-Id+ cells and the anti-Id+ suppress the Id+, then synchronous but aphasic waves of Id and anti-Id activity will appear.

The two schemes outlined above are extreme cases and the evidence implies that idiotype network interactions show limited branching. This problem was investigated by Bona and colleagues using rabbit antibody (Ab1) to the antigen *Micrococcus lysodeikticus* polysaccharide and Ab2, Ab3, Ab4 populations of antibodies raised successively in other rabbits (Fig. 13.2). It was observed that Ab1 and Ab3 molecules both recognized Ab2 and Ab4, but that the idiotype network is not totally symmetrical in this system; this is because the Ab3 population was not able to bind to the antigen, while Ab1 did. It then follows that the anti-Id site present on Ab2 which recognizes Ab1 and Ab3 is not an internal image of the antigen, otherwise it would stimulate antigen-binding antibodies in the Ab3 population. Furthermore, although Ab4 binds to Ab1, it does so with a much lower avidity than binding to Ab3 to which it was originally raised. This shows that each stage in the chain of interactions generates anti-idiotypic antibodies

Antibody population	'Antigen' preparation			
	Ag	Ab1	Ab2	Ab3
Ab2	–	10	–	9
Ab3	–	–	10	–
Ab4	–	3	–	4
$\log_2$ haemagglutinin titres on SRBC-Ab$_n$				

Fig 13.2 Idiotype network interactions. The table shows the reactivities between a series of anti-Ids (Ab2-Ab4) raised successively (see Fig. 13.1) to Ab1, antibody to a micrococcus carbohydrate antigen. Reactions were tested by coating sheep red cells with test antigens and observing the haemagglutinating titre with the anti-Ids: none of the anti-Ids bound to the micrococcus carbohydrate (Ag). Ab2 binds to both the antigen it is raised to (Ab1) and the antibody raised to it (Ab3), indicating the symmetry of the reactivity. As Ab4 recognizes both Ab3 (to which it was raised) and Ab1, this shows that Ab1 and Ab3 share idiotopes, therefore, the degree of heterogeneity between different antibodies at different levels of this system is limited. Data from Wikler and Urbain, 1984.

which are only imperfect images of their corresponding idiotypes. Although the Ab3 population did not contain antigen-binding molecules, it was possible to induce antibodies to the antigen (β2-6 fructosan) by priming with Ab2 followed by antigen. In this case, some of the activated cells produced antibody which cross-reacted with the related antigen β2-1 fructosan. Because Ab1 did not bind to β2-1 fructosan and antigen alone does not induce this specificity, it follows that the priming with Ab2 generates a parallel set of antibodies to the original Ab1. That is to say, the conventional Ab1 binds to β2-6 fructosan, but the Ab2/antigen-induced parallel set binds to β2-6 and β2-1 fructosan.

Analysis of the antibodies induced by Ab2 populations in other systems supports the idea of limited branching within idiotype networks. For example, Ab2 to anti-MHC molecules (Ab1) induces some Ab3 which also bind to MHC, although this is only a small proportion of the Ab3 population specific for MHC (less than 10%). Evidently this is not an Id, anti-Id two-component system, but it does not display unlimited branching either.

Ability to recognize isogeneic idiotopes appears to be more limited than recognition of allogeneic idiotopes. For example, the anti-idiotypic response of BALB/c mice to the isogeneic myeloma protein J558 has been examined by isoelectric focusing. BALB/c mice can produce six to sixteen different clones of anti-Ids which do not cross-react on the myeloma MOPC104E that recognizes the same epitope in dextran as J558. Allogeneic anti-Ids recognize Ids on both these antibodies, indicating that, in this case, isogeneic recognition is more limited, hence of greater specificity.

The degree of branching of the network has certain implications for the way in which networks are controlled. It has been argued that regulatory interactions will only be significant if a large proportion of antigen-specific antibodies express a single idiotope and can, therefore, be regulated concomitantly. This type of common idiotope which may be recognized by T cells is called a 'regulatory idiotope'. The procedure of antibody induction by Ab2 indicates whether there is a close linkage between a particular Id and a particular antigen specificity. If anti-Id induces a large number of Id$^+$ antigen-specific molecules in an individual, this shows that there is a pool of antigen-reactive B cells bearing the Id which could be regulated via that Id. The factors which affect the degree of connection between Id and anti-Id are outlined below.

Whether anti-Id induces antigen-specific antibody depends on the species and strain of animal used, as well as on the nature of anti-Id molecules: if the anti-Id contains a high proportion of internal image idiotopes, then it should induce antigen-specific antibody in all strains of a species, and in other species also, provided that they recognize the same (internal image) epitope on the antigen which is recognized by the original Id. In this case, the anti-Id mimics the antigen, and can thus regulate all cells which are antigen-specific. If, however, the anti-Id (Ab2) is not an internal image of the antigen, its ability to induce antigen-specific antibodies will depend on the B cell repertoire of the animal. If there are B cells which express the Id and are antigen-specific, Ab2 will induce antigen-specific Ab3, but if the animal does not readily generate Id$^+$ antigen-specific B cells, then Ab2 will not induce antigen-specific Ab3. The ability to induce antigen-specific antibody in this instance depends on the V genes of the strain; it also explains why anti-Id (Ab2) generates antigen-specific Ab3 more readily in strains sharing the Ig allotype of the original Id$^+$ strain than in animals of different allotype.

PHYSIOLOGICAL NETWORK INTERACTIONS

The preceding experiments used large quantities of Ids and aggressive immunization regimes to generate anti-Ids. While this is valid for investigating the type of response the immune system is capable of making, the amounts of any particular Id present *in vivo* are generally very low unless it is dominant in a particular response. Additionally, it might be anticipated that the low levels of particular Ids would not induce strong reactions, being self molecules. For these reasons, the demonstration by Kelsoe and colleagues that physiological quantities of syngeneic Ids could markedly affect immune reactions is of particular importance: it was shown that 10µg of anti-Id per mouse significantly suppressed the expression of the cognate Id (i.e. the Id recognized by the anti-Id), while 100ng or even 10ng significantly enhanced Id expression (Fig.13.3). These amounts are equatable with the levels of Ids naturally present in serum. It was also found that injection of minute quantities of idiotype modulated the reactions to some extent, further supporting the theory of a physiologically active network. Interestingly, in these experiments it was noted that, although treatment with anti-Id had a profound effect on Id expression, the overall level of antibody produced to the antigen (NP-CG) was not changed. This is a frequent finding in many idiotypic systems where the expression of a particular Id is suppressed: other Id$^-$ clones specific for the antigen are induced, so that the overall antigen-specific response is little changed. This occurs even in cases where the suppressed Id would normally constitute a major part of the responding antibodies (for example, the anti-arsonate

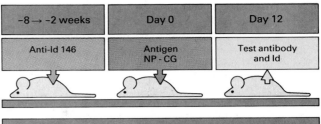

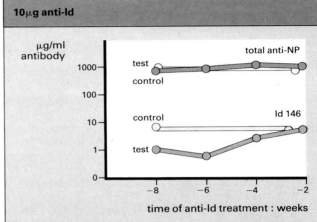

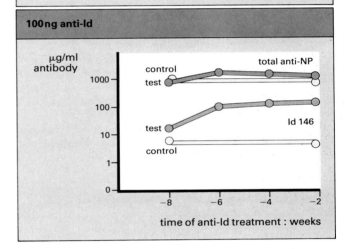

Fig.13.3 Enhancement and suppression induced by anti-Id. C57BL/6 mice were preinjected (two to eight weeks before antigen challenge) with 100ng or 10µg of anti-Id to the antibody B1-8, which is specific for the hapten NP. The 146.Id on Bi-8 is site-associated. The mice were then immunized with the hapten-carrier conjugate NP-CG, and the induced antibodies were tested twelve days later. The levels of total anti-NP and of the 146.Id were measured in control (light pink) and anti-Id pretreated animals (dark pink). Pretreatment with 10µg anti-Id between four and eight weeks before immunization suppressed the Id response, but it did not affect the total response to NP (upper). Pretreatment with 100ng of anti-Id enhanced the Id response, but again it did not alter the total anti-NP (lower). Effects could be observed in this system with as little as 10ng per mouse. Data from Kelsoe, Reth and Rajewsky, 1981.

cross-reactive Id). There is also evidence that anti-Ids arise naturally *in vivo* during immune responses and modulate those responses. This is seen in the waves of T15 Id and anti-Id which follow immunization of BALB/c mice with phosphoryl choline (PC) coupled to a carrier protein. T15 is a dominant idiotype to PC in these mice. The initial demonstration of this was in BALB/c mice injected repeatedly with Pneumococcus R36A vaccine. These animals developed a strong response to PC after seven days, and by twelve weeks there was a response to the T15 which coincided with a small reduction in the number of plaque-forming cells against the antigen. Although it has been more difficult to demonstrate anti-Ids in humans because of the general lack of homozygosity at the Ig V alleles, naturally occurring anti-Ids have been found. These are present after immunization with external antigens including tetanus toxoid and KLH, following the generation of Id-bearing antibodies to these antigens. In each case the Ids present were specific for the individual. It is possible that the overall pattern of natural anti-Id induction is quite different for responses where there is a dominant idiotype and for those where there is not. Maternal antibodies crossing the placenta can also induce anti-Id antibodies in addition to the anti-allotypic specificities which occur more frequently (see below).

Perhaps of greatest interest in this respect is the suggestion that anti-Ids may play a part in human disease. There are reports that patients with systemic lupus erythematosus (SLE) who are in remission have anti-idiotypic antibodies specific for DNA autoantibodies in their serum. These are presumably capable of interfering with DNA/antibody formation in this disease. Typically, the anti-Ids are patient-specific. There is also speculation that anti-receptor antibodies present in some autoimmune conditions (for example, Graves' disease and myasthenia gravis) may have arisen as anti-Ids to antibodies directed against the ligand which binds to the receptor, but this is unproven. A further complication in autoimmunity is the occasional finding of Id/anti-Id complexes contributing to renal pathology.

ID-SPECIFIC T HELPER CELLS AND IDs ON T CELLS

The T cell antigen receptor also expresses idiotypes and can, therefore, participate in network interactions. In some cases, B cell (immunoglobulin) Ids are also present on T cells, which was for many years a cause of controversy as to whether the T cell receptor uses Ig V genes to generate its V regions. Since immunoglobulin and T cell receptor genes are totally separate, it is concluded that the sharing of Ids by B cells and T cells arises by functional, rather than genetic, constraints (cf. recurrent Ids, see Chapter 2). Anti-Id can directly stimulate T cells by substituting for the antigen/MHC signal in the same way that it can substitute for antigen in stimulating B cells. This has been shown by measuring IL-2 production by cloned T cells in the absence of accessory cells when treated with allogeneic anti-Id raised specifically to the T cell clone.

Evidence for similarities between the T cell and B cell idiotypes comes from systems using both natural and synthetic antigens. For example, murine anti-idiotype to C57BL/6 anti-(T,G)-A--L could be used to prime popliteal lymph node cells so that they respond to (T,G)-A--L, and this effect was also seen with nylon wool-enriched T cells. Similar results have been described using anti-idiotype to anti-nuclease in order to prime T cells so as to help the anti-nuclease B cell response. It is also possible to prime autoimmune T cells (for example, to thyroglobulin) by the

use of anti-Id to monoclonal autoantibodies. In these cases, the priming of T cells with anti-idiotype produces an enhancement of the antibody response affecting both the Id+ and Id- responses, but the experiments have not yet been performed with cloned T cells.

The ability to stimulate T helper cells with anti-Id demonstrates that idiotypic interactions involving signalling to T cells can take place. However, of greater physiological importance is the finding that T cells (TH2) recognizing B cell Ids can participate in an immune reaction and modulate their expression. It is important to discriminate between the experiments described above where anti-Id stimulates antigen-specific T cells, and the experiments described below where Id on B cells or antibodies stimulates Id-specific T cells.

It has been conclusively shown in a number of systems that Id-specific T helper cells can be generated, for example in the response to hen egg lysozyme (HEL) (Fig. 13.4). In these experiments, the dominant B cell Id which appears in the secondary response to HEL is virtually absent from the primary response. This dominant Id occurs on a very large proportion of anti-HEL hybridomas generated from mice producing a secondary

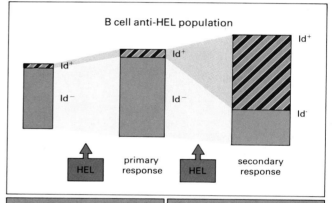

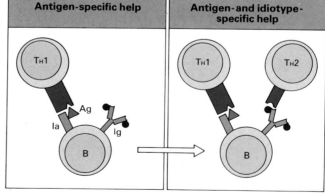

Fig. 13.4 Two types of T helper cell. Primary immunization of A/J mice with the antigen HEL produces a response in which a recurrent Id (termed IdX) constitutes about 1% of the response. The secondary response to this antigen generates antibodies of which the majority express the Id. Other experiments show that this observation is due to the presence of two classes of T helper cell acting as indicated below. A carrier-specific T helper cell (TH1) helps all B cells specific for HEL, while an Id-specific T cell selectively expands the IdX population in the secondary response. The phasing of this reaction suggests that the Id-specific T cells must first be stimulated by B cells expressing the Id during the primary response, before they can deliver help.

anti-HEL response. This shows that it is genuinely a single idiotope regulating the secondary response, so one could consider this to be a regulatory idiotope. Since this Id appears on antibodies of different epitope specificity, it is possible that it is related to a particular V gene framework rather than site-related residues. In this case, the evidence indicates that there are two types of T helper cell: a) the antigen-specific T helper which recognizes carrier determinants and can help B cells recognizing other epitopes on the antigen in an MHC-restricted manner; b) the idiotype-specific T cells which selectively expand B cell populations carrying the dominant Id. Because these two populations often operate sequentially during an immune response, as occurs here, they are referred to as T_H1 (antigen-specific) and T_H2 (idiotype-specific) cells. There are analogous populations of suppressor cells designated T_S1 and T_S2.

In these experiments it was also noted that the dominant Id appeared on antibodies directed to different epitopes on HEL. This Id is not associated with the combining site of the antibodies, therefore it does not present the conceptual

difficulties which would arise if the Id was site-associated. However, these observations have led to the suggestion that antigen is also required for the action of T_H2 cells in some circumstances: antigen would bring together B cells directed towards different epitopes on the molecule, which would then permit Id-specific T cells to act on several populations of B cells in the immediate vicinity.

The effect of idiotype-specific T helper cells can be seen in experiments where these cells are functionally deleted by neonatal tolerization. This tolerization can be effected by treatment with anti-Id, in which case the animal can still generate an immune response to the antigen, but this response lacks the specific idiotype; the response to antigen as a whole may, thus, be substantially reduced due to the loss of the Id^+ component (Fig. 13.5). Idiotypic suppression of adult animals is usually much less effective than in neonates, due to the appearance of new B cell clones which compensate for the disappearance of the dominant Id. There is also evidence that, in neonatally suppressed animals, idiotype-specific suppressor cells may be generated, thereby reinforcing the suppression obtained by deletion of idiotype-specific T helper cells.

Idiotype-specific T helper cells can also be generated during the neonatal period, as has been shown in mice injected with the A48.Id to bacterial levan. This produces an increase in the proportion of Id^+ antibodies in all strains tested. In some strains, however, it also produced some reduction in the anti-levan response. The induction of Id was unrelated to immunoglobulin haplotype or H-2 haplotype (Fig.13.6). The ability to produce an A48.Id

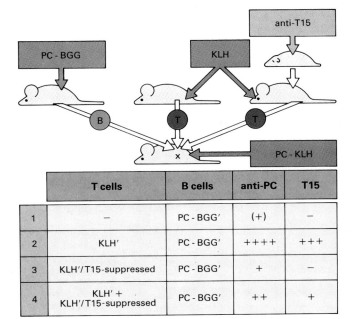

	T cells	B cells	anti-PC	T15
1	–	PC - BGG'	(+)	–
2	KLH'	PC - BGG'	++++	+++
3	KLH'/T15-suppressed	PC - BGG'	+	–
4	KLH' + KLH'/T15-suppressed	PC - BGG'	++	+

Fig.13.5 Requirements for antigen- and idiotype-specific help. Lethally irradiated recipient mice (x) were reconstituted with B cells primed to the hapten phosphoryl choline (PC) by immunization with PC coupled to bovine gamma globulin (BGG), and with T cells from mice primed to KLH. The recipients were then immunized with PC-KLH, and the antibody response to PC was measured along with the T15 component of the response. Animals reconstituted with B cells alone make no response to PC (1), while animals reconstituted with B and T cells from a normal donor make a large response dominated by T15 (2). If the T cell donor is Id-suppressed during the neonatal period by the injection of anti-T15.Id, the anti-PC response is greatly suppressed and the T15 component of it is absent (3). Addition of T cells from a normal donor partly restores the response to PC and allows the emergence of some T15⁺ antibodies (4). This and other experiments imply that the Id-specific T helper cell (T_H2) becomes functionally tolerized in neonates treated with anti-T15, which limits their ability to support an anti-PC response. The observation that the response is restored with normal KLH-primed T cells implies that the lack of reactions is not due to a suppressor cell.

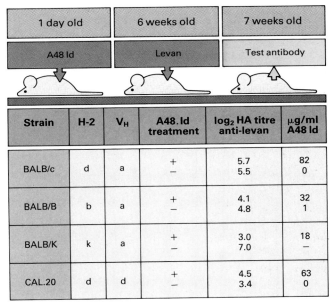

Strain	H-2	V_H	A48.Id treatment	log₂ HA titre anti-levan	µg/ml A48 Id
BALB/c	d	a	+ / –	5.7 / 5.5	82 / 0
BALB/B	b	a	+ / –	4.1 / 4.8	32 / 1
BALB/K	k	a	+ / –	3.0 / 7.0	18 / –
CAL.20	d	d	+ / –	4.5 / 3.4	63 / 0

Fig.13.6 Genetics of idiotype-specific T cell help. Neonatal animals were injected with A48.Id and challenged when adult with the antigen levan which is recognized by the A48 antibody. The total antibody response to levan and the A48 component was tested. Treatment of BALB/c mice in this way resulted in a large increase in the level of A48 by comparison with untreated controls. This effect was also produced in strains with other H-2 and IgV_H haplotypes. In each case, the effect on the total anti-levan response was variable. As the response is transferable with T cells, it appears that the neonatal A48 induced Id-specific T helper cells, but the ability to do this is unrelated to MHC or immunoglobulin gene loci. Data of Bona and Victor, 1984.

response to levan in this system is transferable with $Ly1^+2^+$ cells which directly recognize the A48.Id, since they can be removed with A48 antibody and complement.

The ability to generate T$_H$2 cells in a response depends both on the strain of the animal, as well as on a signal to trigger these cells, this trigger being the Id itself. This means that animals lacking a particular idiotype cannot trigger Id-specific cells and so lack the specific T$_H$2 cells. This has been shown in CBA/NxBALB/c hybrid mice. CBA/N mice have an X-linked B cell defect which precludes them from making a normal response to phosphoryl choline dominated by the T15 idiotype (see Chapter 4). The hybrid male CBA/NxBALB/c mice are also defective, but the females are normal in this respect. Although the female T cells could help the T15$^+$ response of female B cells, the male T cells were unable to do so. As the defect does not affect T cell function directly, it was concluded that the male T cells were unable to produce idiotype-specific help

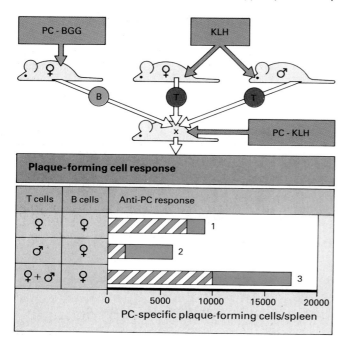

Plaque-forming cell response

T cells	B cells	Anti-PC response	
♀	♀		1
♂	♀		2
♀ + ♂	♀		3

PC-specific plaque-forming cells/spleen

Fig.13.7 Requirement of Id expressing B cells to generate Id-specific T cells. These experiments were performed with (CBA/NxBALB/c) F1 mice. Females of this type are phenotypically normal and produce an anti-PC response dominated by the T15.Id, as does the BALB/c parent. F1 males have the defective CBA/N X-chromosome which prevents the B cells from making a T15-dominated response. Lethally irradiated recipient mice were reconstituted with B cells from female mice and T cells from either male or female mice. They were then immunized with KLH-PC and the anti-PC response was measured (plaque-forming cells per spleen); the proportion of cells expressing the T15.Id was also estimated. Animals reconstituted with female T cells produce a normal response dominated by T15 (hatched area) (1), while those reconstituted with male T cells produce a response not dominated by T15 (2). Addition of female cells partly restores the T15 dominance in the system (3). It appears that it is necessary for the Id-specific T cells to have 'seen' T15 during their development in order to support a T15-dominated response. The third experiment indicates that the failure of male mice to support a response is not due to the presence of Id-specific suppressors.

in this experiment, because the appropriate T$_H$2 cells were not induced in the male animals. This in turn was caused by the absence of T15$^+$ cells capable of inducing them (Fig. 13.7) Other workers have shown, however, that donor cells from mice treated as neonates with anti-T15 (therefore Id-suppressed) can subsequently support a T15$^+$ response in suitable circumstances. Clearly, the cause of the lack of Id expression (that is, genetic or produced artificially) is critical in these experiments.

A different hypothesis to explain idiotype dominance of responses proposes that this is determined by the initial repertoire of B cell receptors in animals. That is to say, if an animal generates a large proportion of its virgin antigen-specific B cells with a particular idiotype, then in an antibody response B cells of that idiotype will predominate to that antigen. The B cell repertoire is determined initially by the immunoglobulin heavy and light chain genes, and it would be anticipated that Ids generated directly from germline V and J genes would be predominant in the unstimulated B cell repertoire. This follows the idea of germline-determined recurrent Ids outlined in Chapter 2. Evidence that this does, in fact, occur is seen when spleen cells of various mouse strains are stimulated with the polyclonal B cell mitogen LPS and the response is analysed for the incidence of cells expressing the M460 Id. It is found that different strains of mice fall into two groups, according to the level of expression of M460 positive clones. In some strains the Id is common (up to $1/10^4$ spleen cells), whereas in others it is vanishingly rare. Animals with the higher levels of Id share the Ig$_H^a$ allotype of BALB/c in which it was originally described, while strains with lower levels of expression have other allotypes. The levels of expression of the Id in these experiments, being the same in nude mice of the same Ig allotype, suggested that the level of expression of a particular Id can be independent of T cells.

An examination of the structural basis of Ids in mouse strains with different Ig allotypes has been made for the A5A Id. This is expressed strongly in the response to streptococcal carbohydrate in Ig$_H^e$ strains and only weakly in the DBA/2, Ig$_H^c$ strain. For this Id the two types of animal produce antibodies with similar heavy chain D regions recognized by the anti-Id, but the remainder of the heavy chains are quite different among the various strains. This, again, emphasizes that anti-Ids recognize epitopes on the Ids which may or may not be derived from particular sets of germline genes. Although there appear to be two separate hypotheses here which can explain idiotype dominance in an immune response, it is quite possible that both mechanisms occur in immune responses *in vivo*. In this case, the virgin state of the B cell repertoire is determined by B cell Ig$_H$ genes and this is reflected in the primary response (or in the LPS-driven polyclonal stimulation), but in the secondary response T$_H$2 cells specific for particular Ids appearing in the primary response can selectively expand them.

A further consideration is the nature of help from an Id-specific T cell. Antigen-specific T helpers are MHC-restricted, that is, they normally only help B cells of their own MHC type. The underlying basis of this reaction is that the T cell is primed by a particular antigen/MHC combination on an antigen-presenting cell; it subsequently interacts with B cells expressing the same antigen/MHC combination, with the B cells effectively acting as an antigen-presenting cell for the cooperating T cell. It is hard to see how an Id might become associated with MHC class II molecules on the B cell surface in the same way as antigen fragments do. It is understandable, therefore, that many instances of Id-specific T cell help are not MHC-restricted. This, however, leaves the problem of how the T cell recognizes the Id on B cells: it is possible that the relatively high density of Id (IgG) on a B cell by comparison with Ia-associated antigen permits T cells to interact with the B cells despite lack of MHC recognition. Alternatively, the Id may mimic an antigen/MHC signal by itself. More recently it has been found that the Id-specific T helper cells which expand the T15 part of the response to phosphoryl choline could bind directly to T15-coated plastic plates. These cells (Ly1$^+$, Thy1$^+$, mIg$^-$) can evidently bind to Id without associate recognition of Ia. Clearly, the underlying immunochemistry requires further clarification.

IDIOTYPE-SPECIFIC SUPPRESSION

As with the interactions mentioned above, suppressive effects can take place at two levels within the idiotype network: there is the direct effect of anti-idiotypic antibody which can suppress the activation of Id$^+$ sets of B cells, and there are Id-specific suppressor T cells, sometimes referred to as the 'Ts2 population'. The clearest examples of suppression are seen in neonatal mice injected with anti-Id, where the suppression is frequently profound and long-lasting. This can be achieved either by direct administration of the anti-Id, or indirectly from the mother transplacentally or in the milk. In general, the use of allogeneic anti-Ids in these experiments tends to produce a wider ranging suppression than isogeneic anti-Ids. This is due to the fact that many allogeneic anti-Ids have wider cross-reactivity on related Ids than isogeneic anti-Ids. For example, isogeneic anti-Id to MOPC104E (an anti-dextran myeloma antibody) administered to neonates caused suppression of clones expressing the Id when the adult animals were subsequently immunized with dextran. It did not, however, produce any effect on the anti-dextran response as a whole. On the other hand, allogeneic anti-Ids raised to this antibody frequently suppress both this clonotype and a number of other anti-dextran clones, thereby reducing the overall anti-dextran response. Here, the range of suppression reflects the range of cross-reactivity of the anti-Ids used.

It is possible to induce neonatal idiotype-specific suppression to the anti-dextran response in nude animals, but it is most difficult to transfer the suppression with spleen cells of mice suppressed in this way. These two results show that the development of idiotype-specific T suppressors is not necessary in this type of suppression where the antigen is T independent. The hypotheses which may be invoked to explain neonatal idiotype-specific suppression in this case reflect the explanations of how B cells become tolerized to antigen during the neonatal period, that is, clonal deletion or abortion of immature B cells at a stage where they are particularly susceptible to tolerization. This is presumably accompanied by a failure to generate new clones carrying this idiotype during later life.

Idiotype-specific suppression has also been produced by immunization of mothers with Ids expressed on antibodies determined by the paternal genotype. An example of this, described by Bona, is the suppression of the anti-inulin response in (C.B20xBALB/c)F1 offspring of a C.B20 mother immunized to the BALB/c Id expressed on EPC109, anti-levan (both antigens are polyfructosans

containing β2-1 linkages). The suppression was observed to be complete when the offspring were immunized with levan at four months. This result is conceptually important, because it shows how immune responses occurring in the mother may affect the development of the immune system in her offspring and, indeed, set particular starting conditions in the idiotype network of the young animal. As the immunological events occurring in immunologically immature animals have profound and long-lasting effects, this kind of maternal/fetal interaction could be one of the most marked outcomes of idiotype network interactions.

It is much more difficult to produce suppression in adult animals. This can be observed when comparing the effect of anti-T15 in adult and neonatal animals. Only a small dose is required in the neonate to suppress the T15 part of the anti-phosphoryl choline response when it reaches maturity, but the T15$^-$ part of the response in these animals is unaffected, since new clones replace what would otherwise be a response dominated by T15. Adult mice require high levels of anti-T15 to affect the expression of the idiotype; nevertheless, in suppressed adult animals the entire anti-PC response is greatly, although temporarily, reduced. This is because new anti-PC clones have had insufficient time to develop, but T15$^-$ antigen-specific clones appear later as suppression wanes (Fig.13.8).

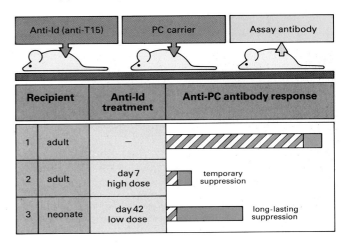

Recipient		Anti-Id treatment	Anti-PC antibody response		
1	adult	–	/////////		
2	adult	day 7 high dose		temporary suppression	
3	neonate	day 42 low dose		long-lasting suppression	

Fig.13.8 Anti-Id induced suppression in neonates and adults. Mice were pretreated with anti-T15.Id, either during the neonatal period or as adults. They were subsequently immunized with the hapten PC coupled to a carrier. The total antibody to PC was measured along with the T15 component of the response (hatched area). Normal adult mice make a good response to PC which is dominated by T15 (1). Adult mice pretreated with anti-Id are temporarily suppressed with the loss of the T15 component, accounting for the reduction in the total anti-PC response (2). Mice treated with anti-Id in the neonatal period undergo long-term suppression of their T15$^+$ B cells, but generate T15$^-$ PC-specific cells to compensate (3).

If idiotypic manipulation does not act by tolerizing B cells, the alternative possibility to explain Id-specific suppression is the occurrence of Id-specific suppressor cells. It might be assumed that if suppression can be transferred to recipients with spleen cells, then T suppressors are responsible; this, however, is not always correct, as in some instances B cells can transfer suppression. An example of this is seen in suppression of the T15 response to phosphoryl choline described by Pollok and colleagues (Fig. 13.9). This can be transferred from neonatally suppressed mice to normal adult mice via spleen cells, but when the spleen cells are subfractionated into T and B cells it is found that the B cells are responsible for the suppression. The explanation for this finding is that, in the suppressed mice, T15$^-$ cells come to dominate the anti-PC response, and this dominance is maintained when the cells are transferred. The T15$^+$ B cells in this case are not actually deleted, as they can still be induced with the mitogen LPS, but they are functionally inactive.

When considering the possible induction of idiotype-specific T suppressors, the experimental evidence indicates that these cells can arise in two ways: in some cases, anti-idiotype induces T suppressors, whereas in other systems it is the idiotype itself which produces suppression. As in the case of antigen-driven immune responses, the means of administration and the dose of idiotype or anti-idiotype are usually critical factors in determining whether help or suppression develops (see (below).

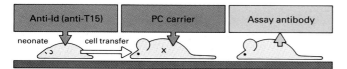

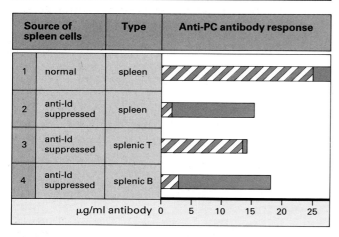

Source of spleen cells		Type	Anti-PC antibody response
1	normal	spleen	
2	anti-Id suppressed	spleen	
3	anti-Id suppressed	splenic T	
4	anti-Id suppressed	splenic B	
	µg/ml antibody		0 5 10 15 20 25

Fig.13.9 Establishing a state of Id dominance by B cells.
Irradiated recipient BALB/c mice were reconstituted with spleen cells from mice treated with anti-T15.Id in the neonatal period. They were then immunized three days later with the hapten PC coupled to a carrier, and the antibody to PC was assayed along with the T15 component of the response (hatched area). Recipients reconstituted with normal spleen make a large anti-PC response dominated by T15 (1), whereas reconstitution with cells from anti-Id-suppressed mice produces a response in which the T15 component is greatly reduced but partly compensated by T15$^-$ PC-specific antibodies (2), as expected. Surprisingly, recipients receiving splenic T cells make a T15-dominated response (3), while animals receiving splenic B cells from the Id-suppressed animals do not make T15 (4). This indicates that B cells can establish their own characteristic level of Id expression (eigen state?), independently of Id-specific T helpers or suppressors. This state may then subsequently determine how other member cells of the network behave. In different circumstances, therefore, idiotype dominance may be determined at the B or T cell level.

The induction of T cell-mediated suppression by anti-Id is most readily explicable by assuming that the anti-Id induces suppressor T cells expressing Id on their surface receptor, and these in turn can interact with T helpers (T$_H$2) expressing a complementary 'anti-Id' receptor. By suppressing the action of Id-specific T helpers, Id representation in the antibody response is reduced. Conversely, the induction of Id-specific suppression by idiotype itself is explicable by stating that the idiotype induces suppressors expressing an 'anti-Id'-bearing receptor. These cells can then interact directly with B cells expressing the Id to cause their suppression. In the first instance, the Ts cells are seen to act on T helpers; in the second, they act directly on the B cells.

The first description of this type of suppression was the demonstration by Eichmann and colleagues that guinea pig IgG2a against the A5A (anti-strep-A carbohydrate) Id suppressed the A5A component of the response in A/J mice. The suppression was chronic and could be transferred with I-J$^+$ T cells, but not with B cells. In this system there was a decrease in specific T$_H$ cell activity, suggesting that the T suppressors were themselves expressing Id and acting on Id-specific helpers. Whether it is the subclass of the anti-Id used or its affinity that influenced the induction of suppression was not determined. Interestingly, IgG1 of similar specificity induced Id-specific help in this system. In a similar system where the anti-arsonate response was suppressed by anti-Id, the active cells were shown to be Ly2,3$^+$, as are most antigen-specific T suppressors.

There are also several examples of Id-specific suppression produced by Id. Again, the effect is often most marked when the idiotype is administered in the neonatal period, but in addition there is evidence for the spontaneous generation of Id-specific suppressors in the response to TNP-levan, where removal of T cells by anti-Thy1 caused an increase in the level of expression of the 460.Id in subsequent in vitro cultures. This would be an example of a suppressor cell acting directly on the 460.Id$^+$B cells, as the suppressor population could also be removed on Id-coated plates. This is also circumstantial evidence that Id-specific T suppressors can recognize Id in isolation, rather than as part of an Id/MHC complex. As regards antigen-specific T cell help and suppression, evidence is accumulating that Id-specific helper and suppressor factors exist, such that the Id-specific cells and their targets need not interact directly, but might communicate by mutual interactions in proximity to Ia$^+$ cells with affinity for the factors.

CONNECTANCE IN THE IDIOTYPE REPERTOIRE

It is now known that the immunoglobulins and T cell antigen receptor are produced from different sets of genes. It may, therefore, be surprising that Id manipulations using anti-Ids raised to Ids on immunoglobulins can also affect T cells. An example of this is the observation that anti-Id raised to anti-staphylococcal nuclease stimulates antigen-specific T cells. Similarly, anti-Id to anti-GAT induces antigen-specific T cell help. There are numerous other instances of this phenomenon. When considering how Ids might recur on different antibodies (see Chapter 2), one explanation was that similar structures (Ids) were required by different antibodies to bind the same antigen. This argument cannot easily be used to explain shared Ids on immunoglobulins and T cell receptors, because T cells recognize antigen/MHC, which is quite different from the epitopes recognized by B cells. Furthermore, in the case of staphylococcal nuclease, the anti-Id which recognizes Ids on both T and B cells does not recognize a site-associated Id. It is, therefore, impossible to explain the presence of shared B and T cell Ids on the grounds of a similar binding specificity-related structure.

Shared B and T cell Ids can be explained in a number of ways. It is possible that interactions between T cell and B cell V genes occur to produce gene convergence, but a more probable explanation is found in the interactions of the immune system as a whole. It was noted above that the ability to generate a particular B cell Id from germline genes affected whether T cells were generated capable of recognizing that Id. Although this finding is not universal, it shows that the expression of the T cell repertoire can be influenced by the B cell repertoire. Thus, the expansion of particular B cell clones following antigen stimulation can subsequently influence the spectrum of T cells. In turn, the presence of Id-specific T$_H$ cells can selectively expand particular populations of B cells in an immune response in spite of whether, as in the HEL system, the B cells are directed towards different antigenic determinants.

The effects of these interactions are most clearly seen in inbred animals which express high levels of dominant Ids, but the findings in outbred rabbits also suggest that the overall number of Id/anti-Id interactions is limited. These findings have led to the idea that there are particular (dominant) regulatory idiotopes found on both T cells and a number of B cells specific for particular antigens. While there is little doubt that some of these idiotopes are important in controlling immune responses to many common antigens which bind to germline-encoded antibodies, it is still an open question whether the majority of immune responses to less common antigens are controlled by idiotypic interactions as well as by antigen.

USING THE NETWORK

While the significance of idiotypic interactions in normal physiology is still debated, manipulation of the immune system via Ids is an accepted proposition. Three main areas of interest have arisen in this respect: a) The examination of Id representation of immune responses. b) The use of anti-Ids to mimic antigen in stimulating or suppressing particular clones of lymphocytes. c) The targeting of toxic molecules to cells expressing particular Ids so as to eliminate them.

Examination of Ids in immune responses has been carried out for a number of pathological conditions with obscure aetiology, in order to determine whether particular Ids are associated with the disease. Given that particular Ids recur in different individuals with the same disease, this can point to either a genetic predisposition based on the individual's immunoglobulin V region genes (including D and J), or to the possibility that a particular antigen is important in inducing a disease. An example of recurrent Ids in autoimmune disease is seen in rheumatoid arthritis where the Id Wa has been demonstrated in 60% of patients, but it is virtually absent from normal pooled immunoglobulin and was not found on 100 other monoclonal antibodies. Since these patients are unrelated, the association of this Id with rheumatoid factors suggests that

it is specifically related to the antiglobulin binding site. In other cases, rheumatoid factors expressing a particular Id recur in different members of the same family, but not generally in other rheumatoid patients. In this case, a particular set of V genes appears to be predisposed to the production of antiglobulin within the family. Yet another idiotype associated with rheumatoid factors appears to identify a subset of antibodies which cross-react with DNA/histone.

A second example of recurrent Ids in autoimmunity has been noted in the MRL.lpr mouse where the Id H130 is found on 40-60% of the serum anti-DNA, and increases in titre as the mice age; however, its association with anti-DNA is only partial, as a large proportion of the Id does not occur on anti-DNA. This is suggestive of coordinate expression of parallel sets of H130 expressing Id, where one of the parallel sets is anti-DNA. This finding can be explained by saying that an Id-specific T helper cell expands the population of H130$^+$ cells, or it may reflect a change in the way the immunoglobulin V genes are expressed as the mice age. In humans, specific idiotypes are also associated with anti-DNA molecules occurring in patients with SLE.

The recurrence of particular Ids has been shown in a great number of other autoimmune diseases and their models, including autoimmune thyroiditis, Hashimoto's disease, autoimmune haemolytic anaemia and, to a lesser extent, myasthenia gravis. Of equal interest are the studies where there is no cross-reactivity among the Ids on antibodies in patients with the same disease. There have been, for example, several studies looking for common Ids on the oligoclonal immunoglobulins which appear in the cerebrospinal fluid of patients suffering from multiple sclerosis. The idea, in this case, is to see whether the antibodies of different patients have some similarities, even though the antigen itself (if it exists at all) is not identified. The finding of recurrent Ids in different patients would implicate a particular antigen. No significant cross-reactivity was shown in these studies, but this offers a possible approach to diseases of unknown aetiology where an infectious agent or immunopathological events are suspected.

Quite apart from any information these studies provide on the aetiology of autoimmune disease, it has been hoped that they might also lead to new ways of treating the conditions. Anti-Id to anti-thyroglobulin causes some reduction of the level of circulating anti-thyroglobulin in rats with autoimmune thyroiditis. Similarly, anti-Ids to anti-acetyl choline receptor cause some amelioration of experimental myasthenia (induced by immunization with the receptor in adjuvant). The fact that these treatments are not more successful can be partly ascribed to the emergence of Id$^-$ autoantibodies, and/or the difficulties associated with suppressing an established immune response. The emergence of Id$^-$ clones when a dominant idiotype is suppressed is a common occurrence in both autoantigenic and conventional antigen systems. Consequently, efforts are now directed towards neonatal Id-specific suppression which is much more permanent (but can still be bypassed), and towards suppressing Id-bearing T cells. It has been suggested that the T cells controlling an immune response are more clonotypically restricted than the B cells, therefore suppression is less easily bypassed with the appearance of new clones. For example, it has been reported that autoreactive T cell lines recognizing thyroglobulin (+Ia) can induce, or in some cases suppress, autoimmune thyroiditis. Here the implication is that the lines induce Id-specific T suppressors which have a broad spectrum of reactivity on other endogenous autoreactive T cell clones.

The manoeuvres described above have been aimed at suppressing immune responses, but one of the most exciting areas of idiotype research is the use of anti-Ids to induce immune responses. In this case, the anti-Ids substitute for antigen where the antigen itself is not readily available or cannot be used for other reasons. Many anti-Ids can induce immune responses in animals of the strain whence the Id was derived, but this is not usually adequate when a universal anti-Id vaccine is required. The anti-Ids inducing responses in animals of a particular strain can often do so because they stimulate B cell clones which are naturally generated in that strain, and they coordinately express the idiotype and the antigen-binding specificity. However, to be able to induce responses in animals with different sets of V genes it is necessary that the anti-Id genuinely mimics an epitope of the antigen; this does not necessarily mean that the anti-Id is structurally identical to the antigen epitope, in terms of an exact match between the amino acids of a hypervariable loop and the epitope. Indeed, in some experiments, anti-Ids act as internal images of carbohydrate antigens where they cannot have identical molecular structures. The meaning of this type of mimicry is that the anti-Id can form a set of secondary bonds with the Id, similar to those formed with the epitope, the Id in this case being the desired antibody response.

Examples of this kind of induced idiotype response are the induction of protective immunity to *Trypanosoma rhodesiense* (the aetiological agent of sleeping sickness), of specific antibodies to the hepatitis B antigen, of protective immunity to *E. coli* infection, and the generation of antibodies to the rabies virus. The inducing Id in each case was a monoclonal antibody to an epitope on the specific antigen. In the case of immunity to *T. rhodesiense*, it was found that the anti-Ids induced little antibody when used alone, nevertheless they could provide protective immunity by priming for a large response when the animals were subsequently challenged with the antigen. This is similar to the results seen in many of the experimental idiotype systems (for example, the induction of antinuclease by anti-Id to antinuclease, described by Miller). More of these anti-Id vaccines are being prepared in the laboratory and may find their way into human use in the future. The advantages of anti-Id vaccines must be balanced against the possibility of using actual antigens prepared by gene cloning in bacteria. Anti-Id vaccines are likely to be of greater use where the antigen is structurally complex and where it is difficult to obtain expression of the cloned gene.

A final use of anti-Ids is in targeting toxic molecules to B cells, and possibly T cells, which has been done for thyroglobulin-reactive T cells. There have been several attempts to treat B cell lymphomas in patients by coupling the cytotoxic A chain of ricin to specifically prepared anti-Id, and injecting the toxic conjugate. Long periods of remission have been obtained by this means, but relapses have occurred as variant lines of the lymphoma have arisen with low levels of surface Id, hence resistant to the toxic conjugate. Two other problems with this approach are the necessity of tailor-making each anti-idiotype for each tumour (until sufficiently large numbers of such reagents are available), and the reactions which naturally occur to a xenogeneic protein: most anti-Ids are prepared in mice or rabbits.

These few examples show that manipulation of immune responses via the idiotype network, or by the use of anti-Ids, is a real prospect and this is an active area of research.

SUMMARY

The immunoglobulin on individual B cells and the specific MHC/antigen receptor on T cells both express particular idiotypes which can be recognized by other lymphocytes. This knowledge leads to the development of the network theory of immune regulation, which states that lymphocytes can exert control over the functions of other lymphocytes via idiotypic interactions. Idiotypic regulation is seen as an adjunct to the regulation exerted by antigen. It is most readily detected in systems where particular Ids dominate the response to the antigen, when the germline genes of an animal are predisposed to the production of precursor B cells expressing that Id.

In experimental systems, the numbers of idiotopes which an animal recognizes on its own antibodies are limited. Thus, it appears that idiotypic interactions primarily occur through a few 'regulatory idiotopes'. Idiotype regulation may either help or suppress an immune response, and may act at the level of B cells or T cells. Indeed, in several instances it is found that B cells and T cells specific for a particular antigen share a common Id, or at least are capable of corregulation by a single anti-Id. Idiotype interactions include: a) the expansion of Id$^+$ B cells by an Id-specific T helper cell population; b) the suppression of antibody responses by Id-specific T suppressor cells acting either on antigen-specific T helpers or directly on the B cells; c) the modulation of cell-mediated responses with Id-specific T cells acting on other T cells; d) the alteration of immune responses by anti-Id or Id either administered exogenously or acquired from the mother in fetal and neonatal life. This last type of Id-mediated immunoregulation often has profound and long-lasting effects.

Quite apart from the physiological significance of idiotype network interactions, the system offers several opportunities for the investigation and external manipulation of the immune response, including immunization by internal image anti-Ids, as well as the possibility of up- or down-regulating particular clones of lymphocytes.

FURTHER READING

Bona C. (1981) *Immune response: Idiotype anti-idiotype network.* CRC Critical Reviews in Immunology **2**, 33.

Bona C., Heber-Katz E. & Paul W.E. (1981) *Idiotype- anti-idiotype regulation I. Immunization with a levan binding myeloma protein leads to the production of auto-anti-(anti-idiotype) antibodies and the activation of silent clones.* J. Exp. Med. **153**, 951.

Bottomley K. & Mosier D.E. (1979) *Mice whose B-cells cannot produce the T15 idiotype also lack an antigen-specific helper T cell required for T15 expression.* J. Exp. Med. **150**, 1399.

Dunn E.B. & Bottomley K. (1985) *T-15 specific helper T cells: analysis of idiotype specificity by competitive inhibition analysis.* Eur. J. Immunol. **15**, 728.

Etlinger H.M. & Heusser C.H. (1983) *Lack of requirement for idiotype matching: T cells from mice which cannot produce idiotype support idiotype-positive antibody response.* Eur. J. Immunol. **13**, 851.

Hahn B.H. (1984) *Suppression of autoimmune diseases with anti-idiotypic antibodies: Murine lupus nephritis as a model.* Springer Sems Immunopathology **7**, 25.

Idiotypy In Biology and Medicine. Ed.Kohler H., Urbain J. & Cazenave P.-A. (1984) Pub. Academic Press Inc., Orlando, Florida USA.

Infante A.J., Infante P.D., Gillis S. & Fathman C.G. (1982) *Definition of T cell idiotypes using anti-idiotypic antisera produced by immunization with T cell clones.* J. Exp. Med. **155**, 1100.

Jerne N.K. (1974) *Towards a network theory of the immune system.* Ann.Immunol. (Paris) **125c**, 373.

Juy D., Primi D., Sanchez P. & Cazenave P. A. (1983) *The selection and maintenance of the V region determinant repertoire is germline encoded and T cell independent.* Eur. J. Immunol. **13**, 326.

Kelsoe G., Isack D. & Cerny J. (1980) *Thymic requirement for cyclical idiotype and anti-idiotypic immune responses to a T dependent antigen.* J. Exp. Med. **151**, 289.

Kelsoe G., Reth M. & Rajewsky K. (1981) *Control of idiotope expression by monoclonal anti-idiotope and idiotope-bearing antibody.* Eur. J. Immunol. **11**, 418.

Lifshitz R., Parhami B. & Mozes E. (1981) *Enhancing effect of murine anti-idiotypic serum on the proliferative response for (T,G)-A--L.* Eur. J. Immunol. **11**, 27.

Male D.K (1986) *Idiotypes and Autoimmunity.* Clin. Exp. Immunol. **65**, 1.

Metzger D.W., Furman A., Miller A. & Sercarz E.E. (1981) *Idiotypic repertoire of anti-hen eggwhite lysozyme antibodies probed with hybridomas.* J. Exp. Med. **154**, 701.

Miller G.D., Nadler P., Asano Y., Hodes R. & Sachs D. (1981) *Induction of idiotype bearing nuclease specific helper T cells by in vivo treatment with anti-idiotypes.* J. Exp. Med. **154**, 24.

Paul W.E. & Bona C. (1982) *Regulatory idiotopes and immune networks: a hypothesis.* Immunology Today **3**, 230.

Roitt I.M., Male D.K., Cooke A. & Lydyard P.M. (1983) *Idiotypes and autoimmunity.* Springer Sems Immunopathology **6**, 51.

Sacks D.L., Kelsoe G.H. & Sachs D.H. (1983) *Induction of immune responses with anti-idiotypic antibodies: Implication for the induction of protective immunity.* Springer Sems Immunopathology **6**, 79.

Sercarz E.E. & Metger D.W. (1980) *Epitope specific and idiotope specific cellular interactions in a model protein antigen system.* Springer Sems Immunopathology **3**, 145.

CELLULAR TRAFFIC IN VIVO

14 Lymphocyte and APC Traffic

Most of our detailed knowledge of the workings of the immune system has come from *in vitro* experiments, where the activation of immunologically relevant cells is examined in a variety of liquid culture media. Such conditions are very different from those in which immune interactions occur *in vivo*. Although lymphocytes can be found free-floating in blood, lymph and tissue exudates, immune responses are initiated and generated in specific lymphoid organs. The lymphoid system is organized so that each lymphoid organ drains a defined tissue or vascular compartment. Antigen entering any particular part of the body will be transported to the appropriate local lymphoid organ where the primary immune response is initiated. For example, the lymphatic system transports antigen from most intercellular spaces to lymph nodes. Antigens in blood are processed in the spleen whereas those entering the gastrointestinal tract are dealt with by a special set of organs, including the Peyer's patches, appendix, tonsils, adenoids and colonic patches, which are collectively referred to as the gut-associated lymphoid system (GALT).

Most lymphocytes are constantly recirculating from blood through secondary lymphoid organs and back into the bloodstream. Millions of lymphocytes pass through each lymphoid organ daily. Thus, wherever an antigen enters the body tissues it will be exposed to the full repertoire of lymphocyte antigen receptor specificities. Accessory cells, such as macrophages and dendritic cells within the lymphoid organ, process and present the antigen to specific lymphocytes, thus initiating the immune response. Non-activated cells merely pass through the tissue in a few hours and are returned to the blood where they spend just a few minutes before migrating into another lymphoid organ. Although the majority of lymphocyte traffic passes through the secondary lymphoid tissue, a small, but nevertheless significant number of lymphocytes pass through most other tissues in the body where they may be activated by antigen presented by local accessory cells. Accessory cells themselves do not constantly recirculate in the way that lymphocytes do, but they can migrate locally to carry antigenic material to lymphoid tissues. These accessory cells should be distinguished from resident tissue cells which may be induced to present antigen when stimulated to express Ia antigens by IFN.γ from activated T cells.

It is important to point out at the outset that progress in the field of lymphocyte traffic has been very slow because of the difficulties involved in studying *in vivo* phenomena. For example, many studies have used lymphocytes labelled *in vitro* with radioisotopes or, more recently, fluoresceinated compounds, and then followed the fate of these cells *in vivo*; cells were often seen to migrate to lymph nodes. However, since cells are very easily damaged by any *in vitro* treatment, their apparent specific migration to lymph nodes may merely reflect removal of cells perceived as effete by phagocytes within the node. Furthermore, many experimental situations are stressful to the recipient, and corticosteroids released during stress are known to be potent in modifying lymphocyte traffic. Nevertheless, it is clear that the traffic of lymphocytes within the body is not random but is a well orchestrated process which enables immune defence strategies to be efficiently deployed.

Mechanisms of lymphocyte and APC trafficking and the response of this dynamic system to antigenic stimulation will be examined in this chapter. The principles will be illustrated at the end by a short discussion of lymphocyte traffic through the gut.

ORGANIZATION OF SECONDARY LYMPHOID TISSUES

Lymphatics

Blood capillaries continually leak plasma into tissue spaces. The primary function of the lymphatic system is to prevent life-threatening tissue oedema by removing the excess fluid

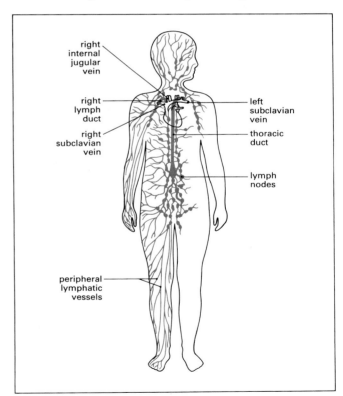

Fig.14.1. The lymphatic system. Peripheral lymphatic vessels drain interstitial fluid and cells to lymph nodes which 'filter out' particulate matter from the lymph. Efferent lymphatics carry concentrated lymph and recirculating lymphocytes, either directly or indirectly via further nodes, to the blood. Most of the lymphatic channels drain into the left subclavian vein via the thoracic duct. However, lymphatics of the upper right side drain via the right lymph duct into the blood at the junction between the right subclavian and right internal jugular veins.

and transporting it back into the bloodstream. Secondarily, the lymphatics transport erythrocytes and other cells, bacteria and a variety of debris to the local lymph node. Lymphatic capillaries within the tissue are similar to blood capillaries but larger, flatter and much more permeable. Fluid (and cells) enters these capillaries through gaps between adjacent endothelial cells. This fluid is termed 'lymph', although at this stage it differs little from blood plasma. Lymphatic capillaries join to form collecting lymphatics which merge to form larger pre-nodal (afferent) lymphatic trunks, where much of the water and small molecules return to the blood via sinuses. Particulate material, including antigenic substances, is processed by phagocytic and other accessory cells in the lymph node. The protein-rich lymph then enters post-nodal (efferent) lymphatic trunks which return it to the venous blood system. Lymph from most of the lower body and from the left side of the upper torso is returned to the left subclavian vein via the large thoracic duct. Lymph from the right side of the upper body, the diaphragm and most of the lungs is transported in the smaller right lymph duct to the junction of the right subclavian and right internal jugular veins (Fig.14.1; see previous page).

Smooth muscle in the walls of lymphatic vessels and one-way valves allow lymph to be actively pumped through the system. This pumping action creates a negative pressure in the tissue spaces which draws more fluid into the lymphatic capillaries. The rate of lymph flow can also be modulated by a variety of nervous, hormonal and physical influences, and in this way the system is able to cope with fluctuations in the volume of tissue fluid to be transported.

Lymph Nodes

Histologically, lymph nodes consist of three recognized areas: the cortex, paracortex and medulla. B lymphocytes are mainly found in the cortex, whereas the paracortex is primarily a T cell area. In the resting, unstimulated lymph node, the cortex has a collection of primary, B cell-containing follicles. Following antigenic stimulation, these enlarge and form secondary follicles containing areas of active proliferation termed 'germinal centres'. The medulla contains relatively fewer cells, but these are of both B and T cell lineages. In addition, the majority of plasma cells in the node accumulate on strands of connective tissue fibres termed 'medullary cords' (Fig.14.2).

Afferent lymphatics (or central lymphatics if supplying second or other nodes in a chain) drain into the subcapsular sinus of the node, which is lined with phagocytic cells. In some species (including rodents and humans, but not sheep) the majority of recirculating lymphocytes (both B and T cells) enter the node via specialized post-capillaries called high endothelial venules (HEV) in the deep zone of the cortex. They then migrate to the B and T cell areas and, in most species including man, subsequently leave the node in the efferent lymphatic vessels. However, in the pig, very few cells enter the efferent lymph; they return directly to the blood in the node. T cells generally have a longer transit time and, thus, lymph nodes are relatively T cell-rich lymphoid organs.

Spleen

The spleen contains two major types of tissue: the red pulp which is primarily concerned with destroying effete red blood cells, but which can also serve a secondary haemopoietic function, and the white pulp which contains the lymphoid tissue (see Fig.14.2). Most of the white pulp is found in the form of periarteriolar lymphatic sheaths (PALS); these are separated from the red pulp by the marginal zone which is the major site of antigen localization and contains specialized APCs (marginal zone macrophages). Lymphocytes enter the spleen in the marginal zone sinuses by passing through post-capillary venules (there are no specialized HEV in the spleen). T and B cells then migrate to their respective areas and subsequently cross into the red pulp to return to the venous effluent. B cells generally take longer than T cells to pass through the spleen. Lymphocytes, and particularly plasma cells, are also found in the red pulp where they are presumed to be in transit to post-capillary venules of the splenic vein.

Gut-Associated Lymphoid Tissue (GALT)

The lymphoid tissues associated with the gastrointestinal tract include the tonsils, Peyer's patches, appendix and colonic patches, and they differ from other lymphoid organs in that they lack a defined capsule and afferent lymphatics. The Peyer's patches have been the most extensively studied but, apart from minor differences, the other members of GALT have similar features. These lymphoid patches were first demonstrated by Peyer in 1667; they are found on the small intestine, particularly towards the distal end, and their numbers vary between species (approximately 200 in man, 12 in the mouse). Sheep and pigs also have a long stretch of Peyer's patch tissue at the end of the ileum, which appears to have functions of a primary lymphoid organ. That is, like the bone marrow, it generates virgin B cells. This tissue also involutes as the animal reaches sexual maturity.

Each Peyer's patch consists of a small aggregation of lymphoid follicles, each with a germinal centre, which contain predominantly B cells. Interfollicular areas, particularly those nearer the intestinal lumen, are rich in T cells. Between the lumen and the follicles are the Peyer's patch domes which are comprised of epithelial and subepithelial regions (see Fig.14.2). The epithelial layer is distinct from that found elsewhere in the gut, being flat rather than columnar and having very few goblet cells or microvilli. The epithelium also has a specialized cell, the M or microfold cell, actively engaged in sampling the lumenal contents of the intestine and interacting with immunologically active cells in the subepithelial layer of the dome.

Recirculating lymphocytes enter the Peyer's patch through HEV (when present) in the interfollicular regions, and migrate to the T and B cells areas of the tissue. Some of these cells may migrate to the dome epithelial layer which is interspersed with intraepithelial lymphocytes, and may then pass into the intestinal lumen. The traffic of lymphocytes to the intestinal lumen via the dome epithelium appears to be increased following antigenic stimulation. Most recirculating cells leaving the Peyer's patches travel in afferent lymphatics to the mesenteric lymph nodes, which then return them to the blood via the thoracic duct.

Other Lymphoid Tissues

Other collections of lymphoid tissues occur throughout the body, particularly associated with mucosal surfaces. For example, the bronchus-associated lymphoid tissues (BALT) and tissues associated with the urogenital tract perform a similar function to the GALT in sampling and responding to antigens entering via their relevant mucosal surfaces. In certain diseases, secondary lymphoid tissue can develop in peripheral tissues (for example, the synovium in patients with rheumatoid arthritis).

Fig.14.2. Organization of peripheral lymphoid tissues. The structures of a lymph node, spleen and gut-associated lymphoid tissue (GALT), exemplified here by a Peyer's patch, are illustrated. Recirculating lymphocytes enter the tissues from the blood in post-capillary venules, some of which are specialized as HEV (lymph node and Peyer's patch). They then enter distinctive T and B cell areas, each having distinctive APCs, before leaving again in efferent (lymph node) or afferent (Peyer's patch) lymph, or in the blood (spleen).

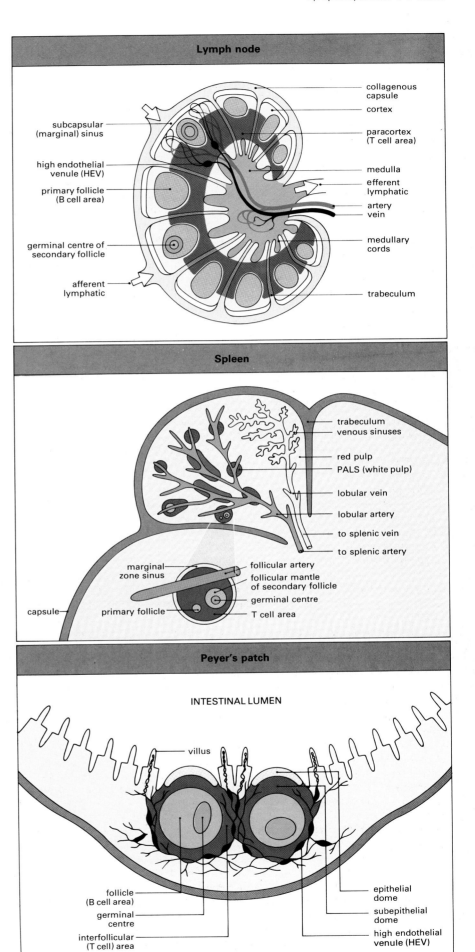

Lymph node

collagenous capsule
cortex
paracortex (T cell area)
medulla
efferent lymphatic
artery
vein
medullary cords
trabeculum

subcapsular (marginal) sinus
high endothelial venule (HEV)
primary follicle (B cell area)
germinal centre of secondary follicle
afferent lymphatic

Spleen

trabeculum
venous sinuses
red pulp
PALS (white pulp)
lobular vein
lobular artery
to splenic vein
to splenic artery

marginal zone sinus
capsule
primary follicle

follicular artery
follicular mantle of secondary follicle
germinal centre
T cell area

Peyer's patch

INTESTINAL LUMEN

villus

follicle (B cell area)
germinal centre
interfollicular (T cell) area

epithelial dome
subepithelial dome
high endothelial venule (HEV)

LYMPHOCYTE RECIRCULATION

The first definitive evidence of lymphocyte recirculation came from the pioneering work of Gowans nearly thirty years ago. He showed that the majority of lymphocytes in the efferent lymph from a rat lymph node came from the blood and were not merely a product of lymphocyte proliferation within the node. Much of our subsequent knowledge was gained through the study of larger animals, such as sheep, where afferent and efferent lymphatics to individual lymph nodes can be easily cannulated.

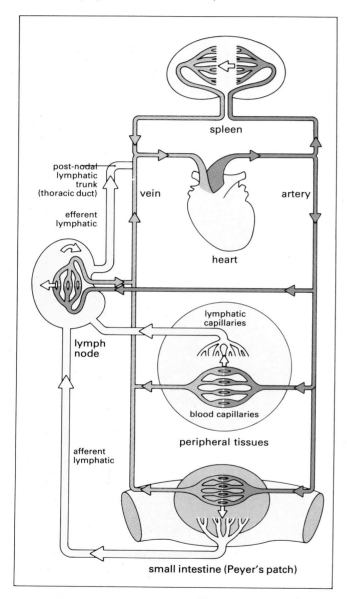

Fig. 14.3. The major routes of lymphocyte recirculation.
Cells in the blood migrate primarily into secondary lymphoid tissues, here exemplified by lymph node, spleen and Peyer's patches. Traffic also occurs through most peripheral tissues, where migrating lymphocytes travel to local (peripheral) lymph nodes in afferent lymphatics. Peyer's patch lymphocytes also travel to lymph nodes (mesenteric) in afferent lymphatics. From lymph nodes, cells travel in efferent lymphatics and re-enter the circulation via post-nodal lymphatic trunks. Routes of flow of lymphocytes are indicated (arrows).

Lymphocytes appear to be unique in that they not only leave the blood to enter tissues (as other blood-borne cells, such as the polymorph, do) but also return to the blood, repeating this process many times. This recirculation is clearly independent of antigen, as it has been shown to occur vigorously in fetal sheep. Secondary lymphoid tissues are the major sites of recirculatory lymphocyte traffic (Fig. 14.3). For example, it has been estimated that, in the rat, over fifty percent of lymphocytes leaving the blood enter the splenic white pulp; in sheep, a lymph node may extract twenty-five percent of all lymphocytes which enter it in the blood. Although lymphocyte recirculation through peripheral, non-lymphoid tissues is much lower than through secondary lymphoid tissues, it nevertheless plays an important role in immunological surveillance. For instance, the brain has one of the lowest levels of lymphocyte traffic, and yet experiments by Hasek and colleagues showed that even here efficient immune responses could be mounted in order to reject allogeneic lymphoma cell grafts. Lymphocyte traffic passes through peripheral tissues in only a few hours; this is as fast or faster than traffic through secondary lymphoid tissues.

Long-lived recirculating lymphocytes consist primarily of memory T and B cells, and virgin T cells. Although NK cells are also thought to recirculate, very little information is available on the traffic of these cells. Under normal circumstances, most virgin B cells have a short lifespan and do not enter the recirculating pool. Studies by MacLennan and colleagues have shown that, following their release from the bone marrow, virgin B cells can enter the recirculating pool in two circumstances. During the first few days of a primary response to antigen, virgin B cells with appropriate antigen specificity will be activated, and their progeny then enter the recirculating pool. If the pool is depleted experimentally (for example, by chronic suppression of B cell development with anti-IgM and anti-IgD injections), mature B cells are unable to divide sufficiently to replenish the pool which then becomes repopulated with virgin B cells. The mechanisms which normally determine the appropriate recirculatory pool size are unknown.

As stated earlier, routes of recirculation are not random. For example, although B and T cells enter secondary lymphoid tissues to the same degree, traffic to peripheral tissues is primarily a T cell phenomenon. This is shown by examining the T and B cell content of peripheral lymph in afferent lymphatics. Lymphocytes also demonstrate a preference for the type of secondary lymphoid organ which they will enter: from peripheral lymph nodes they will preferentially return to similar nodes, whereas GALT cells show a preference for returning to GALT tissues. A possible basis for such observations will be discussed later.

The mechanisms of lymphocyte traffic through a secondary lymphoid organ can be analysed in three distinct phases. First, lymphocytes must bind to the surface of the vascular endothelium in the appropriate post-capillary venules, before migrating into the tissue by opening up tight junctions between endothelial cells. This appears to take only five to ten minutes. The second phase takes place over the following few hours and involves selective migration of T and B lymphocytes into their distinctive areas within the tissue. Finally, most of the cells leave the tissue in order to re-enter the blood. Most lymphocytes are actively motile cells and are thought to simply migrate along the line of least resistance to their exit point. The mechanisms involved in the first two phases, which have been the subject of active research recently, will be discussed in the following section.

MECHANISMS OF LYMPHOCYTE MIGRATION

Lymphocyte Homing Receptors

The migration of recirculating lymphocytes from blood into specific lymphoid tissues has been called 'homing'; much emphasis has been placed recently on characterizing complementary adhesion molecules present on lymphocytes (homing receptors), and on the endothelial cells of HEV. Much of the work on lymphocyte homing receptors has come from the laboratories of Woodruff (on the rat) and Weissman (on the mouse). The interaction of lymphocytes with HEV was studied *in vitro* by incubating lymphocytes on thin sections of lymphoid tissues under critically controlled conditions. In this assay, recirculating lymphocytes bind specifically to HEV and not significantly to other blood vessels. It was found that B lymphocytes bound preferentially to Peyer's patch HEV, whereas T cells bound preferentially to peripheral lymph node HEV. Mesenteric lymph node HEV appeared to bind both T and B cells equally well. These binding preferences clearly reflected the homing preferences of the cells, since Peyer's patches are relatively B cell-rich and lymph nodes are T cell-rich. Some murine lymphomas were found to selectively bind only to Peyer's patch HEV, and others only to lymph node HEV. A minority of normal lymphocytes also appear to have similar specific HEV binding properties. It was proposed that the observed preferential migrations

could be best accounted for by the presence of two distinct homing receptors: one specific for lymph node HEV, the other for Peyer's patch HEV (Fig.14.4). It was presumed that these receptors bound to specific complementary adhesion molecules on the appropriate HEV cells, thus commencing the events leading to migration of the lymphocyte into the lymphoid tissue.

Subsequently, monoclonal antibodies have been produced which bind specifically to one or other of the homing receptors, and which block not only binding of lymphocytes to the appropriate HEV but also *in vivo* homing of cells (treated with antibody *in vitro*) to the appropriate tissues (Fig.14.5).

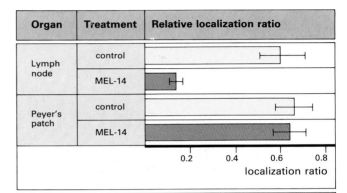

Organ	Treatment	Relative localization ratio
Lymph node	control	
	MEL-14	
Peyer's patch	control	
	MEL-14	

0.2   0.4   0.6   0.8
localization ratio

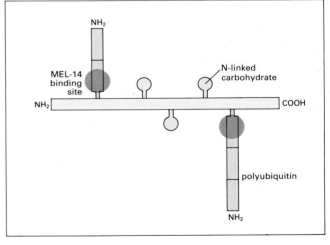

Fig.14.5. The peripheral lymph node homing receptor detected by monoclonal antibody MEL-14. The upper panel shows that treatment of lymphocytes (from mesenteric nodes) with the antibody MEL-14 blocks the localization of the cells in lymph nodes but not Peyer's patches. Before injection, the lymphocytes were labelled with a fluorescent dye so that they could be identified later in the appropriate tissues. The lower panel shows a model of the putative lymph node homing receptor detected by MEL-14. One or more (two shown here) polyubiquitins are covalently linked to a glycosylated 'core' protein. MEL-14 appears to bind to the C-terminal 13 amino acids of ubiquitin only when it is bound to this specific core protein.

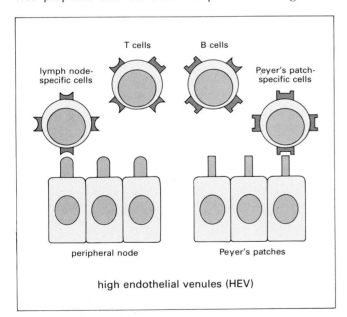

Fig.14.4. Hypothetical model for the molecular basis of lymphocyte migration. It is proposed that lymphocytes can bear two (or more?) distinct 'homing' receptors for high endothelial venules (HEV) in peripheral lymph nodes and Peyer's patches, which are also presumed to bear different molecules interacting with recirculating lymphocytes. Although both B and T cells can bear both of these receptor molecules, their preferential migration to gut and peripheral lymphoid tissues respectively may be explained by the relative number of each homing receptor. Some mature cells and immunoblasts may only have one of these receptors, and thus will only migrate to the appropriate tissue. Although not shown, subsets of T cells may bear different levels of homing receptors, since they also show different relative migratory patterns.

For example, antibodies to mouse (MEL-14) and rat (A.11) peripheral lymph node homing receptors have been described. The homing receptor recognized by MEL-14 has been the most extensively characterized. It appears to have lectin-like activity in that its binding is blocked by mannose-6-phosphate. This implies that the adhesion molecule on the high endothelial cells involves sugar residues.

Biochemical analyses revealed that the MEL-14 defined homing receptor has a molecular weight of approximately 80kD and is a single glycosylated polypeptide chain. Recent analyses using cDNA clones derived from a lymphoma expressing MEL-14 determinants have shown that MEL-14 actually recognizes a conformational epitope on the protein ubiquitin, which is only revealed when ubiquitin is bound to the appropriate peptide chain. None of the other internal or cell-surface ubiquitinated molecules (which are, as the name implies, present in all cells) are detected by MEL-14. Since the cDNA clones encoded large, tandem head-to-tail ubiquitin transcripts which are probably translated as polyubiquitins, it has been suggested that the lymph node homing receptor defined by MEL-14 consists of a unique 'core' protein to which one or more polyubiquitins are covalently attached (see Fig.14.5). This suggestion is supported by the observation that the purified homing receptor protein from the lymphoma cell has at least two N termini. It has also been speculated that other homing receptors might be of a similar structure but with different 'core' proteins. Very recently, human lymphocytes have also been shown to possess very similar receptors for HEV.

Although the data discussed above suggest that homing receptors recognizing specific HEVs account for the migration of lymphocytes to appropriate tissues, it is not yet clear how general and important this mechanism really is. Since lymphocytes can recirculate through many tissues (for example, skin and spleen) which do not have specialized HEV, and recirculation through secondary lymphoid organs occurs normally in species completely lacking HEV, it would appear that such homing receptors are not critical. However, it is conceivable that a similar receptor system could mediate binding to normal post-capillary venules in these tissues and species. The resolution of this dilemma may have to wait for a long time as the appropriate experiments are very difficult to do. The nature of the molecules on the endothelial cells which are recognized by migrating lymphocytes is virtually unknown. As mentioned

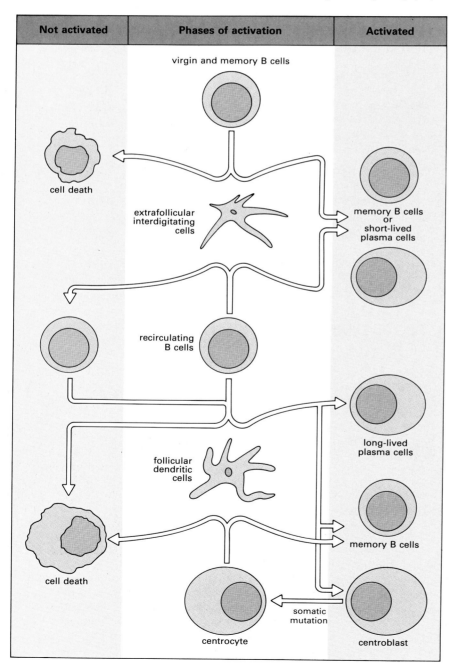

Fig.14.6. Proposed phases of B cell activation by T dependent antigens.
Both virgin and memory B cells can be activated on extrafollicular interdigitating cells, to become memory cells or short-lived plasma cells. Non-activated virgin B cells die, but recirculating B cells may progress to follicular dendritic cells where they can be activated, if their antigen is present, to induce germinal centre formation involving the formation of centroblasts (as well as long-lived plasma cells and memory B cells). Somatic mutation to give altered receptors may occur in centroblasts which are then subjected to immediate selection on the follicular dendritic cell. Based on MacLennan and Grey, 1986.

above, sugar residues such as mannose-6-phosphate may be involved. Other work has suggested that sulphated glycoconjugates made by HEV of lymph nodes are important. Cited in support of this suggestion has been the observation that sulphated polysaccharides will modify lymphocyte migration *in vivo*. However, as mentioned at the beginning of this chapter, the validity of such observations is doubtful because of the ease of artefactually modifying migratory patterns *in vivo*.

Selective Distribution of Lymphocytes to T and B Areas

Each secondary lymphoid organ has easily recognizable, distinct areas containing predominantly T or B cells. Yet both these cell types enter the tissue in the same area, usually via post-capillary venules (HEV if present) in the T cell area. How do these cells follow separate routes of migration to their appropriate area? The mechanism is still completely unknown, but a few suggestions have been made. One possibility is that B and T cells move randomly but have differential adhesive properties for their distinctive areas, and they are thus retained longer in these regions. The basis for such a model could be their relative binding affinity for the distinct, non-lymphoid stromal cells in each region. B cell areas have follicular dendritic cells, whilst T cell areas have dendritic interdigitating cells. Curtis and de Sousa have described soluble factors produced by T and B cells which can inhibit their respective aggregation; this might prevent the accumulation of cells in the wrong domain.

EFFECT OF ANTIGEN ON THE LYMPHOID SYSTEM

Antigen Transport and Localization

If an antigen gains direct access to the blood, it will initially localize primarily to macrophages in the marginal zone of the spleen. Antigens present in the gut may be directly sampled by Peyer's patch M cells and intraepithelial lymphocytes which can transport them through the short distance to T and B areas of the patch. Similar events may occur in the bronchus-associated tissue of the lung. Antigens entering most other peripheral tissues will be transported to local lymph nodes either free in the lymph or by cells. Most antigen free in the lymph will localize first to phagocytes present in the subcapsular sinus before reaching other areas of the node. Antigens will localize to extra-follicular interdigitating cells before follicular dendritic cells, which require specific antibody to bind antigen. Both mature and virgin lymphocytes gain access to antigen on interdigitating cells in the T cell area, but only mature recirculating cells will reach follicular dendritic cells where, if activated by T dependent antigen, they participate in the formation of germinal centres (Fig.14.6; see also page 14.8). Antigen can be transported in the afferent lymph on cells such as macrophages or on lymphocytes in the form of immune complexes bound to Fc or complement receptors. Such lymphocyte-fixed antigens can be passed to follicular dendritic cells.

In the skin, specialized Ia-positive APCs, called Langerhans cells, continually leave the epidermis through afferent lymphatics where they change morphology and are often referred to as 'veiled' cells because of their distinctive appearance. On reaching the lymph node, these veiled cells migrate to the T cell area where they change morphology again to form interdigitating cells in the paracortex (Fig.14.7). In the epidermis, circulating precursor cells leave the blood to form new Langerhans cells. Many antigens entering the skin will localize to Langerhans cells and be transported to the local node on veiled cells (sometimes then referred to as 'antigen-laden' cells), where they can present the antigen to T cells migrating through the paracortex. Similar migrant veiled cells have been found in intestinal lymph destined for mesenteric lymph nodes, and it seems likely that such APC traffic may also occur in other peripheral tissues. *In vitro*, veiled cells and dendritic cells (interdigitating cells) appear as non-phagocytic cells, but this may be an artefact since they have been seen to be actively phagocytic *in situ*.

Although efferent lymph is normally virtually devoid of macrophages and other APCs (except B cells), under some conditions Ia-negative, antigen-laden, macrophages have been found in thoracic duct lymph. The functional relevance of such cells is not known, but they may serve the role of transporting antigen to the spleen in order to further disseminate the immune response.

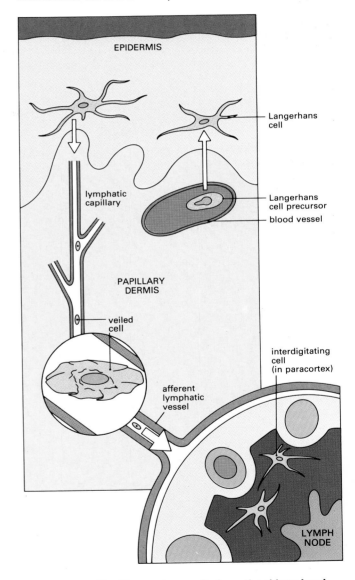

Fig. 14.7. Traffic of Langerhans cells from the skin to local lymph nodes. Langerhans cells regularly leave the skin, sometimes carrying antigen, to enter the afferent lymphatics where they change morphology and are recognized as veiled cells. These carry antigen to T cell areas in the paracortex where they form interdigitating cells.

Lymphocyte Traffic

The response of a lymph node to antigen is reflected in the output of cells into the efferent lymph from that node (Fig.14.8). This can be separated into four arbitrary, overlapping phases. Within a few hours of antigen stimulation, a local inflammatory response develops producing an increase in blood flow to the node of up to twenty-five times. This gives rise to a concomitant increase in lymphocyte traffic into the node. With some antigens there is a simultaneous 'shut-down' of cell exit from the node (but no change in the rate of flow of the lymph itself). Experiments by McConnell and colleagues indicated that complement activation or PGE2 production in the node can cause this shut-down. How lymphocytes are prevented from leaving is not known, but one suggestion has been that cell adhesiveness is increased to form a lymphocyte 'plug' in the node. Adhesion molecules such as LFA-1 (see Chapter 6) might be involved in such a process.

The second phase takes place one to two days following antigen stimulation, and is seen as a marked increase in the output of small lymphocytes into the efferent lymph. This output is devoid of antigen-specific lymphocytes, which are recruited into the immune response and retained within the node. These cells are thought to be trapped through their recognition of antigen on appropriate APCs. This probably also explains the phenomenon of antigen-stimulated lymphocytes preferentially localizing to antigen-triggered lymph nodes, since entry of cells into the node is antigen-independent. During this antigen-triggered, non-migratory phase there is a localized proliferation and differentiation of cells. The activated cells transiently lose their HEV homing receptors and therefore fail to stain with antibodies such as MEL-14.

After about two days, cell proliferation has increased markedly and, coincidently with this, blast cells begin to appear in the efferent lymph; this emigration peaks at about four days (earlier in the secondary response). These blasts show specific homing properties. For example, gut IgA precursors migrate specifically to mucosal areas, blasts triggered in lymph nodes return to other lymph nodes. It has been suggested that this specific homing is mediated by blast cells which are only reexpressing the homing receptor they initially used in order to enter the lymphoid tissue where they were triggered. This still remains to be substantiated. In secondary responses, many B cell blasts migrate to the bone marrow or mucosal surfaces where they undergo terminal differentiation to plasma cells which, in contrast to plasma cells in secondary lymphoid tissue, are long-lived (at least twenty days).

Finally, after four to five days, blast cell output begins to decline and small sensitized (memory) cells start to emerge. These then enter the blood to become part of the re-circulating pool, having reexpressed homing receptors.

Germinal Centre Formation

In a primary response to a T dependent antigen, B cells are recruited non-specifically to the antigen-stimulated lymphoid tissue, and antigen-specific B cells activated on follicular dendritic cells in primary follicles form germinal centres where differentiation events (such as class switching and somatic mutation) are thought to occur. The majority of antigen-binding cells (B cells) are to be found within germinal centres in stimulated lymphoid tissues. Since only T dependent antigens induce germinal centre formation, it is not surprising that proliferating B cells within the follicle are found in association with T cells. These T cells are predominantly of the TH phenotype, in contrast to T cell areas which normally consist of less than fifty percent of TH cells (for lymph nodes).

Shortly after antigen administration, there is a dramatic increase in the frequency and total number of IgM^+D^- B cells within a lymph node (in Peyer's patches they are IgA^+D^-, and in a secondary response of lymph nodes the cells are IgG^+D^-). This lack of IgD is specific to germinal centre cells, and the loss of this surface molecule seems to be one of the earliest events in germinal centre formation. Germinal centre cells express high levels of binding sites for the lectin peanut agglutinin (PNA) which binds to terminal galactosyl residues. This expression has proved very useful in the isolation and further study of germinal centre cells.

Germinal centre cells (centroblasts: pale-staining, rapidly proliferating B cell blasts) appear three days following primary immunization. They have low levels of surface immunoglobulin and no IgD, but are high in class I and II MHC molecules and can subsequently give rise to memory B cells. It has been suggested by MacLennan and colleagues that somatic mutation of Ig V regions occurs primarily in

Fig. 14. 8. Effect of antigenic stimulation on efferent lymph from a local lymph node. Shortly following antigen exposure, there is a marked decrease ('shut down') of cells leaving the node, but a marked increase in cells entering it. Following this, the outflow of lymphocytes resumes and increases to several times higher than normal. However, the lymph is devoid of antigen-specific cells which are retained within the node. As this period wanes, blast cells begin to appear and this is later followed by the appearance of sensitized, specific memory cells.

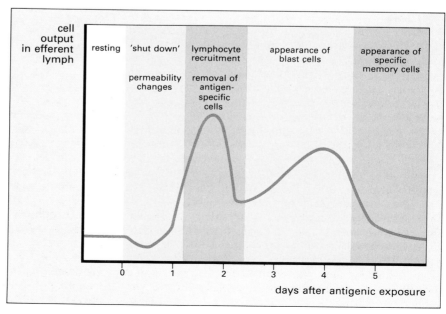

these centroblasts, and that B cells (centrocytes) with newly mutated Ig molecules are subject to immediate selection by antigen on the follicular dendritic cells (see Fig. 14.6). Since antigen on follicular dendritic cells is in the form of immune complexes, epitopes recognized during the early part of the response will be largely masked and only B cells with higher affinity receptors will be reactivated. Other cells die within the germinal centres where their debris is ingested by phagocytic cells, forming the characteristic tingible bodies of germinal centre macrophages.

LYMPHOCYTE TRAFFIC THROUGH THE GUT

Antigen present within the intestinal tract is first encountered by M cells which actively sample lumenal contents, and intraepithelial lymphocytes present in the dome epithelium of Peyer's patches. These cells can transport antigen to the underlying B and T cell areas also containing macrophages which may process and present the antigen. B cells themselves might also present antigen to T cells directly and subsequently become activated in response to helper signals from the T cell (see Chapter 6). Triggered cells differentiate and travel in draining lymphatics from the GALT to the regional mesenteric lymph node. Unlike lymph nodes and spleen, very little antibody synthesis occurs within the Peyer's patch. APCs, including highly Ia-positive veiled cells, also travel in the afferent lymph from the gut mucosa to the mesenteric lymph node.

Antigen presentation in GALT often leads to the generation of antigen-specific suppressor cells, which subsequently also appear in the mesenteric nodes and spleen. At the same time, local immune responses to the antigen take place unabated. This suggests that the suppressor cells migrate out of the GALT to act peripherally (oral tolerance), perhaps in order to prevent systemic responses to gut antigens which gain access to the blood.

On leaving the mesenteric lymph node, activated B and T cells migrate to the blood and may then spend some time in the spleen before seeding to the lamina propria of the intestine and other mucosal exocrine sites. Within the lamina propria, only T lymphoblasts localize to the epithelial layer. B blasts terminally differentiate into plasma cells, most of which secrete IgA. Since cells activated in the gut also migrate to other mucosal sites, it has been proposed that the term GALT be expanded to the mucosa-associated lymphoid tissue (MALT) system. This includes the gut, lungs, lactating mammary glands, salivary and lacrimal glands, and also the urogenital tract (Fig. 14.9). The mechanism for selective homing of gut-derived lymphocytes to this variety of mucosal tissues is not known. Some evidence suggests that it may be due to locally produced chemotactic factors. For example, a globulin fraction of milk whey has been shown to have chemoattractive activity for IgA$^+$ and IgG$^+$ lymphocytes from mesenteric but not from other peripheral lymph nodes.

For the concept of MALT to be accepted, the homing to the gut of cells activated in other mucosal sites needs to be demonstrated. Clearly, such a system would be advantageous for protecting against microorganisms invading the body at different mucosal sites. It might also be exploited in the treatment of certain infectious diseases. For example, oral immunization might be an effective route for protecting against infections of the genital tract, such as herpes or gonorrhoea.

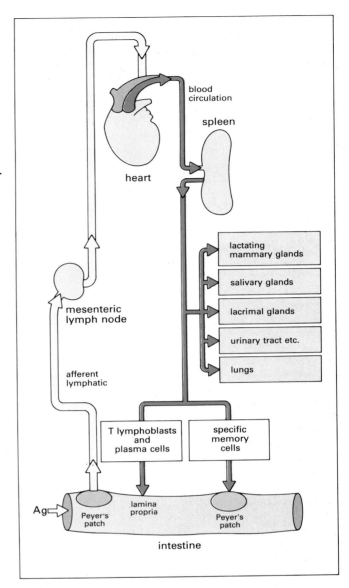

Fig. 14.9. Illustration of the traffic of lymphocytes through gut-associated lymphoid tissues and other exocrine mucosal sites.

SUMMARY

Most lymphocytes continually recirculate throughout the various tissues of the body. The majority of lymphocyte traffic occurs through the secondary lymphoid tissues, such as the lymph nodes, spleen and GALT. A small, but nevertheless significant, number of lymphocytes pass through most other tissues of the body. This serves to ensure that wherever foreign antigenic material enters the body, it will encounter the full range of receptor specificities and thus quickly trigger an immune response.

Cells leave the blood via post-capillary venules which, in some lymphoid tissues (of some species) such as lymph nodes and Peyer's patches, are specialized into high endothelial venules (HEV). Most lymphocytes appear to have one or more specific homing receptors which may allow them to migrate through HEV of specific lymphoid tissue. Upon entering the lymphoid tissue, T and B cells migrate to distinct areas where, if they do not encounter specific antigen, they spend a few hours before leaving to re-enter the blood. In the spleen, cells return directly to the blood in the red pulp, whereas in other lymphoid tissues they travel along lymphatics, sometimes passing through other lymph nodes before entering the blood.

APCs circulate locally, to carry antigen from peripheral tissues to local lymph nodes. Events within the lymphoid tissue ensure optimal interaction of specific cells with their antigen. In the case of B cells, this leads to germinal centre formation where differentiation events probably occur, such as class switching and somatic mutation. Activated

blast cells first leave the tissue and migrate to specific sites. Following this migration, specific memory cells return to the recirculating pool to re-enter lymphoid tissue, often of the same type. That is, progeny of cells activated in lymph nodes often show preference for returning to other lymph nodes. Such preferential migratory patterns increase the efficiency of the system, since individual invading micro-organisms will also have preferential sites of entry into the body. Thus, defence of the body by the immune system does not rely on chance encounters of specific cells with antigen, but it is an efficiently orchestrated process.

FURTHER READING

Adair T.H. & Guyton A.C. (1985) *Introduction to the lymphatic system.* In Experimental biology of the lymphatic circulation (page 1). Johnston M.G. (ed.), Research monographs in cell and tissue physiology **9.** Elsevier, Amsterdam.

Bell E.B. & Botham J. (1982) *Antigen transport. I. Demonstration and characterization of cells laden with antigen in thoracic duct lymph and blood.* Immunology **47,** 477.

Bienenstock J. & Befus D. (1984) *Gut- and bronchus-associated lymphoid tissue.* Am. J. Anat. **170,** 437.

Blood Cells and Vessel Walls: functional interactions. (1980) CIBA Foundation Symposium **71.** Excepta Medica, Amsterdam.

Butcher E.C. & Weissman I.L. (1984) *Lymphoid tissues and organs.* In Fundamental Immunology (page 109). Paul W. (ed.), Raven Press, New York.

Chin Y.-H., Corey G.D. & Woodruff J.J. (1983) *Lymphocyte recognition of lymph-node high endothelium. V. Isolation of adhesion molecules from lysates of rat lymphocytes.* J. Immunol. **131,** 1368.

Chin G.W., Pearson L.D. & Hay J.B. (1985) *Cells in sheep lymph and their migratory characteristics.* In Experimental Biology of the lymphatic circulation (page 141). Johnston M.G. (ed.), Research monographs in cell and tissue physiology **9.** Elsevier, Amsterdam.

Chin Y.-H., Rasmussen R., Cakiroglu A.G. & Woodruff J.J. (1984) *Lymphocyte recognition of lymph node high endothelium. VI. Evidence of distinct structures mediating binding to high endothelial cells of lymph nodes and Peyer's patches.* J. Immunol. **133,** 2961.

Curtes A.S.G. & de Sousa M. (1975) *Lymphocyte interactions and positioning. I. Adhesive interaction.* Cell Immunol. **19,** 282.

Czinn S.J. & Lamm M.E. (1986) *Selective chemotaxis of subsets of B lymphocytes from gut-associated lymphoid tissue and its implications for the recruitment of mucosal plasma cells.* J. Immunol **136,** 3607.

De Sousa M.A.B. (1981) *Lymphocyte Circulation. Experimental and Clinical Aspects.* John Wiley, Chichester.

Drexhage H.A., Mullink H., de Groot J., Clake J. & Balfour B.M. (1979) *A study of cells present in peripheral lymph of pigs with special reference to a type of cell resembling the Langerhans cell.* Cell. Tiss. Res. **202,** 407.

Ermak T.H. & Owen R.L. (1986) *Differential distribution of lymphocytes and accessory cells in mouse Peyer's patches.* Anatomical Record **215,** 144.

Essays on the anatomy and physiology of lymphoid tissues (1980). Trnka Z. & Cahill R.N.P. Monographs in Allergy **16.** S. Karger, Basel.

Gallatin W., St. John T.P., Siegelman M., Reichart R., Butcher E.C. & Weissman I.L. (1986) *Lymphocyte homing receptors.* Cell **44,** 673.

Gallatin W.H., Weissman I.L. & Butcher E.C. (1983) *A cell surface molecule involved in organ-specific homing of lymphocytes.* Nature **304,** 30.

Gowans J.L. (1959) *The recirculation of lymphocyte from blood to lymph in the rat.* J. Physiol. (Lond.) **146,** 54.

Gowans J.L. & Knight E.J. (1964) *The route of recirculation of lymphocytes in the rat.* Proc. R. Soc. London (Biol.) **159,** 257.

Hall J.G. (1985) *The functional anatomy of lymph nodes.* In Lymph Node Biopsy Interpretation (page 1). Stansfield A.G. (ed.), Churchill Livingstone, London.

Hasek M., Chutna J., Sladocek M. & Lodin Z. (1977) *Immunological tolerance and tumour allografts in the brain.* Nature **268,** 68.

Heinen E., Braun M., Coulie P.G., Van Snick J.V., Moeremans M., Cormann N., Kinet-Denoël & Léon J. Simar (1986) *Transfer of immune complexes from lymphocytes to follicular dendritic cells.* Eur. J. Immunol. **16,** 167.

Hopkins J., McConnel I. & Pearson J.D. (1981) *Lymphocyte traffic through antigen-stimulated lymph nodes. II. Role of prostaglandin E_2 as a mediator of cell shutdown.* Immunology **42,** 225.

Jalkanen S., Bargatze R., Hsu M., Wu N., & Butcher E.C. (1985) *Surface receptors involved in lymphocyte homing in man.* Fed. Proc. **44,** 1177.

Kraal G., Hardy R.R., Gallatin W.H., Weissman I.L. & Butcher E.C. (1986) *Antigen-induced changes in B cell subsets in lymph nodes: analysis by dual fluorescence flow cytofluorometry.* Eur. J. Immunol. **16,** 829.

Liu H. & Splitter G.A. (1986) *Localization of antigen-specific lymphocytes following lymph node challenge.* Immunology **58,** 371.

MacLennan I.C.M. & Gray D. (1986) *Antigen-driven selection of virgin and memory B cells.* Immunological Reviews **91,** 61.

Mayrhofer G., Holt P.G. & Papadimitriou J.M. (1986) *Functional characteristics of the veiled cells in afferent lymph from the rat intestine.* Immunology **58,** 379.

McConnel I. (1982) *Lymphocytes and the lymphoid system.* In Lachman & Peters (page 72).

McConnel I. & Hopkins J. (1981) *Lymphocyte traffic through antigen-stimulated lymph node. I. Complement activation within lymph nodes initiates cell shutdown.* Immunology **42,** 217.

Pals S.T., Kraal G., Horst E., de Groot A., Sheper R.J. & Meijer C.J.L.M. (1986) *Human lymphocyte-high endothelial interaction: organ-selective binding of T and B lymphocyte populations to high endothelium.* J. Immunol. **137,** 760.

Parrott D.M.V. (1986) *The structure and organization of lymphoid tissue in the gut.* In Food Allergy and Intolerance. Brostoff J. (ed.), Bailliere Tindall.

Rasmussen R.A., Chin Y.-H., Woodruff J.J. & Easton T.G. (1985) *Lymphocyte recognition of lymph node high endothelium. VII. Cell surface protein involved in adhesion defined by monoclonal anti-HEBF$_{LN}$ (A.11) antibody.* J. Immunol. **135,** 19.

Rouse R.V., Reichert R.A., Gallatin W.H., Weissman I.L. & Butcher E.C. (1984) *Localization of lymphocyte subpopulations in peripheral lymphoid organs: directed lymphocyte migration and segregation into specific microenvironments.* Am. J. Anat. **170,** 391.

Smith M.E. & Ford W.L. (1983) *The recirculating lymphocyte pool of the rat: A systematic description of the migratory behaviour of recirculating lymphocytes.* Immunology **49,** 83.

Sprent J. (1973) *Circulating T and B lymphocytes of the mouse. I. Migratory properties.* Cell. Immunol. **7,** 10.

Tomasi T.B., Larson L., Challacombe S. & McNabb P. (1980) *Mucosal immunity: the origin and migration patterns of cells in the secretory system.* J. Allergy Clin. Immunol. **65,** 12.

Weissman I.L., Warnke R., Butcher E.C., Rouse R. & Levy R. (1978) *The lymphoid system. Its normal architecture and the potential for understanding the system through the study of lymphoproliferative diseases.* Human Pathology **9,** 25.

15 Inflammation

Inflammation is the process by which leucocytes and serum molecules are diverted towards areas of damage in the body. Inflammatory reactions often occur quite independently of the immune system, following physical injuries. The plasma enzyme kinin, clotting and plasmin systems as well as mast cells, may all be activated in inflammation, interacting in association with the autonomic nervous system to produce the characteristic inflammatory responses. When antigenic stimuli are present, the immune system can also recruit these effector systems either directly or via the action of the complement system. Indeed, the prime function of the complement system is to provide a link between immune reactions and various effector systems.

There are three principal components of an inflammatory reaction: a) increased blood flow to the affected area, accompanied by b) increased capillary permeability in the local vasculature, and c) increased migration of cells from the blood vessels into the affected area. The first two factors lead to a rise in the passage of the larger serum molecules out of the vessels, thereby forming a protein-rich exudate which contains leucocytes called in to the inflammatory area by chemotactic stimuli. The cell types seen in different inflammatory foci vary widely depending on the nature of the antigenic stimulus, its persistence and the type of immune reaction it elicits.

Acute inflammatory foci contain mostly polymorphonuclear leucocytes, whereas regions of chronic inflammation contain a higher proportion of lymphocytes and macrophages, and possibly also epithelioid and giant cells. In other circumstances, such as the Jones Mote delayed hypersensitivity reaction, large numbers of basophils are seen, and eosinophils are particularly prevalent in the reactions to some intestinal helminth infections. This chapter examines how different cell populations accumulate at sites of immunological inflammation, and the way in which different stimuli attract different cells and activate the various effector systems. This is superimposed on a background of increased passage of serum molecules into the region and transport of antigens out of the area to the regional lymph nodes. Particularly important in this respect are the antibodies and complement components arriving at the site. Macrophages too are most important, both in limiting the damage caused by pathogens and in transporting antigen to the local lymph nodes to present it to lymphocytes. Lymphocytes and macrophages also interact with the resident tissue cells, via interferons and interleukins, increasing their antiviral resistance and enhancing major histocompatibility complex expression. Ultimately, the outcome of the reactions depends largely on whether the antigenic stimulus is eliminated so that resolution of the damage and tissue regeneration can proceed, or whether the stimulus persists, in which case the agent may be walled off by a ring of fibrosis or it may induce chronic inflammatory reactions. Chronic immune reactions can be as damaging as the original pathogen, and this is seen as hypersensitivity.

CHEMOTAXIS

Chemotactic Factors and Receptors

Cells arrive at sites of inflammation under the influence of chemotactic molecules. These molecules induce directional migration of cells, which can be observed *in vitro* as the movement of cells up increasing concentration gradients of the molecule. Chemotaxis should be distinguished from chemokinesis, the increased random movement of cells, since many inflammatory mediators are chemokinetic but not chemotactic. Histamine is an example of this type of molecule. Chemotactic factors are generated at sites of inflammation and diffuse towards the local capillaries, inducing leucocytes to traverse the endothelium and enter the tissues. In general, they are mostly small short range signalling molecules which are relatively labile. A large number of molecules are chemotactic for leucocytes. Some, such as fibronectin or peptides of fibrin and thrombin, can act independently of any immunological processes. Of primary interest to immunologists are those generated by macrophages and lymphocytes, by the pathogens themselves, or by the interaction of the immune system (antibody) and the complement system. The effects of chemotactic molecules are not confined to cell motility, as many of them also activate leucocyte cytotoxic and microbicidal activities when present at higher concentration.

The first such factor to be identified was the C5a glycopeptide which is released form the N terminus of the α chain of C5 by the action of classical or alternative pathway C5 convertases (C3b2b4b and C3bBb3b or a variety of other enzymes, such as tissue hydrolases and bacterial proteases, which may be released at sites of tissue damage or infection. Human C5a has 74 amino acid residues with a C-terminal Arg residue. Intact C5a is chemotactic for neutrophils and macrophages at concentrations as low as 1nM; however, it is rapidly degraded *in vivo* by serum carboxypeptidases which remove the Arg residue to produce a molecule (C5a desArg) only one-tenth of the same potency, but constituting the major proportion of the active C5 peptides. Further removal of C-terminal residues leaves a molecule which is chemotactically inactive but still blocks C5a binding to its receptor. This shows that the activity of C5a is not wholly dependent on its C-terminal residues. Since the C-terminal pentapeptide does not bind to the receptor, this suggests that C5a contains both a receptor binding site in the bulk of the peptide, and a cell activation site at its C terminus. Human neutrophils have 100,000-300,000 C5a receptors per cell, while the number on macrophages varies greatly, with four- to five-fold fewer receptors on inflammatory macrophages. This means that the sensitivity of an activated macrophage for the C5a chemotactic stimulus is reduced.

Macrophages, monocytes and neutrophils also recognize and are attracted by low concentrations (1nM) of formylmethionyl peptides, of which the most active is fMet-Leu-Phe. These peptides are released by bacteria. Since prokaryotes initiate protein translation with an fMet residue while eukaryotes do not, these peptides provide a specific chemotactic signal marking the presence of invading bacteria. The receptor (which on SDS PAGE has a molecular weight of 50-60kD) occurs in two different forms, with high and low affinities, which are interconvertible. For example, guanine nucleotides reduce the proportion of high affinity receptors. This is thought to occur indirectly by acting on cellular enzymes. The physiological regulation of affinity also appears to be indirectly determined by the degree of occupancy of the receptor, with fMet-Leu-Phe increasing the proportion of high affinity form. For different cell preparations the number of receptors ranges from 10-100,000 per cell, with the high affinity form being in the minority. So, as with the activity of the C5a receptor, the chemotactic receptivity of the cells depends on the strength of the stimulus and the activation state of the cells.

Factor	Characteristic	Source	Action on
C5a	77 amino acid peptide	N terminus of C5 α chain	neutrophils eosinophils macrophages
f.Met-Leu-Phe	tripeptide with blocked N terminus	prokaryotes	neutrophils eosinophils macrophages
LTB4	arachidonic acid metabolite via lipoxygenase pathway	mast cells basophils macrophages	neutrophils macrophages eosinophils (present in ECF)
Neutrophil Chemotactic Factor (NCF)	750kD protein	mast cells	neutrophils
Eosinophil Chemotactic Factor (ECF)	ECF-a 70kD	mitogen-activated T cells	eosinophils

Fig. 15.1 Chemotactic factors. List of chemotactic factors which are highly active at low concentrations, and which are thought to be active *in vivo*. Other active molecules include fibrinopeptide B and thrombin of the blood clotting system, as well as nerve growth factor and a variety of less well-defined lymphokines.

Human monocytes, neutrophils and eosinophils also have receptors for leukotriene B4 (LTB4), the neutrophil receptor again having high and low affinity forms. LTB4 is both chemotactic and chemokinetic, and its activity is greatly enhanced in the presence of some other eicosanoids, especially PGE2 which is not itself chemotactic. LTB4 was probably first identified as having chemotactic activity in preparations of eosinophil chemotactic factor of anaphylaxis (ECF-A). A major source of LTB4 at sites of inflammation are the macrophages themselves, thus, the first cells to arrive at a reaction site can induce further immigration. C5a, fMet peptides and LTB4 do not block each others' receptors, which shows that the receptors are different; nevertheless they can act synergistically *in vitro*, and would presumably do so *in vivo* also.

One problem with studies of chemotactic molecules is that an observation of *in vitro* activity does not necessarily imply that the factor is active *in vivo*. For example, it has

been noted that although LTB4 and C5a desArg are equally potent *in vitro* on a molar basis, *in vivo* C5a desArg appears to be 80-fold more active. Other workers investigating this problem consider that C5a desArg is normally only very weakly chemotactic, and that its activity *in vivo* is enhanced by the presence of a cofactor, present in serum at 4μg/ml, with which the chemotaxin forms a unimolar complex.

Many of the leucocyte-derived chemotactic factors are not fully characterized. In spite of this, some of them may be of great importance, since they appear to have selective action on particular populations of effector cells. For example, macrophage chemotactic factor c (MCF-c) released at sites of delayed hypersensitivity by purified protein derivative causes selective chemotaxis of Ia-positive macrophages. Another example is eosinophil chemotactic factor A (ECF-A), which is released by mast cells and contains two specific chemotactic tetrapeptides as well as less specific factors. Some of the better characterized molecules are listed in Figure 15.1.

It is interesting that different sites of inflammation contain markedly variant populations of inflammatory cells. This may be partly explained in terms of the proportions of cells available in the pool of blood leucocytes, and partly in terms of the blend of chemotactic stimuli acting sequentially on different cells. For example, neutrophils respond more rapidly to C5a than monocytes, and neutrophils which have entered the tissues release a chemotactic factor for monocytes. One might also anticipate an increase in the relative proportions of macrophages at sites of inflammation with time, since they live longer than the polymorphs. It therefore appears that a combination of factors is required to explain the shift in the cell populations during the development of an inflammatory reaction.

Cellular Migration

Exposure of granulocytes to chemotactic stimuli results in a rapid membrane depolarization, associated with an increase in intracellular Ca^{++} and cAMP. Shortly thereafter (5-10 seconds), pseudopodia start to extend and elastase is released. At the same time other markers of cell activation can be detected, such as increased superoxide generation and arachidonic acid release from membrane phospholipids. The signal for movement involves a transmethylation reaction in both neutrophils and macrophages, as judged by reduced locomotion in the presence of methylation inhibitors. The precise mode of action is uncertain, but alterations in methylation reactions affect both affinity of the chemotactic receptors and the lipid composition of the cell membrane. Remodelling of the plasma membrane phospholipids accompanies chemotaxis, but this alone does not account for directional movement which involves the coordinated activation of the cytoskeleton. Leucocytes are extremely sensitive to variations in the concentrations of chemotactic factors across their length, which may vary by as little as 0.1% and still induce directional migration. During cellular locomotion there is a reorientation of the cells' chemotactic receptors towards the leading edge, and continuous recycling of the receptors into the cytoplasm and back again to the leading edge as the cell moves.

In vivo, the neutrophil response to chemotactic stimuli is seen as margination along the walls of the capillaries followed by increased adhesion to the endothelial cells. The migrating cells then extend pseudopods into the junction between two endothelial cells and move through the gap by amoeboid movement. Finally, they break through the basement membrane to enter the tissues. The process of migration from the vessels and movement through damaged tissues congested with debris is facilitated by secretion of neutral proteases (for example, elastase, collagenase, cathepsins) which are released soon after triggering by chemotactic stimuli. The importance of neutrophil chemotaxis is demonstrated in the lazy leucocyte syndrome. In this condition the neutrophils fail to respond to chemotactic stimuli, such as C5a, possibly due to being desensitized to the stimuli by very low doses of the agonist during development. This results in repeated infections with pyogenic bacteria.

ACTION OF EFFECTOR CELLS

Macrophage Activation
Although neutrophils form the majority of the cell population at sites of acute inflammation, macrophages are at least as important because of the large number of different functions they can perform (see Fig. 15.2). Macrophages are a heterogeneous population of cells, but the differences between various macrophages are due more to their distinct developmental stages than to individual differentiation pathways. Macrophages develop by a series of stages during which they acquire additional receptors, metabolic functions and enhanced microbicidal and cytotoxic capacities. This process is called macrophage activation. Based on surface markers and functions, a developmental scheme has been proposed in which the blood monocyte can enter the tissues either to become a resident tissue macrophage or as an immature macrophage responsive to chemotactic stimuli. The responsive cell reacts to inflammatory mediators and is attracted to sites of tissue damage. Inflammatory macrophages are larger than resident tissue macrophages. They have increased responses to chemotactic agents, increased phagocytic abilities and higher levels of certain granule enzymes and secretory capacities. In this scheme

Characteristic	Particular* regulatory stimulus	Activation stage			Effects
		immature macrophage	primed macrophage	activated macrophage	
Fc receptors	interferons	+	+ +	+ +	increased phagocytosis and ADCC
C3 receptors CR1, CR3	chemotactic factors & T cell lymphokines	+	+	+ ⌇	increased phagocytosis and ADCC
Mannose-Fucose receptor	MAF	+ +	+	+	decreased phagocytosis of carbohydrate-containing particles
C5a receptors	C5a	+ +	+	+	decreased sensitivity to chemotactic stimuli
F-Met - - receptor		+	+	+	
LTB4	(receptor not sufficiently well-characterized for analysis)				
Surface Ia	IFNγ	±	+ +	+ + +	antigen presentation to T cells
Lysosomal hydrolases	phagocytosis & lymphokines	+	+ + +	+ + +	increased microbicidal and cytotoxic ability
Secretory neutral proteases		+	+ +	+ + +	breakdown of inflammatory debris
Lysozyme	constitutive	+ +	+ +	+ +	enzymolysis of bacterial cell walls
Tumour Necrosis Factor	IFNγ & LPS	−	−	+ +	cytotoxic for tumour cells
Eicosanoids		+	+ +	+	regulate inflammatory reactions
Reactive Oxygen Intermediates (ROIs)	IFNγ some protein antigens	−	+	+	cytotoxic and antimicrobial activities
Complement		+	+	+ +	local supplement to complement levels
IL-1	many antigens	+ or −	+ or −	+ or −	activates T cells pyrogen induces acute phase proteins

* many inflammatory stimuli increase the various characteristics – only particularly active stimuli are noted
⌇ increased activity

Fig. 15.2 Characteristic activities of macrophages.
Macrophages have a very large number of functions which summate to produce their overall activity, and these are modulated by various stimuli during development of the cells from immature macrophages to activated macrophages. Many inflammatory mediators increase the activity of the various functions, but only particularly active stimuli are noted. An increase in the activity of surface receptors may be due to an increase in the overall number of receptors (as occurs with the Fc receptors), or to modulation of receptor affinity (as occurs with some of the complement receptors).

the resident tissue macrophages may subsequently be primed to respond to appropriate stimuli, but they are generally only weakly responsive. It had been thought that resident macrophages were an intermediate stage between monocyte and inflammatory macrophage, but this now appears less likely.

Macrophage effector functions depend on a number of different cellular activities, and these may be viewed under three headings: a) the expression of cell surface proteins, b) the intracellular activity, including that of the cytoskeleton and mitochondria and the levels of intracellular enzymes, and c) the secretory capacity of the cell. More than 30 different macrophage surface receptors and over 75 different secretory proteins have been identified, and they are not all regulated concomitantly. Naturally, complicated functions such as phagocytosis or tumoricidal activity depend on numerous cellular activities, consequently only the most important capacities affecting effector functions and immune regulation are discussed below, and are listed in Figure 15.2.

Opsonization and Internalization

Opsonization is the process by which particles are coated with molecules which render them more readily phagocytosed. All opsonins appear to act by immobilizing the particle on the surface of the phagocyte. Macrophages can recognize particles non-specifically via the action of surface carbohydrate receptors, and specifically by their Fc receptors. After classical pathway complement activation, antigens may also be opsonized by fragments of C3 deposited on the immune complex. The carbohydrate receptors are

thought to be important in recognition of bacteria (for example, *Staphylococcus aureus* and *Micrococcus luteus*), and possibly also in recognition of tumour cells. Particles with surface carbohydrates can bind to phagocytes either directly to lectin-like receptors, or by the action of extracellular lectins cross-bridging oligosaccharides on the bacteria and phagocyte. Interestingly, one of the carbohydrate receptors which is specific for mannose-fucose is down-regulated on activated macrophages in the presence of MAF or IFN$_\gamma$, while the number of Fc receptors and the activity of the complement receptors (especially CR3) increase under similar circumstances. In essence, the T cells can signal to incoming macrophages to make them less non-specifically adherent and increase their capacity for immune adherence.

Mouse macrophages have separate receptors for different classes of IgG. FcRI recognizes γ_{2a} while FcRII recognizes γ_1 and γ_{2b}. Some human macrophages have receptors for IgE as well as IgG. There have also been reports that C1q could act as a macrophage Fc receptor, since C1q binds specifically to macrophages and neutrophils via its collagenous tail, but the binding is normally weak so that the receptor site would not usually be occupied by C1q. It might, however, be involved in the uptake of larger complexes coated with several C1q molecules due to the potentially higher avidity binding with several ligands. It appears that different classes of Fc receptor are under different regulatory controls, and may be coupled to various signal transduction systems. BCG stimulation causes mouse macrophages to express more FcRI and less FcRII, while both are increased on inflammatory macrophages.

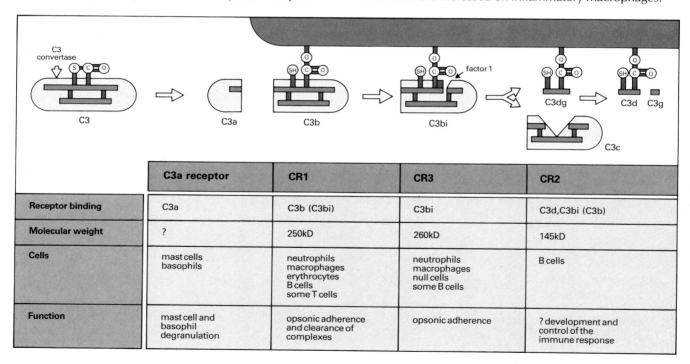

	C3a receptor	CR1	CR3	CR2
Receptor binding	C3a	C3b (C3bi)	C3bi	C3d, C3bi (C3b)
Molecular weight	?	250kD	260kD	145kD
Cells	mast cells basophils	neutrophils macrophages erythrocytes B cells some T cells	neutrophils macrophages null cells some B cells	B cells
Function	mast cell and basophil degranulation	opsonic adherence and clearance of complexes	opsonic adherence	? development and control of the immune response

Fig. 15.3 C3 products and receptors. Complement C3 is cleaved by C3 convertases and several other proteases which split C3a from the α chain. C3a receptors are present on mast cells and basophils. Activation of C3 causes the exposure of an internal thioester bond which is highly active and can link to a number of chemical groups. The active form is highly unstable and decays within milliseconds so that, ordinarily, C3b may only become covalently attached to molecules in the immediate vicinity of the reaction site – usually close to the antigen/antibody

reaction, or on the alternative pathway activator surface. C3b is inactivated by factor I in the presence of factor H to yield C3bi which is further degraded enzymatically, as indicated. Receptors for C3 products are not totally specific for a single ligand. For example, receptor CR1 present on neutrophils has been referred to as the C3b receptor, although it also binds C3bi albeit less avidly. The most likely functions of the receptors are listed, but the function of CR2 on B cells is still debated.

Human macrophages express two different receptors for C3 products. These are CR1 and CR3. CR1 is the C3 receptor which is present also on polymorphs, B cells and erythrocytes. It is normally present at about 5000 receptors per cell, but chemotactic agents (C5a, LTB4 etc.) can increase expression ten-fold. Cocapping experiments show that Fc receptors and CR1 are interlinked via the cytoskeleton, such that they normally act synergistically, but C3 alone can act as an opsonin especially on activated cells where the receptors have increased lateral mobility in the membrane. In this case the receptors can act coordinately so that the particle is zippered onto the membrane. The CR1 receptors only become associated with the cytoskeleton after they have become crosslinked during phagocytosis. CR3 is confined to phagocytes, large granular lymphocytes and a minority of B cells. Its specificity is for inactivated C3b (C3bi) and possibly also for C3d. Increasing evidence points towards CR3 being the Mac-1 surface antigen recognized by the monoclonal antibody OKM1. Although the CR3 level is relatively higher than CR1 on tissue macrophages compared with inflammatory macrophages, it is uncertain whether its function is essentially different from that of CR1. It has been noted that patients deficient in Mac-1 are susceptible to repeated bacterial infections, but since other deficiencies sometimes accompany this condition failure to clear the bacteria cannot unequivocally be attributed to CR3 deficiency. The formation of the various C3 components and the location of their receptors are listed in Figure 15.3.

The process of endocytosis of opsonized particles by macrophages involves internalization via Fc receptors centred on clathrin-coated pits in the plasma membrane. Unoccupied Fc receptors are recycled to the surface again, while immune complexes are vectored towards phagolysosomal destruction. This is not the end of the matter, however, since partially degraded antigens may subsequently become associated with MHC class II molecules in antigen-presenting macrophages. This implies that they can be directed to another intracellular compartment. Clearly, the pathways of antigen breakdown and reexpression on macrophages and other antigen-presenting cells will have a major role in determining how an immune response will develop following antigen uptake.

Microbicidal Activity of Macrophages and Polymorphs
Bacteria and parasites taken into the phagosomes of macrophages and polymorphs are usually killed by a combination of enzymes and other antibacterial proteins from the lysosomes and granules, in association with reactive oxygen intermediates (ROIs). Which of these systems will be most important depends on the type of organism and the state of activation of the cell. Researchers have used macrophages from patients with chronic granulomatous diseases to resolve whether O_2-dependent or O_2-independent mechanisms are more important. These macrophages generate very few reactive oxygen products, due to an enzyme deficiency (usually an NADPH-linked oxidase or its cofactor). For example, lymphokines enhance the microbicidal activity of macrophages from these patients to Leishmania parasites, but do not affect the metabolic deficiency. This implies that in this case the O_2-independent systems are toxic. In spite of the debate on the relative importance of various mechanisms, it is notable that organisms which can inhibit phagosome/lysosome fusion (for example, M. tuberculosis), as well as organisms which fail to trigger the cells' respiratory burst, often escape destruction also. In other words, the importance of the

different systems depends on the organism. The potential microbicidal effector mechanisms include:

1. Reactive oxygen intermediates (.OH, O·, O_2^- and H_2O_2). The phagosomal membrane is originally derived from the plasma membrane, and binding of particles to receptors on the plasma membrane initiates a burst of respiratory activity along with an increase in the activity of the hexose monophosphate shunt providing NADPH. Oxygen is activated by an NADPH oxidase sited in the phagosomal membrane which produces the various ROIs, O_2^-, .OH and singlet oxygen O·. The superoxide ion is converted into H_2O_2 by the action of superoxide dismutase. Each of these products is highly reactive and potentially lethal for cells (for instance, singlet oxygen oxidizes double bonds); for this reason, the polymorphs and macrophages protect themselves from ROIs escaping from the phagosome by a chain of redox reactions involving glutathione. It seems likely that microorganisms may also attempt to use this kind of system to escape destruction by ROIs, as has been noted with experimental T. brucei infections of mice. In this case, using inhibitors of glutathione synthesis led to a rapid clearance of parasites from the blood.

2. Toxic oxidants produced by the interaction of H_2O_2 on halides in the presence of peroxidase or catalase. H_2O_2 is the starting material for the next step of the reactions. In the presence of myeloperoxidase and halides such as Cl^- or I^- toxic halide, compounds such as hypohalites are generated. H_2O_2 in the presence of myeloperoxidase can also act on amino acids to generate aldehydes, thus damaging the bacterial surface; aldehydes are themselves toxic. The myeloperoxidase for these reactions may be released into the phagosome from neutrophil azurophilic granules (macrophage lysosomes do not contain myeloperoxidase), or may be taken up into the cell by endocytosis. Macrophages may also be able to carry out these reactions using catalase from peroxisomes, although it is not certain that catalase-catalysed reactions would be as effective as those catalysed by myeloperoxidase, particularly since many of the more pathogenic bacteria secrete catalase themselves, presumably as a protective measure. Eosinophils also generate H_2O_2 and contain very high levels of eosinophil peroxidase. They are especially effective at damaging multicellular parasites and trypanosomes, the toxic activity being greatly enhanced in the presence of halide ions. This leads to the conclusion that the pathways mentioned above are also active in eosinophils. In addition, it has been observed that secreted eosinophil peroxidase can sensitize tumour cells to the toxic effects of H_2O_2 secreted by macrophages. Neutrophils and macrophages stimulated into phagocytosis emit small amounts of light (chemiluminescence) which is thought to be caused by the decay of ROIs to the ground state, hence this is a marker of the reactions listed above.

3. Cationic proteins of polymorphs, active at neutral pH. Cationic proteins are present in neutrophil granules but are not generally found in macrophages, although lymphokine-inducible cationic proteins have been demonstrated in rabbit alveolar macrophages. Cationic proteins are most effective at alkaline pH, that is, before acidification of the phagolysosome, and have been shown to damage Candida. Eosinophils also contain at least seven cationic proteins (which have not yet been localized to granules), as well as major basic protein (MBP) which forms the main component of the crystalloid core of eosinophil-specific granules.

These proteins have a major effect in promoting eosinophil adherence to schistosomules, and MBP is directly toxic for these parasites. The eosinophil cationic proteins also affect the activity of plasma enzyme systems (fibrin formation and plasmin). It therefore seems likely that neutrophil and eosinophil cationic proteins perform different functions.

4. Phagosome acidification. Phagosome acidification occurs at the time of lysosome fusion; this enhances the activity of myeloperoxidase and favours the peroxidatic action of catalase. Acidification of the phagolysosome may by itself damage some microorganisms. Typically, the pH falls to 3.5-4.0, and parasites such as *T. gondi* are sensitive to these conditions. In addition, the pH optimum of the majority of the lysosomal enzymes is acid.

5. Lysosomal enzymes, mostly active at acid pH. The importance of macrophage lysosomal and secreted enzymes in bacterial killing is uncertain, and it is quite possible that the lysosomal hydrolases and cathepsins are primarily

complement lytic components or lysosomal cationic proteins. Lysozyme is secreted constitutively, regardless of the activation state of the cell.

6. Growth inhibitors, including lactoferrin and arginase. In some circumstances, the ability to prevent bacterial growth by the secretion of molecules which break down or sequester trophic substances is important. For example, arginase limits the availability of arginine, and while this presents little problem to most bacteria, it has been shown that schistosomicidal activity of macrophages correlates with their arginase secretion; tumour cells are also susceptible to the action of this enzyme. Lactoferrin binds to macrophages by a specific receptor, it is endocytosed, and may enter phagolysosomes where it is active at acid pH. Neutrophils can synthesize lactoferrin themselves, which is found in their granules. Lactoferrin sequesters iron, and loading neutrophils with iron reduces their ability to kill some bacteria. The antimicrobial activity of macrophages is set out in Figure 15.4.

Fig. 15.4 Antimicrobial systems of macrophages. Bacteria and other particles may be opsonized by antibody or complement and become attached to macrophages via their Fc and C3 receptors. Attachment precipitates phagocytosis and the particle is internalized. Unoccupied receptors are recycled back to the cell membrane, while the phagocytosed material proceeds along another course towards degradation. Phagocytosis initiates activity of the hexose monophosphate shunt which supplies electrons to an enzyme in the phagosomal membrane (probably a cytochrome), and this generates toxic oxygen metabolites (see text) which can damage microorganisms. In the second stage of the process the pH of the phagosome is transiently increased, during which time cationic proteins from granules may be active. The pH of the phagolysosomal vacuole subsequently falls, and acid hydrolases and lactoferrin start to exert their cytotoxic activities. Peroxidase or catalase under these conditions causes H_2O_2 and halide ions to generate toxic oxidants, such as hypohalites, which may further damage the phagocytosed particle or organism.

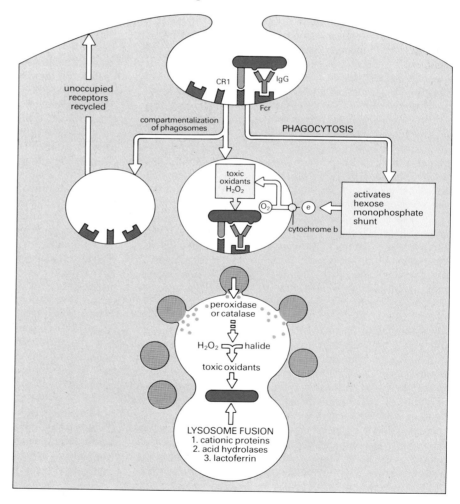

involved in the ultimate breakdown of the phagocytosed material, rather than as a killing mechanism. Lysozyme constitutes up to 2.5% of the macrophage protein, and can act both within the phagolysosome and as a secreted protein. It breaks the bond between MurNac and GlcNac in the bacterial cell wall peptidoglycan. This may damage Gram-positive bacteria, but gaining access to the cell wall of Gram-negative bacteria (which have an outer lipid bilayer) requires synergistic action with other systems, such as the

Secretory Products

Lysozyme (see above) is the major secretory product of macrophages, but other lysosomal hydrolases may be released following phagocytosis of particles and in response to IFN_γ. However, the secreted neutral proteases are more likely to be important in the extracellular milieu and, unlike the lysosomal hydrolases, their level of secretion varies markedly depending on the activation state of the macrophage. Collagenase, elastase, plasminogen activator and a cytotoxic proteinase are included in this group. The secretion occurs in two stages, mirroring the steps required to produce activation. MAF primes the cells and enzyme release is triggered by phagocytosis, high levels of lymphokines and endotoxin.

Activated macrophages can also secrete complement components, C1q, C2, C4, C3, C5, FB and FD. Although the background level of complement in the body is produced by liver and gut epithelium (C1q), local 'topping up' of the levels of complement occurring at sites of inflammation allows the complement-mediated reactions to continue in circumstances where the components are being continually consumed.

Eicosanoids, interleukin-1 and IFN_β are also secreted by macrophages. The immunoregulatory functions of IFNs and IL-1 are discussed in Chapter 9, and the inflammatory and antiviral functions of these molecules are outlined below. In conclusion, the activation of macrophages is a complex event, and not all receptors and functions are up-regulated; however, the general activity of the cell shifts from being a non-specific effector, becoming responsive to lymphokines and capable of interaction with lymphocytes as an antigen-presenting cell. Neutrophils and eosinophils are potent but short-lived effector cells, responsive primarily to chemotactic and opsonic stimuli. Which of these cells will be most effective in antimicrobial activity depends largely on the organism and its ability to withstand the battery of enzymes, active proteins and cytotoxic metabolites produced.

INFLAMMATORY MEDIATORS

This section considers the effects of various mediators on the local blood supply and on the cells of the immune system (Fig.15.5). The molecules which mediate inflammatory reactions come from the complement system, lymphocytes, granulocytes, mast cells and platelets, causing the observed alterations in blood flow and capillary permeability. Their actions affect both the local arterioles

Fig. 15.5 Mediators of inflammation. List of some of the major inflammatory mediators along with their principal sources and effects.

Mediator	Sources	Activators	Principal effects
Bradykinin	high molecular weight kininogen	factor XIIa/ kallikrein other proteases	vasodilation ↑ vascular permeability pain
Histamine	mast cell and basophil granules	IgE and antigen anaphylatoxins	vasodilation ↑ vascular permeability spasmogen chemokinesis
C3a and C5a	complement system	C3 and C5 convertases other proteases	spasmogens mast cell degranulation C5a-chemotaxis ↑ vascular permeability
Platelet Activating Factor (PAF)	basophils neutrophils macrophages	depends on cell type	platelet factor release spasmogen neutrophil activation ↑ vascular permeability
Eicosanoids (see below)	macrophages monocytes endothelial cells mast cells basophils etc	many inducers	modulate effects of other mediators vasoactive
PGE2	cyclooxygenase pathway	many inducers	vasodilation potentiates effects of histamine, bradykinin, C5a and LTB4
PGI2	cyclooxygenase pathway	many inducers	vasodilation blocks platelet aggregation and bronchoconstriction
TxA2	cyclooxygenase pathway	many inducers	vasoconstriction platelet aggregation bronchoconstriction
LTB4	lipoxygenase pathway	many inducers	neutrophil and macrophage chemotaxis modulates increase in vascular permeability
LTD4	lipoxygenase pathway	many inducers	spasmogen ↑ vascular permeability LTB4 and LTD4 produces bronchospasm
IL-1	macrophages	macrophage activators (e.g. C5a)	pyrogen, PG production induces acute phase proteins activation of T cells
IFN_γ (MAF)	T cells	antigen	macrophage and K cell activation modulates inflammatory reactions

and capillaries, and are not confined to leucocytes, as an inflammatory reaction involves the whole tissue. For example, OAF released from T cells acts on osteoclasts to increase bone remodelling and, conversely, factors such as kinins and tissue enzymes released by damaged tissues are important in initiating the leucocyte infiltration.

C3a and C5a were both initially identified as inflammatory mediators by their actions in causing smooth muscle contraction. They are referred to as anaphylatoxins because they mimic some of the reactions of anaphylaxis, and it was subsequently found that they both cause mast cell degranulation. The spasmogenic action of these mediators is now thought to be primarily due to histamine release from the mast cell granules; however, since not all of the activity is blocked by histamine receptor inhibitors (H1 and H2), leukotrienes are also implicated. Surprisingly, the receptors on mast cells for C3a and C5a are different, as evidenced by the fact that they fail to produce tachyphylaxis to each other although they do produce it to themselves. C4a also weakly activates mast cells, but this is probably insignificant physiologically. As with the chemotactic activity of C5a, removal of the C-terminal Arg residue by carboxypeptidases drastically reduces the spasmogenic activity of C3a and C5a. C5a has been reported to increase vascular permeability independently of mast cell histamine release, which is enhanced in the presence of LTD4 and PGE2. The data on the effect of C3a and C5a on the immune response are confused, with reports that the former suppresses mitogen stimulation of peripheral blood lymphocytes, while the latter augments primary plaque formation of mouse spleen cells. In each case it is possible that the effects were secondary to action on basophils or macrophages in the cultures, and the question of any direct effect requires resolution.

Mast Cells, Basophils and Platelets

Mast cells are important sources of mediators, being located close to blood vessels, which suggests that their effects may be localized. They can be activated by immune reactions, both directly via sensitization with IgE, and indirectly via C3a and C5a. Mast cells are also activated by tissue damage independently of immune reactions. Triggering of mast cells produces an influx of Ca^{++} followed by a rise in intracellular cAMP. This induces granule release (exocytosis), and activates phospholipase to release arachidonic acid from membrane phospholipids. Arachidonic acid is converted into eicosanoids (prostaglandins, leukotrienes and thromboxanes) via the cyclooxygenase and lipoxygenase pathways, as will be discussed in the next section. The mast cell granules contain histamine, proteolytic enzymes, heparin and a high molecular weight neutrophil chemotactic factor (NCF). Basophils, which in many respects are similar to mast cells, also contain vasoactive amines. Platelet-activating factor, which is newly synthesized after triggering, is also found in basophils, neutrophils and monocytes.

Histamine has a powerful effect on the local vasculature, causing smooth muscle contraction, increased blood flow and capillary permeability, but it also has a number of negative feedback effects on leucocytes. These include the suppression of lysosomal enzyme release from neutrophils and the activation of non-specific T suppressor cells. The function of the neutrophil chemotactic factor present in the granules is not certain. Since it has a high molecular weight, its speed of diffusion and action will be less than that of C5a and LTB4, but there is some evidence that it contributes towards the cellular accumulation in the bronchi which is

seen in the late phase of allergic asthma. Enzymes released from the granules include tryptic enzymes which can directly generate C3a and plasmin, and can activate kininogenase which causes the release of bradykinin from high molecular weight kininogen. Bradykinin is another extremely potent vasoactive mediator. The enzymes must also contribute to the clearance of debris from around the inflammatory focus, allowing access for neutrophils and macrophages.

Platelets, which are also sources of vasoactive amines, especially 5-hydroxytryptamine (5HT), are activated following vascular damage, but they also have receptors for Fc and can be triggered by immune complexes. There are two major types of platelet granules: the alpha granules containing proteolytic enzymes and cationic proteins, and the so-called dense bodies containing 5HT and ADP. Alterations in vascular permeability caused by 5HT can promote the deposition of complexes on the endothelium. This occurs in immune complex disease, and it is notable that treatment of animals with methysergide, which blocks 5HT formation, ameliorates the immune complex disease which develops spontaneously in NZB/W mice.

Eicosanoids

Prostaglandins (PGs) and leukotrienes (LTs) are produced by many of the effector cells involved in an immune response, with mast cells, basophils and macrophages being the most important sources. Arachidonic acid is the initial substrate for all these products, and is released from membrane phospholipids either by the action of phospholipase A or indirectly by the sequential activation of phospholipase C.

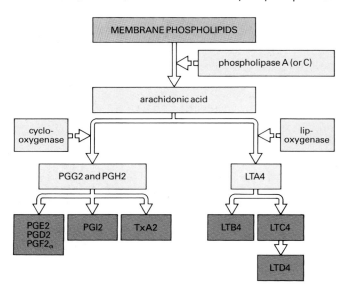

Fig. 15.6 Eicosanoids. The eicosanoids are generated from arachidonic acid which is released from membrane phospholipids, either directly by phospholipase A or indirectly via phospholipase C. Arachidonic acid may then be metabolized, either via the cyclooxygenase pathway to yield the prostaglandins and thromboxanes, or via the lipoxygenase pathway to yield the leukotrienes. The most active intermediates are shaded dark pink. Some of the molecules induce inflammatory reactions, while others inhibit them; seen as a whole, therefore, the eicosanoids modulate inflammation particularly by potentiating the actions of other mediators. Steroids exert part of their anti-inflammatory effect by inhibiting the generation of arachidonic acid, while salicylate and indomethacin inhibit the cyclooxygenase pathway.

Arachidonic acid may be converted by cyclooxygenase into the unstable endoperoxides PGG2 and PGH2 which are the precursors of prostaglandins (PGE2, PGD2, PGF2α and PGI2) and thromboxanes (TxA2 and TxB2). Alternatively, the enzyme 5-lipoxygenase generates LTA4 which is the precursor of the other leukotrienes (LTB4, LTC4 and LTD4) (Fig.15.6).

PGE2 is detectable in inflammatory exudates, with a maximum accumulation time six to twenty-four hours after the early mediators, histamine and bradykinin. PGE2 enhances the chemotactic and vasoactive properties of other mediators (for example C5a, LTB4, bradykinin and histamine), although it is difficult to show effects caused by PGE2 alone. PGE2 by itself causes pyrexia and increased blood flow. The question of the role of prostaglandins in inflammation is complicated by several studies which have shown PGE1 to suppress inflammatory reactions, ameliorate immune complex disease and reduce the sensitivity of neutrophils for C5a. It therefore appears that prostaglandins are comediators which modulate the developing reactions, where the regulation depends on the blend of prostaglandins produced.

Leukotrienes LTC4 and LTD4 also affect the vasculature. Generally speaking, they directly caused an increase in vascular permeability, while the effect on blood flow varies for different species and dosages. LTC4 and LTD4 are now known to be the most important components of SRS-A (Slow Reacting Substance of Anaphylaxis) which causes smooth muscle contraction, and are responsible for the bronchospasm which often occurs after the immediate response in allergic asthma. Leukotrienes have been shown to inhibit

lymphocyte transformation and mitogen responsiveness *in vitro*, and very low doses of LTB4 induce non-specific T suppressor cells. Whether leukotrienes released at sites of inflammation would have any effect on lymphocytes *in vivo* is debatable, since specific immune responses often occur at some distance from the site, in the local lymph nodes. Nevertheless, the shutdown in traffic through responding lymph nodes is mediated by prostaglandins, hence eicosanoids have several functions at different locations in immune and inflammatory reactions, even if their effects are localized.

Interferons, Lymphokines and Monokines

Interferons were originally identified as glycoproteins which interfere with viral replication, although they also have numerous other roles, including that of an inflammatory mediator. Interferons fall into three main groups: IFN$_\alpha$, IFN$_\beta$ and IFN$_\gamma$. There are at least 20 different types of human IFN$_\alpha$ including allelic and non-allelic variants. IFN$_\alpha$ is produced primarily by virally infected leucocytes and IFN$_\beta$ by infected fibroblasts, although this division is not absolute. IFN$_\gamma$ is primarily produced by mitogen- or antigen-activated T cells, and so it is an additional link between the immune system and inflammatory reactions.

IFN$_\alpha$ and IFN$_\beta$ have about 30% amino acid homology and are, therefore, related, while IFN$_\gamma$ also has some similarities, particularly at the N terminus, and is probably also distantly related. Two types of IFN receptor have been discovered, one binding IFN$_\alpha$ and IFN$_\beta$ and the second binding IFN$_\gamma$. Generally, the IFNs do not bind to the other type of receptor, although IFN$_\beta$ has been shown to bind

Fig. 15.7 Antiviral actions of interferons. Interferons bind specifically to one of two types of IFN receptor. The IFNs have numerous effects, of which two are illustrated here. They cause the synthesis of antiviral proteins, including 2′,5′ Adenosine synthetase and a protein kinase. Both of these are activated by dsRNA, an intermediate of viral replication. The synthetase induces formation of 2′5′ppp-oligo A which activates an endonuclease capable of causing mRNA degradation. The protein kinase phosphorylates the initiator of protein translation eIF2, thereby inactivating it. It is possible that the action of IFN in this way partly uses the cell's own regulatory faculty to exert its antiviral action.

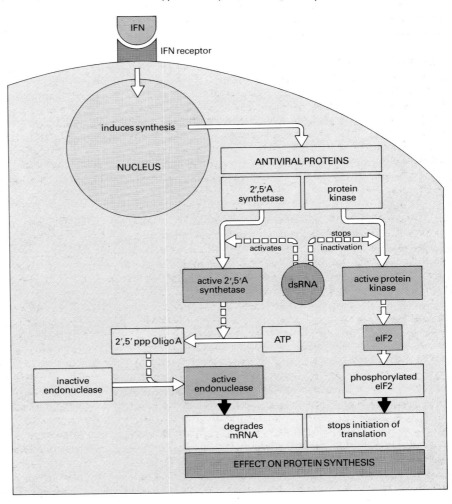

weakly to the IFN$_\gamma$ receptor in one study. It was once thought that IFNs were totally species-specific, based on species specificity of their binding to receptors, but it is now known that this is not wholly true. In spite of this, they all induce synthesis of a group of proteins in common, while IFN$_\gamma$ induces some unique proteins. The inducers of interferons include the viruses themselves, as well as several bacteria (*B. abortus, H. influenzae* and others), rickettsials, mycoplasmas and bacterial products such as LPS. Naturally, antigens from any of these sources can induce IFN$_\gamma$ (immune interferon) in a population of sensitized T cells. However, the most potent synthetic inducer of IFN has been found to be dsRNA. dsRNA is thought to be an intermediate produced in cells during the replicative cycle of many viruses, and viruses which generate dsRNA are particularly effective inducers of IFN.

The proteins induced in the target cells are responsible for inhibition of viral replication, but there is no single mechanism. For instance, IFN-treated fibroblasts inhibit the replication of vesicular stomatitis virus at the level of viral nucleic acid replication, while retrovirus production is inhibited at the stage of virion assembly. One of the induced proteins is a protein kinase which phosphorylates several cellular proteins. Synthesis of the kinase is induced by interferon, but it becomes activated by binding to dsRNA. Thus the cell is put into a state of 'alert' by IFN, but the active antiviral state only develops as viral proteins are encountered — a case of cellular brinkmanship. The kinase phosphorylates the initiator of protein translation eIF2, thus inhibiting protein translation. Several other proteins are phosphorylated, including a protein of ~70kD found in virally resistant cells, but their function is not known. A second induced protein is 2'5' adenylate synthetase. This too is activated by dsRNA and causes synthesis of 2'5' adenosine polymers from ATP. This in turn activates an endogenous endonuclease which causes mRNA breakdown, also inhibiting protein synthesis. The antiviral effects of interferons are illustrated in Figure 15.7 (see previous page). Interferons cause slowing of protein synthesis, and at high levels the cytostatic effect may progress to cytotoxicity. The effects of

IFNs in modulating the immune response and their actions in inducing MHC molecules are discussed more fully in Chapters 10 and 11. In addition, IFN$_\beta$ has been shown to induce Fc$_\gamma$ receptors on human lymphocytes, but reduces Fc$_\mu$ receptors. IFNs increase Fc receptors on macrophages and thus enhance phagocytosis. Interestingly, different types of IFN$_\alpha$ have differential effects on the induction of Fc receptors. IFN$_\gamma$ is relatively less effective at inducing Fc receptors when compared with its strong antiviral activity. There are associated changes in the cytoskeleton of IFN-treated cells, including an increase in the number of actin filaments. It is perhaps surprising in view of the general up-regulation of many inflammatory reactions that the maturation of monocytes to macrophages is delayed by IFN$_\alpha$, but this may be seen in the context of IFN cytostatic activity. One consequence of this is that monocyte cytotoxic activity, which usually decays rapidly in culture, is retained longer in the presence of IFN. A further function of both IFN$_\gamma$ and IFN$_\alpha$ is to enhance IL-1 release.

IL-1, released by macrophages, has numerous effects on immune reactions, but it was initially identified as an endogenous pyrogen, a mediator causing fever. Several other cells produce IL-1-like molecules; as with the IFNs, the effects on cells outside the immune system may be as important as the immunoregulatory actions. These effects include neutrophil mobilization from bone marrow (a peptide produced by C3 breakdown is thought to do this also), chemotaxis of neutrophils and macrophages, and the induction of PGE2 release from several cell types. It also induces bone resorption and cartilage breakdown and, most surprisingly, sleep. Fever is caused by action on hypothalamic temperature control centres by a mechanism involving PGE2 induction. Also, IL-1 acts on hepatocytes causing the synthesis and release of acute phase proteins. With this wide spectrum of regulatory activity on the more primitive elements of the host defence system, it seems probable that IL-1 was an evolutionarily primitive mediator of inflammation which has developed more specific functions, concomitantly with the development of the adaptive immune system (cf. the complement system).

Fig. 15.8 Immune system-mediated inflammation: summary. The immune system can initiate inflammatory reactions either via the complement classical pathway activated by IgG or IgM and antigen, or by recruiting mast cells sensitizing them with IgE so that they are triggered following contact with antigen. The anaphylatoxins C3a and C5a also trigger mast cells and basophils. C5a is also chemotactic and activates macrophages. Eicosanoids released from the mast cells affect the local vasculature, and LTB4 is itself chemotactic. Additional eicosanoids are produced by the macrophages themselves, as well as by the local endothelium. Once present at the site of inflammation, inflammatory cells come under the additional controls of lymphokines including IFN$_\gamma$ and MIF in the presence of lymphocytes. The latter are of greater importance in chronic inflammatory reactions.

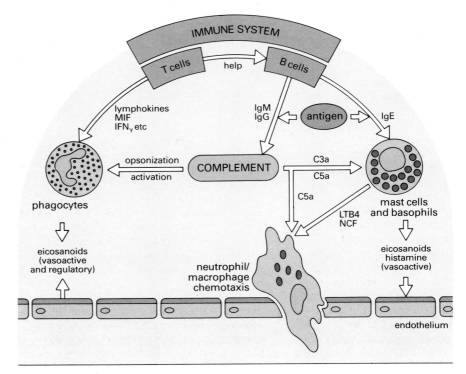

The various lymphokines released by activated T cells are the major controlling mediators of the immune response, but are also particularly important in causing macrophage activation, thereby facilitating destruction of intracellular parasites. Lymphokines are thought to be the major controllers of chronic inflammatory reactions, and of particular importance are macrophage arming factor (MAF) and migration inhibition factor (MIF). For example, fluids extracted from granulomas induced by antigen coupled to sepharose beads in sensitized individuals contain high levels of MIF and IFN_γ. MAF consists of several components of which the major one is IFN_γ. In this role it causes macrophage activation as detailed in a previous section. Migration inhibition factor (MIF) is thought to be responsible for the accumulation of macrophages at sites of chronic inflammation, along with some of the less well-defined chemotactic factors mentioned above. They are, therefore, particularly important in mediating delayed hypersensitivity reactions, although many of them are only poorly characterized. They are also responsible for the differences seen in the handling of intracellular parasites during a primary and secondary immune response (for example, the Koch phenomenon). The differences between the acute and chronic inflammatory responses and the ways in which different mediators regulate these responses are discussed in the next section, and Figure 15.8 summarizes the ways in which the immune system can activate the inflammatory processes.

THE DEVELOPMENT OF INFLAMMATION

The preceding section has described the factors which mediate inflammatory reactions without reference to the type of reaction seen, but inflammatory reactions precipitated by immunological events can either occur as an acute reaction, or develop into a chronic condition. Although acute inflammation is effected by systems which contain a number of positive feedback loops, the actions of these systems are set against a background level of inhibitory activity. Serum enzyme inhibitors (for example α_2-macroglobulin, α_1-antitrypsin) are essential in controlling the actions of the effector systems and ensuring that their activity is localized to the inflammatory site. The complement system is controlled by the actions of C4bp, FH and FI, which cause the breakdown of C4b and C3b, while the C3 and C5 convertases are inherently labile enzymes and decay over a relatively short time span. The rate of decay of the alternative pathway C3 convertase C3bBb is controlled by the acute phase protein FP (properdin), such that the decay of the convertase is slowed in the presence of FP. Hence the activity of the amplification loop may be up-regulated during inflammation. Other systems are similarly controlled by specific inhibitors (for instance the recently described IL-1 inhibitor), the decay of active intermediates and the consumption of substrate molecules. Most important of all, the outcome of immunologically mediated inflammation is largely determined by whether antigen (the primary stimulator of the immune system) is eliminated, or whether it persists. However, if the stimulus is removed, the lesion may resolve with the removal of the exudate and cellular debris which are phagocytosed and transported away from the site by macrophages. Fibrin is degraded by plasmin, and active macrophages can generate a plasminogen activator. The eventual outcome depends on the degree of damage to the tissue and on whether the cells

of the tissue are able to regenerate. In some cases there may be complete regeneration of the tissue, but if the cells are unable to regenerate fully, the lesion is repaired by fibroblasts which lay down collagen.

Sites of chronic immunologically mediated inflammation contain a wide variety of cells, but there are usually greater numbers of macrophages and fewer neutrophils than in acute lesions. Lymphocytes also accumulate relatively late in the reactions. At some inflammatory sites, particularly in autoimmune diseases, the lymphocytes may be organized into structures resembling lymphoid follicles, with germinal centres. This can occasionally be seen in the rheumatoid synovium or in the thyroid in Hashimoto's thyroiditis. Chronic inflammation may be an extension of the acute reaction due to the persistence of the initiating antigen, but in many cases delayed hypersensitivity reactions occur, so that the damage caused by the immune system is at least as detrimental as the original stimulus. The most extreme forms of these reactions produce immunological granulomas, of which the tuberculoid granuloma is the classic example. Macrophages and lymphocytes are the most abundant cells, with epithelioid and multinucleate giant cells often present. The latter are thought to be derived from macrophages. Epithelioid cells have a flattened appearance and lack the phagocytic capacities of macrophages, while the giant cells are polykaryons formed by the fusion of up to 100 cells. In granulomas, the macrophages usually predominate in the centre of the site, while lymphocytes tend to accumulate on the periphery. The development of the reaction is primarily controlled by factors released by antigen-activated T cells in the periphery, including macrophage arming factor and migration inhibition factor. Another lymphokine, the macrophage fusion factor (MFF), may be responsible for the formation of giant cells.

As stated above, the progression to chronic inflammation is due to the persistence of the antigenic stimulus. Broadly speaking, persistent antigens are of two types: autoantigens, and microbial antigens from organisms capable of resisting the actions of the immune system. Microorganisms may adopt one of two main strategies for avoiding elimination. They either evade immune recognition, or resist the effector arm of the immune response. For example, trypanosomes continually alter their surface antigens to evade recognition, and in this case the 'chronic' reactions are more akin to repeated primary or acute reactions. On the other hand, *Mycobacterium leprae* can resist the macrophage killing mechanisms and proliferate within the cells, thus evading the effector arm of the response. Different organisms stimulate various inflammatory mechanisms to different extents, hence mycobacteria (which have strongly adjuvant properties) generate lesions resembling chronic reactions even from the outset. Thus, the type of organism is ultimately most important in determining the outcome of inflammatory reactions, but the immune status of the individual is also relevant. This is seen in the different forms of leprosy, varying from lepromatous leprosy with large numbers of organisms present and weak cell-mediated immunity, to the opposite case of tuberculoid leprosy.

An individual cannot eliminate his own autoantigens, which are the stimuli for the chronic inflammatory reactions occurring in autoimmune diseases. One problem here is that persistent tissue damage causes the release of more autoantigen, thereby producing a vicious circle. It is notable that patients with Goodpasture's syndrome (autoantibodies to renal basement membranes and thence kidney damage) sometimes recover following plasmaphaeresis. It appears that removal of the autoantibody for a period breaks the cycle of destruction, thus allowing the kidney to recover and so reducing stimulation of the immune system. Again, in these chronic reactions the majority of cell populations are macrophages and lymphocytes, and the reactions are presumably mediated primarily by lymphokines.

Finally, while this chapter has considered the many interacting systems involved in inflammation, it must be remembered that the most important factor of all is the antigen. Antigen is the initiator of the response; its removal is the signal for the termination of the immune reactions and therefore of the effector arm of the immune response, this being mediated by the inflammatory mechanisms and inflammatory cells.

SUMMARY

The immune system aims to eliminate antigen by activating a number of effector systems which produce inflammatory reactions. Antibody and lymphokines can either act directly on the target systems and tissues, or indirectly by activating complement. Inflammation is seen as alterations in blood supply to the affected area accompanied by changes in vascular permeability and immigration of leucocytes. The cells migrate under the influence of chemotactic factors (C5a, LTB4 and others). Once they have arrived at the site of inflammation, phagocytes take up antigenic particles under the direction of opsonizing antibody and complement components. Lymphokines and microbial products cause the incoming macrophages to become activated by enhancing their phagocytic, cytotoxic and secretory capacities. Lymphokines also signal to the tissue cells, causing a variety of effects such as the induction of class II MHC molecules.

The main sources of inflammatory mediators are the plasma enzyme systems, mast cells, basophils, platelets, lymphocytes and macrophages. Particularly important in the initiation of acute inflammation are the anaphylatoxins C3a and C5a, bradykinin, the vasoactive amines and the eicosanoids which modulate the actions of the others as well as being active in their own right. Lymphokines, leukotrienes and IFNs are likely to be more important in chronic reactions. The outcome of the response as a whole is largely determined by the nature of the antigenic stimulus and type of immune response which it induces in a particular individual, and this in turn is largely related to the persistence of the antigen.

FURTHER READING

Adams D.O. & Hamilton T.A. (1984) *The cell biology of macrophage activation.* Ann. Revs. Immunol. **2,** 283.

Anderson P., Yip T.K. & Vilcek J. (1984) *Specific binding of human interferon-γ to high affinity receptors on human fibroblasts.* J. Biol. Chem. **257,** 11301.

Bar-Shavit R., Kahn A., Mudd M.S., Wilner G.D., Mann K.G. & Fenton J.W. (1984) *Localization of a chemotactic domain in human thrombin.* Biochem. **23,** 397.

Becker S. (1984) *Influence of interferon on human monocyte to macrophage development.* Cell Immunol. **84,** 145.

Bell D.M., Roberts N.J. & Hall C.B. (1983) *Different anti-viral spectra of human macrophage interferon activities.* Nature **305,** 319.

Boyle M.D., Lawman M.J.P., Gee A.P. & Young M. (1985) *Nerve growth factor: a chemotactic factor for polymorphonuclear leukocytes in vivo.* J. Immunol. **134,** 564.

Chenoweth D.E. & Hugli T.E. (1980) *Human C5a and C5a analogs as probes of the neutrophil C5a receptor.* Mol. Immunol. **17,** 151.

Davies P., Bailey P.J., Goldenberg M.M. & Ford-Hutchinson A.W. (1984) *The role of arachidonic acid products in pain and inflammation.* Ann. Revs. Immunol. **2,** 335.

Durum S.K., Schmidt J.A. & Oppenheim J.J. (1985) *Interleukin 1: An immunological perspective.* Ann. Revs. Immunol. **3,** 263.

Fearon D.T. (1984) *Cellular receptors for fragments of the third component of complement.* Immunol. Today **5,** 105.

Fearon D.T. & Wong W. (1983) *Complement ligand receptor interactions that mediate biological responses.* Ann. Revs. Immunol. **1,** 243.

Friedman R.M. & Vogel S.N. (1983) *Interferons with special emphasis on the immune system.* Adv. Immunol. **34,** 97.

Goldman D.W. & Goetzl E.J. (1984) *Heterogeneity of human polymorphonuclear leukocyte receptors for leukotriene B4.* J. Exp. Med. **159,** 1027.

Harashima M., Tashiro K., Sakata K. & Harashima M. (1984) *Isolation of an eosinophil chemotactic lymphokine as a natural mediator for eosinophil chemotaxis from concanavalin-A induced skin reaction site in guinea pigs.* Clin. Exp. Immunol. **57,** 211.

Interferon Nomenclature. (1983) Arch. Virol. **77,** 283.

Kobayashi K., Allred C., Cohen S. & Yoshida T. (1985) *Role of interleukin 1 in experimental pulmonary granulomas.* J. Immunol. **134,** 358.

Krust B., Galbru J. & Hovanessian F. (1984) *Further characterization of the protein kinase activity mediated by interferon in mouse and human cells.* J. Biol. Chem. **259,** 8494.

Larsen G.L. & Henson P.M. (1983) *Mediators of inflammation.* Ann. Revs. Immunol. **1,** 335.

Nathan C. (1983) *Mechanism of macrophage antimicrobial activity.* Trans. Royal Soc. Trop. Med. & Hyg. **77,** 620.

Rook G. (1985) *Cell-mediated immunity.* In Immunology, Ed. Roitt I., Brostoff J. & Male D.K., Gower Medical Publishing, London.

Sen G., Herz R., Davatelis V. & Pestka S. (1984) *Antiviral and protein inducing activities of recombinant human leukocyte interferons and their hybrids.* J. Virol. **50,** 445.

Snyderman R. & Pike M.C. (1984) *Chemoattractant receptors on phagocytic cells.* Ann. Revs. Immunol. **2,** 257.

Taussig M.J. (1984) *Processes in pathology and microbiology;* Chapter 1, Blackwell Scientific Publications.

Toy J.L. (1983) *The interferons.* J. Interferon Res. **54,** 1.

Yoshimura T., Honda M. & Hayashi H. (1984) *Selective chemotaxis of Ia-positive blood monocytes in response to a macrophage chemotactic lymphokine extractable from PPD-induced delayed hypersensitivity reaction site in guinea pigs.* Immunol. **52,** 269.

Glossary

Acute phase proteins: Serum proteins whose levels increase during infection or inflammatory reactions.

ADCC (antibody-dependent cell-mediated cytotoxicity): A cytotoxic reaction in which Fc receptor-bearing killer cells recognize target cells via specific antibodies.

Adherent cells: Cells which bind to a particular substrate during fractionation procedures. This often refers to macrophages, which adhere to plastic.

Adjuvant: A substance which non-specifically enhances the immune response to an antigen.

Agretope: The antigen's recognition structure which allows an antigen or antigen fragments to link to class II MHC molecules.

Affinity: Measure of the binding strength between an antigenic determinant (epitope) and an antibody-combining site (paratope).

Affinity labelling: A technique to identify the amino acid residues involved in a binding site, by using a molecule capable of entering the binding site and then being activated to covalently link to adjacent amino acid residues.

Affinity maturation: The increase in average antibody affinity frequently seen during a secondary immune response.

Allele: Intraspecies variance at a particular gene locus.

Allergy: Originally defined as altered reactivity on second contact with antigen, now usually refers to a Type 1 hypersensitivity reaction.

Allogeneic: Refers to intraspecies genetic variations.

Allotype: The protein product of an allele which may be detectable as an antigen by another member of the same species.

Altered self: The concept that the combination of antigen and a self MHC molecule interacts with the immune system in the same way as an allogeneic MHC molecule.

Alternative pathway: The activation pathways of the complement system involving C3 and factors B, D, P, H and I, which interact in the vicinity of an activator surface to form an alternative pathway C3 convertase.

Amplification loop: The alternative complement activation pathway, which acts as a positive feedback loop when C3 is split in the presence of an activator surface.

Anaphylatoxin: Complement peptides (C3a and C5a) which cause mast cell degranulation and smooth muscle contraction.

Anaphylaxis: An antigen-specific immune reaction mediated primarily by IgE, which results in vasodilation and constriction of smooth muscles, including those of the bronchus, and which may result in death of the animal.

Antibody: A molecule produced by animals in response to antigen, which has the particular property of combining specifically with the antigen which induced its formation.

Antigen: A molecule which induces the formation of antibody.

Antigen bridge: A concept explaining the way in which lymphocytes recognizing different parts of an antigen interact. Originally this was seen as the antigen bridging between the antigen-reactive cells, but now it is thought that antigen fragments present on the surface of one cell are recognized by the other.

Antigen presentation: The process by which certain cells in the body (antigen-presenting cells) express antigen on their cell surface in a form recognizable by lymphocytes.

Antigen processing: The actions which a cell makes to convert antigen into a form in which it can be recognized by lymphocytes.

Antigen suicide: A technique for selectively depleting antigen-reactive cells by supplying them with a toxic form of their specific antigen.

Antiviral proteins: Proteins induced by interferons which render a cell resistant to viral replication.

Associate recognition: The idea that antigen and MHC molecules are recognized by T cells as a single unit.

Atopy: The clinical manifestation of Type 1 hypersensitivity reactions including eczema, asthma and rhinitis.

Autologous: Part of the same individual.

Avidity: The functional combining strength of an antibody with its antigen, which is related to both the affinity of the reaction between the epitopes and paratopes and the valencies of the antibody and antigen.

β_2 microglobulin: A monomorphic polypeptide encoded outside the MHC, which is non-covalently associated with the MHC-encoded polypeptides of class I molecules.

B/B rat: A strain in which a proportion of the animals develop autoimmune diabetes and thyroid autoimmunity.

BCG (Bacille Calmette Guerin): An attenuated strain of *Mycobacterium tuberculosis* used as a vaccine, an adjuvant or a biological response modifier in different circumstances.

BCGF (B cell growth factor): One of the molecules produced by T cells required in the early stages of B cell activation.

BSF (B cell stimulating factors): A group of compounds required for B cell maturation and proliferation.

Biozzi mice: Lines of mice selectively bred to produce low or high responses to particular antigens (originally sheep erythrocytes).

bm mutants: A series of mice derived from a haplotype H-2^b strain, which have mutations in the H-2 region.

Bradykinin: A vasoactive nonapeptide, which is the most important mediator generated by the kinin system.

Bursa of Fabricius: A lymphoepithelial organ found at the junction of the hind gut and cloaca in birds, which is the site of B cell maturation.

Bystander lysis: Complement-mediated lysis of cells in the immediate vicinity of a complement activation site, which are not themselves responsible for the activation.

C1 – C9 complement: The components of the complement classical and lytic pathways, responsible for mediating inflammatory reactions, opsonization of particles and lysis of cell membranes.

C domains: The constant domains of antibody and the T cell receptor. They do not contribute to the antigen-binding site, and show relatively little variability between receptor molecules. The variants are isotypic.

C genes: The gene segments which encode the constant portion of the immunoglobulin heavy and light chains and the α and β chains of the T cell antigen receptor.

C3b inactivator: A factor of the complement system, recently renamed Factor 1.

CD markers: Cell surface molecules of lymphocytes, including:
CD1: A cortical thymocyte differentiation marker.
CD2: A receptor involved in antigen – non-specific T cell activation (E receptor).
CD3: A constant portion of the T cell antigen receptor.
CD4: A marker of T helper cells involved in MHC class II recognition.
CD5: A T cell marker also present on a subpopulation of B cells.
CD8: A marker of T cytoxic cells involved in MHC class I recognition.
CD25: The IL-2 receptor present on activated T cells and on some activated B cells.

CDR (complementarity determining regions): The sections of an antibody or T cell receptor V region, responsible for antigen or antigen/MHC binding.

Capping: A process by which cell surface molecules are caused to aggregate (usually using antibody) on the cell membrane.

Carrier: An immunogenic molecule, or part of a molecule, which is recognized by T cells in an antibody response.

Carrier priming: Selectively sensitizing an animal or population of T cells to carrier determinants of antigen.

Cell cycle: The process of cell division which is divisible into four phases: G$_1$, S, G$_2$ and M. DNA replicates during the S phase and the cell divides in the M (mitotic) phase.

Chemokinesis: Increased random migratory activity of cells.

Chemotaxis: Increased directional migration of cells, particularly in response to concentration gradients of certain chemotactic factors.

Class I, II, III MHC molecules: Three major classes of molecule coded within the MHC. Class I molecules have one MHC-encoded peptide associated with β_2 microglobulin. Class II molecules have two MHC-encoded peptides which are non-covalently associated, and class III molecules are complement components.

Class I/II restriction: The observation that immunologically active cells will only cooperate effectively when they share MHC haplotypes at either the class I or class II loci.

Class switching: The process by which an individual B cell can link new immunoglobulin heavy chain C genes to its recombined V gene, to produce a different class of antibody with the same specificity. This process is also reflected in the overall class switch seen during the maturation of an immune response.

Classical pathway: The pathway by which antigen/antibody complexes can activate the complement system, involving components C1, C2 and C4, generating a classical pathway C3 convertase.

Clone: A family of cells or organisms having a genetically identical constitution.

Clonal abortion: A process in which lymphocytes are rendered incapable of reacting to antigen, resulting in tolerance.

Clonal deletion: The hypothesis that particular clones of autoreactive cells are physically destroyed during ontogeny to maintain self tolerance, or the removal of particular sets of clones during the development of tolerance in adults.

Clonal exhaustion: A mechanism for the development of tolerance in which mature lymphocytes are forced into exhaustive terminal differentiation, leaving no mature cells available to mount a subsequent response.

Clonal selection: The fundamental basis of lymphocyte activation, in which antigen selectively stimulates only those cells which express receptors for it to divide and differentiate.

Cold agglutinins: Antibodies which agglutinate at temperatures below 37°C only.

Con A (concanavalin A): A mitogen for T cells.

Congenic: Referring to animals bred to be genetically identical at every but one defined region of the genome.

Constant regions: The relatively invariant parts of immuno-globulin heavy and light chains and the α and β chains of the T cell receptor; effectively this means all but the N-terminal domains.

Contrasuppression: The action of a group of T cells which renders T helper cells resistant to the action of T suppressors.

CR1, CR2, CR3: Receptors for activated C3 fragments. CR1 is an immune adherence receptor present on cells of the monocyte macrophage lineage, some antigen-presenting cells and erythrocytes. CR2 is present on B cells. CR3 is present on macrophages and some other phagocytes.

Cyclophosphamide: A cytotoxic drug frequently used as an immunosuppressive.

Cyclosporine: An immunosuppressive drug which is particularly useful in suppression of graft rejection.

Cytophilic: Having a propensity to bind to cells.

Cytostatic: Having the ability to stop cell growth.

Cytotoxic: Having the ability to kill cells.

D genes: Sets of gene segments lying between the V and J genes in the immunoglobulin heavy chain genes, and in the T cell receptor α and β chain genes, which are recombined with V and J genes during ontogeny.

Degranulation: Exocytosis of granules from cells such as mast cells and basophils.

Dendritic cells: A set of antigen-presenting cells present in lymph nodes, spleen and at low levels in blood, which are particularly active in stimulating T cells.

Desetope: The part of an MHC molecule responsible for linking to antigen or processed antigen.

DNP (dinitrophenol): A commonly used hapten.

Domain: A region of a peptide having a coherent tertiary structure. Both immunoglobulins and MHC class I and class II molecules have domains.

Dominant idiotypes: Individual idiotypes which are present on a large proportion of the antibodies generated to a particular antigen.

Epstein-Barr virus (EBV): Causal agent of Burkitt's lymphoma and infectious mononucleosis. It has the ability to transform human B cells into stable cell lines.

ECF (eosinophil chemotactic factor): A factor produced at sites of inflammation by T cells, which attracts eosinophils. Other ECFs are produced by triggered mast cells.

Education of T cells: The process by which pre-T cells are educated in the thymus to recognize antigen only in association with self MHC molecules.

Effector cells: A functional concept which in context means those lymphocytes or phagocytes which produce the end effect.

Eicosanoids: Products of arachidonic acid metabolism, including prostaglandins, leukotrienes and thromboxanes.

ELISA (enzyme-linked immunosorbent assay): A group of techniques for measuring antigen or antibody levels, in which one of the reagents is coupled to an enzyme generating a coloured reaction product.

Endothelium: Cells lining blood vessels and lymphatics.

Endotoxin: Lipopolysaccharide component of the cell wall of several species of Gram-negative bacteria, which is a B cell mitogen.

Enhancement: Prolongation of graft survival by treatment with antibodies directed towards the graft alloantigens.

Epitope: A single antigenic determinant. Functionally it is the portion of an antigen which combines with the antibody paratope.

Exon: Gene segment encoding protein.

Fab: The part of an antibody molecule which contains the antigen combining site, consisting of a light chain and part of the heavy chain. It is produced by enzymatic digestion.

Factors B,P,D,H and I: Components of the alternative complement pathway, their names have superseded the old nomenclature: $FP = Properdin$; $FH = \beta_1 H$; $FI = C3b$ inactivator.

Fc: The portion of an antibody which is responsible for binding to antibody receptors on cells and the C1q component of complement.

Forbidden clones: The theory that clones of autoreactive lymphocytes are deleted during development.

Framework segments: Sections of antibody V regions which lie between the hypervariable regions.

Freund's adjuvant: An emulsion of aqueous antigen in oil. Complete Freund's adjuvant also contains killed *Mycobacterium tuberculosis,* while incomplete Freund's adjuvant does not.

FTS (Facteur Thymique Serique): A 9 amino acid residue thymic hormone, also called thymulin.

GALT (gut-associated lymphoid tissue): This refers to the accumulations of lymphoid tissue associated with the gastrointestinal tract, including the tonsils and Peyer's patches.

Gene conversion: A process by which segments of DNA can become converted to share the same sequence as other segments separated in the genome.

Genetic association: A term used to describe the condition where particular genotypes are associated with other phenomena, such as particular diseases.

Genetic restriction: The term used to describe the observation that lymphocytes and antigen-presenting cells cooperate most effectively when they share particular haplotypes.

Germline: The genetic material which is passed down through the gametes before it is modified by somatic recombination or mutation.

Giant cells: Large multinucleated cells, sometimes seen in granulomatous reactions and thought to result from the fusion of macrophages.

Groups, subgroups: A classification of antibodies according to similarities in their V region frameworks.

GvH (graft-versus-host disease): A condition caused by allogeneic donor lymphocytes reacting against host tissue in an immunologically compromised recipient.

H-2: The mouse major histocompatibility complex.

Haplotype: A set of genetic determinants located on a single chromosome.

Hapten: A small molecule which can act as an epitope but which is incapable by itself of eliciting an antibody response.

Helper cells: A functional subclass of T cells which can help to generate cytotoxic T cells and cooperate with B cells in the production of an antibody response. Helper cells usually recognize antigen in association with class II MHC molecules.

Helper factors: Molecules which can deliver T cell help to other lymphocytes. The term is usually reserved for antigen-specific factors, as opposed to non-specific mediators such as the interferons and interleukins.

Heterologous: Refers to interspecies antigenic differences.

HEV (high endothelial venule): An area of venule from which lymphocytes migrate into lymph nodes.

High zone tolerance: Supraoptimal doses of antigens which can tolerize B cells.

Hinge: The portion of an immunoglobulin heavy chain between the Fc and Fab regions. This allows flexibility within the molecule and allows the two combining sites to operate independently. The hinge region is usually encoded by a separate exon.

Histamine: A major vasoactive amine released from mast cell and basophil granules.

Histocompatibility: The ability to accept grafts between individuals.

HLA: The human major histocompatibility complex.

hnRNA (heteronuclear RNA): The fraction of nuclear RNA which contains primary transcripts of the DNA prior to processing to form messenger RNA.

Homologous: The same species.

Humoral: Pertaining to the extracellular fluids, including the plasma and lymph.

H-Y: A minor histocompatibility antigen of mice encoded on the Y chromosome.

Hybridoma: Cell lines created *in vitro* by fusing two different cell types, usually lymphocytes, one of which is a tumour cell.

5-HT (5-hydroxy tryptamine): A vasoactive amine present in platelets and a major mediator of inflammation in rodents.

Hypervariable region: The most variable areas (3) of the V domains of immunoglobulin and T cell receptor chains. These regions are clustered at the distal portion of the V domain and contribute to the antigen-binding site.

Idiotope: A single antigenic determinant on an antibody V region.

Idiotype: The antigenic characteristic of the V region of an antibody.

Immune complex: The product of an antigen-antibody reaction which may also contain components of the complement system.

Immunogen: An antigen which elicits a strong immune response, particularly in the context of protective immunity to a pathogen.

Immunofluorescence: A technique used to identify particular antigens microscopically in tissues or on cells by the binding of a fluorescent antibody conjugate.

Immunopotentiation: Up-regulation of an immune response which may be effected by adjuvants and many other biological response modulators.

Independent recognition: The hypothesis that T cells independently recognize processed antigen and MHC molecules on the surface of antigen-presenting cells and target cells.

Interferon (IFN$_\alpha$, IFN$_\beta$ and IFN$_\gamma$): A group of mediators which increase the resistance of cells to viral infection, by altering the activities of the cells' metabolic machinery. IFN$_\alpha$ is produced by leucocytes, IFN$_\beta$ by fibroblasts and IFN$_\gamma$ by activated T cells. IFN$_\gamma$ has numerous other effects in modulating immune responses.

Interleukins (IL-1, IL-2, IL-3, IL-4): A group of molecules involved in signalling between cells of the immune system. IL-1 is released by numerous cells in the body, including macrophages. It has a wide variety of effects including activation of T cells to express IL-2 receptors. IL-2 is released by activated T cells, and is required for T cell proliferation. IL-3 is released by activated T cells and acts as a panspecific haemopoietin. The designation IL-4 has been provisionally allocated to the B cell growth factor BCGF I.

Internal image anti-idiotype: An anti-idiotype reacting to an antibody specific for a particular antigen, which expresses idiotopes resembling the antigen.

Intron: Gene segment between exons not encoding protein.

Ir gene: A group of immune response (Ir) genes, determining the level of an immune response to a particular antigen or foreign stimulus. A number of them are found in the major histocompatibility complex.

Isoelectric focusing: Separation of molecules on the basis of the charge. Each molecule will migrate to the point in a pH gradient where it has no net charge.

Isologous: Of identical genetic constitution.

Isotype: Refers to genetic variation within a family of proteins or peptides such that every member of the species will have each isotype of the family represented in its genome (e.g. immunoglobulin classes).

J chain: A monomorphic polypeptide present in, and required for the polymerization of, polymeric IgA and IgM.

J genes: Sets of gene segments in the immunoglobulin heavy and light chain genes and in the genes for the α and β chains of the T cell receptor, which are recombined during lymphocyte ontogeny and contribute towards the genes for variable domains.

K cell: A group of lymphocytes which are able to destroy their targets by antibody-dependent cell-mediated cytoxicity. They have Fc receptors.

$\varkappa$ chains: One of the immunoglobulin light chain isotypes.

Kinins: A group of vasoactive mediators produced following tissue injury. Bradykinin, generated from high molecular weight kininogen by kallikrein, is the most important of the group.

Kupffer cells: Phagocytic cells which line the liver sinusoids.

Langerhans cells: Antigen-presenting cells of the skin which emigrate to local lymph nodes to become dendritic cells. They are particularly active in presenting antigen to T cells.

Large granular lymphocytes (LGL): A group of morphologically defined lymphocytes containing the majority of K cell and NK cell activity. They have both lymphocyte and monocyte/macrophage markers.

λ chains: One of the immunoglobulin light chain isotypes.

L3T4: The marker molecule on mouse T cells which defines the helper (CD4$^+$) subset.

L cells: Designation of the null (non-T, non-B) cells which may express K cell and NK cell activity.

LCM (lymphocytic choriomeningitis): A viral disease of mice.

Leukotrienes: A collection of metabolites of arachidonic acid which have powerful pharmacological effects.

Line: A collection of cells produced by continuously growing a particular cell culture *in vitro*. Such cell lines will usually contain a number of individual clones.

Linkage: The condition where two genes are both present in close proximity on a single chromosome and are usually inherited together.

Linkage disequilibrium: A condition where two genes are found together in a population at a greater frequency than that predicted simply by the product of their individual gene frequencies.

Low zone tolerance: Subimmunogenic doses of T dependent antigens which can tolerize T cells.

LPR (lymphoproliferation gene): A gene found in MRL mice which is involved in the generation of autoimmune phenomena.

LPS (lipopolysaccharide): A product of some Gram-negative bacterial cell walls, which can act as a B cell mitogen.

Ly antigens: Two series of mouse lymphocyte cell surface markers. Ly1 is present on T helper cells, but also on some immature lymphocytes and B cells. It appears to correspond to the CD5$^+$ group. Ly2 3 are two closely linked markers identifying T cytotoxic cells corresponding to the CD8$^+$ set. Lyb5 identifies a subset of B cells which recognize type II T independent antigens.

Lymphokines: A generic term for molecules other than antibodies which are involved in signalling between cells of the immune system and are produced by lymphocytes (cf. interleukins).

Lytic pathway: The complement pathway effected by components C5-C9, which is responsible for lysis of sensitized cell plasma membranes.

MAC (membrane attack complex): The assembled terminal complement components C5b-C9 of the lytic pathway, which becomes inserted into cell membranes.

MAF (macrophage arming factor): Factors released by activated T cells which cause macrophage activation, of which IFN., is a major component.

MALT (mucosa-associated lymphoid tissue): Generic term for lymphoid tissue associated with the mucosa of the gastrointestinal tract, bronchial tree etc.

MDP (muramyl dipeptide): The smallest adjuvant-active subunit of the mycobacterial cell wall.

MHC (major histocompatibility complex): A genetic region found in all mammals whose products are primarily responsible for the rapid rejection of grafts between individuals, and which function in signalling between lymphocytes and cells expressing antigen.

MHC restriction: A characteristic of many immune reactions, in which cells cooperate most effectively with other cells sharing an MHC haplotype.

Microglial cells: Phagocytic cells of the brain, which are probably derived from the monocyte lineage and can present antigen.

MIF (migation inhibition factor): A group of peptides produced by lymphocytes, which are capable of inhibiting macrophage migration.

Mitogen: Substances which cause cells, particularly lymphocytes, to undergo cell division.

MLR/MLC (mixed lymphocyte reaction/culture): Assay system for T cell recognition of allogeneic cells, in which response is measured by proliferation in the presence of the stimulating cells.

Monoclonal: Derived from a single clone, for example, monoclonal antibodies which are produced by a single clone and are homogeneous.

MRL.lpr: A spontaneously autoimmune strain of mouse which has been used as a model of rheumatoid arthritis.

Myeloma: A lymphoma produced from cells of the B cell lineage.

NCF (neutrophil chemotactic factor): A protein mediator released by mast cells, causing neutrophil chemotaxis.

Nef (nephritic factor): An autoantibody to the alternative pathway C3 convertase, which stabilizes the enzyme and potentiates the action of the alternative pathway amplification.

Neoplasm: A synonym for cancerous tissue.

Network theory: A proposal, first put forward by Jerne and since developed, which states that T cells and B cells mutually interregulate by recognizing idiotopes on their antigen receptors.

NIP (4-hydroxy, 5-iodo, 3-nitrophenylacetyl): A commonly used hapten.

NK (natural killer) cell: A group of lymphocytes which have the intrinsic ability to recognize and destroy some virally infected cells and some tumour cells.

Non-responder: Refers to strains of animals which fail to make an immune response to antigens which are immunogenic in others.

NP (4-hydroxy, 3-nitrophenylacetyl): A hapten which partially cross-reacts with NIP.

Nude mouse: A genetically athymic mouse. It also carries a closely linked gene producing a defect in hair production.

Null cells: Blood lymphocytes which fail to express B cell or T cell surface markers.

Nurse cells: Cells which can be isolated from the thymus, and are found closely surrounded by developing T cells. They may be involved in thymic education.

NZB, NZB/W: Two spontaneously autoimmune strains of mouse. The NZB is used as a model of autoimmune haemolytic anaemia. The (NZBxNZW)F1 (NZB/W) develops autoantibodies to DNA and develops a nephritis resembling that seen in systemic lupus erythematosus.

Obese chicken: Strain of chicken which develops autoimmune thyroiditis.

OKT markers: A series of monoclonal antibodies recognizing human T cell surface antigens. OKT6 = CD1; OKT3 = CD3; OKT4 = CD4; OKT8 = CD8.

Opsonization: A process by which phagocytosis is facilitated by the deposition of opsonins (e.g. antibody and C3b) on the antigen.

PAF (platelet activating factor): A factor released by basophils, which causes platelets to aggregate.

PALS (periarteriolar lymphatic sheath): The accumulations of lymphoid tissue constituting the white pulp of the spleen.

Parallel sets: This refers to different antibodies which share idiotopes but have different antigen-binding specificity, and may be regulated concomitantly through idiotypic interactions.

Paratope: The part of an antibody molecule which makes contact with the antigenic determinant (epitope).

Passenger cells: Cells in a graft which migrate into the recipient lymphoid tissue and are particularly effective at producing allogeneic sensitization.

Pathogen: An organism which causes disease.

PC (phosphoryl choline): A commonly used hapten which is also found on the surface of a number of microorganisms.

PCA (passive cutaneous anaphylaxis): The technique used to detect antigen-specific IgE, in which the test animal is injected intravenously with the antigen and dye, the skin having previously been sensitized with antibody.

PFC (plaque forming cell): An antibody-producing cell detected *in vitro* by its ability to lyse antigen-sensitized erythrocytes in the presence of complement.

PHA (phytohaemagglutinin): A mitogen for T cells.

Phagocytosis: The process by which cells engulf material and enclose it within a vacuole (phagosome) in the cytoplasm.

Phagosome, phagolysosome: The membrane-bound vacuole formed by phagocytosis and containing the phagocytosed material. After fusion of lysosomes with the phagosome, it is referred to as a phagolysosome.

Pinocytosis: The process by which liquids or very small particles are taken into the cell.

Plasma cell: An antibody-producing B cell, which has reached the end of its differentiation pathway.

Pokeweed mitogen: A mitogen for B cells.

Polyclonal: A term which describes the products of a number of different cell types (cf. monoclonal).

Prausnitz-Kustner reaction: A way of detecting antigen-specific IgE, in which antigen is injected into skin previously sensitized with IgE antibody.

Primary response: The immune response (cellular or humoral) seen following an initial encounter with a particular antigen.

Primary transcript: Direct transcripts of genomic DNA, before excision of introns to produce mRNA.

Primary lymphoid tissues: Lymphoid organs in which lymphocytes complete their initial maturation steps, including the fetal liver, adult bone marrow and thymus, and the Bursa of Fabricius in birds.

Prime: To give an initial sensitization to antigen.

Private specificities: Epitopes unique to a particular MHC haplotype.

Privileged sites: Tissues in which graft rejection reactions are very weak or absent following implantation of allogeneic tissue.

Properdin pathway: Original designation of the alternative pathway of complement activation, named after the molecule properdin (factor P) which stabilizes the alternative pathway C3 convertase.

Prostaglandins: Pharmacologically active derivatives of arachidonic acid. Different prostaglandins are capable of modulating cell mobility and immune responses.

Protein-A: A cell wall component of certain strains of staphylococci, which binds to a site in the Fc region of most IgG isotypes.

Pseudoalleles: Tandem variants of a gene: they do not occupy a homologous position on the chromosome (e.g. C4).

Pseudogenes: Genes which have homologous structures to other genes but which are incapable of being expressed (e.g. Jx3 in the mouse).

Public specificities: Epitopes common to MHC molecules of several different haplotypes.

Qa genes: A mouse gene locus adjacent to the MHC which encodes a considerable number of class I-like molecules.

Radioimmunoassay: A number of different, sensitive techniques for measuring antigen or antibody titres, using radiolabelled reagents.

Receptor: A cell surface molecule which binds specifically to particular proteins or peptides in the fluid phase.

Recombinant strain: A strain of animal in which a genetic cross-over has occurred at a defined chromosomal location.

Recombination: A process by which genetic information is rearranged during meiosis. This process also occurs during the somatic rearrangements of DNA which occur in the formation of genes encoding antibody and T cell receptor molecules.

Recurrent idiotype: An idiotype present in the immune response of different animals or strains to a particular antigen.

Respiratory burst: Increase in oxidative metabolism of phagocytes following uptake of opsonized particles.

Reticuloendothelial system: A diffuse system of phagocytic cells derived from the bone marrow stem cell which are associated with the connective tissue framework of the liver, spleen, lymph nodes and other serous cavities.

Rosetting: A technique for identifying or isolating cells by mixing them with particles or cells to which they bind (e.g. sheep erythrocytes to human T cells). The rosettes consist of a central cell surrounded by bound cells.

Secondary response: The immune response which follows a second or subsequent encounter with a particular antigen.

Secretory component: A polypeptide produced by cells of some secretory epithelia, which is involved in transporting secreted polymeric IgA across the cell and protecting it from digestion in the gastrointestinal tract.

Self tolerance: The idea that, although the immune system recognizes the body's own proteins, it does not react against them.

Site-associated idiotopes: Idiotopes present in the antibody-combining site. This is usually defined functionally, by inhibiting antigen binding with anti-idiotype or vice versa.

SLE (systemic lupus erythematosus): An autoimmune disease of humans, usually involving anti-nuclear antibodies.

Somatic mutation: A process which occurs during B cell maturation and affects the antibody gene region. It permits refinement of antibody specificity.

Spectrotype: The characteristic pattern generated by a set of molecules (e.g. antibody), separated according to their pI by isoelectric focusing.

Suppressor factors: Mediators which can suppress an immune response. The term is usually reserved for antigen-specific suppressors rather than non-specific mediators such as prostaglandins.

Synergism: Cooperative interaction.

Syngeneic: Strains of animals produced by repeated inbreeding so that each pair of autosomes within an individual is identical.

T15: An idiotype associated with antiphosphoryl choline antibodies, named after the TEPC 15 myeloma prototype sequence.

TAC: The human IL-2 receptor (CD25).

Tachyphylaxis: The process by which subsequent doses of a pharmacological reagent produce decreasing effects.

Tandem duplicates: Adjacent copies of related genes linked together on a chromosome.

T cell bypass: The theory that autoimmunity develops because self tolerance at the T cell level is bypassed.

T dependent/T independent antigens: T dependent antigens require immune recognition by both T and B cells to produce an immune response. T independent antigens can directly stimulate B cells to produce specific antibody.

THY: A cell surface antigen of mouse T cells which has allotypic variants.

Thymic epithelial cells: Thymic antigen-presenting cells, expressing high levels of class II MHC antigens, thought to be important in the development of T cell immune recognition.

Thymic hormones: A group of molecules, including thymosin, thymulin, thymopoietin and thymostimulin, produced by the thymus, which help to maintain T cell function and development in secondary lymphoid tissues.

TLA locus: A gene locus linked to the mouse MHC which encodes class I-like molecules.

Tolerance: A state of specific immunological unresponsiveness.

Transformation: Morphological changes in a lymphocyte associated with the onset of division. Also used to denote the change to the autonomously dividing state of a cancer cell.

TNF (tumour necrosis factor): A mediator released by activated macrophages, which is toxic for a number of cells including some tumours.

Triggering of mast cells: Stimulation of mast cell degranulation, effected by crosslinking of surface bound IgE, direct triggering by C3a and C5a, or by drugs.

Vasoactive amines: Products such as histamine and 5-hydroxytryptamine released by basophils, mast cells and platelets, which act on the endothelium and smooth muscle of the local vasculature.

V domains: The N-terminal domains of antibody heavy and light chains, and the α and β chains of the T cell receptor which vary between different clones and form the antigen-binding site.

V genes: Sets of genes which encode the major part of the V domains of antibody heavy and light chains and the α and β chains of the T cell receptor, and which become recombined with appropriate sets of D and J genes during lymphocyte ontogeny.

Veiled cells: Cells found in lymph which develop into dendritic cells in the T cell areas of secondary lymphoid tissues.

White pulp: The lymphoid component of spleen, consisting of periarteriolar sheaths of lymphocytes and antigen-presenting cells.

Xenogeneic: Referring to interspecies antigenic differences (cf. heterologous).

Index